Essentials in Ophthalmology

Series Editor
Arun D. Singh

For further volumes:
http://www.springer.com/series/5332

Khalid F. Tabbara
Ahmed M. Abu El-Asrar
Moncef Khairallah
Editors

Arun D. Singh
Series Editor

Ocular Infections

Springer

Editors
Khalid F. Tabbara, MD, ABO,
FRCOphth
Department of Ophthalmology
The Eye Center
Riyadh
Saudi Arabia

Ahmed M. Abu El-Asrar, MD, PhD
Department of Ophthalmology
King Abdulaziz University Hospital
Riyadh
Saudi Arabia

Moncef Khairallah, MD
Department of Ophthalmology
Fattouma Bourguiba University Hospital
Monastir
Tunisia

ISSN 1612-3212
ISBN 978-3-662-43980-7 ISBN 978-3-662-43981-4 (eBook)
DOI 10.1007/978-3-662-43981-4
Springer Heidelberg New York Dordrecht London

Library of Congress Control Number: 2014958020

Printed on acid-free paper

Springer is part of Springer Science+Business Media (www.springer.com)

Preface

Infections of the eye continue to cause serious ocular morbidity and loss of vision. It is, therefore, highly desirable to maintain a high level of awareness on new developments in the diagnosis and management of infectious diseases of the eye. Both classic infections and emerging infections pose serious threats to man. Many kinds of ocular infections may stay mysterious and sometimes are hard to diagnose. As medical scientists, we have the unique role to dispel the mystery of infections of the eye and replace speculations with certainty and fiction with fact.

This book is an attempt to provide an update on the topic of infections of the eye and adnexae and provide simplified information that would keep the ophthalmologist and the eye care practitioner abreast of the recent advances in antibiotics and in the management of infectious diseases of the eye and adnexae. Certain infections have been eradicated by mass vaccinations, and others have been controlled by public health measures, but the resilience of viruses and the tenacity of bacteria have led to the changes in the pattern of ocular infections and led to the evolution of old diseases and the emergence of newly discovered disorders.

In the past two decades, there have been a number of infectious diseases, and new pathogens have been discovered. Barry and Marshall received the Nobel Prize for medicine in 2005 for their discovery of *Helicobacter pylori* as a cause of peptic ulcer. *Bartonella henselae* has been identified as the cause of Bacillary *angiomatosis* (cat scratch disease) or Bartonellosis. Herpes virus type 8 was discovered as a cause of Kaposi sarcoma in patients with AIDS. Human immunodeficiency virus (HIV) 1 and 2 are now well known to cause AIDS. T-cell lymphoma is caused by human T lymphocyte virus type 1, and Lyme disease is, caused by *Borrelia burgdorferi*. In addition, Whipple disease became known to be caused by *Trophyrema whippelii*. Similarly, severe acute respiratory syndrome (SARS) and Avian influenzae are diseases caused by Corona virus and H5 N1 virus, respectively and Ebola virus is emerging as a cause of Ebola fever. Infections can cause diseases by invasion of tissues and destruction of the architecture of visually important structures in the eye. Infections may lead to immune dysregulation and trigger immune-mediated inflammation of the eye.

Strifes and natural disasters come and go, but infections are going to be with us forever. Certain infections may cause blindness, and therefore, ophthalmologists should remain updated on these disorders.

This book is divided into 16 chapters, making it an easy reference to find a rapid source for the management of infections of the eye. The book is illustrated by figures showing different ocular pathologies and is loaded with tables summarizing the findings.

The book is clinically oriented with a focus on prospects of infections of the eye that are important to the clinicians, including the essentials for diagnosis, laboratory workup, and management. The treatment is a simple evidenced-based approach with detailed information on antibiotics use and dosages. The chapter on antimicrobial agents in ophthalmology summarizes the antibiotics that are available commercially for infections of the eye, as well as the compounded topical medications that are not available in the market. Antimicrobial agents are commonly used in ocular infections and are among the most commonly prescribed drugs in community-based physician offices and hospitals. The use of these antimicrobial agents are outlined in all the chapters of this book.

Despite our enormous effort and progress in the quest to conquer infections, there is significant threat from resistant microorganisms.

The information provided in this book is an update on ocular infections, placing in the hands of ophthalmologists and health practitioners a shortcut and an easy access to the management of ocular infectious diseases.

Khalid F. Tabbara, MD, ABO, FRCOphth
Riyadh, Saudi Arabia
Baltimore, MD, USA

Ahmed M. Abu El-Asrar, MD, PhD
Riyadh, Saudi Arabia

Moncef Khairallah, MD
Monastir, Tunisia

Contents

Molecular Diagnosis of Ocular Infections

1

Jolanda D.F. de Groot-Mijnes

1.1 Introduction

The rapid identification of ocular infections can be crucial since treatment regimens and visual prognosis may be entirely different from noninfectious disorders. The fast identification of specific infectious agents is particularly important in immunocompromised patients [1, 2]. In the clinical practice, the presumed diagnosis of an ocular infection is based on specific clinical features; however, laboratory data may be helpful to confirm a suspected diagnosis, since similar clinical features might be caused by different infectious agents. Laboratory tests based on the analysis of peripheral blood alone are often of limited value, since these may not be informative on ocular processes and positive results may be coincidental [3–5]. Negative peripheral blood results may render a specific diagnosis unlikely but do not rule out the possibility of infection. For a definitive diagnosis of ocular infections, investigation of ocular fluids and biopsies is recommended.

Molecular diagnostics, of which the polymerase chain reaction (PCR) is the most applied procedure, has taken a prominent position within the laboratory diagnostic repertoire, also within the field of ophthalmology. Molecular assays can be highly sensitive and specific, and theoretically, molecular diagnosis can be performed on all types of ocular materials, provided the procedure for a particular pathogen is available. For many viral infections, PCR analysis has replaced the less sensitive culture technique. However, in case of bacterial and fungal infections culture is still preferred over molecular methods, for instance, in orbital cellulitis, mycotic keratitis, and endophthalmitis. Viral conjunctivitis is often a self-limiting disease, questioning the necessity to perform molecular diagnosis even though PCR assay is available for among other adenovirus, herpes viruses, and enteroviruses. However, in case of bilateral blepharoconjunctivitis in children, herpes viral PCR analysis of tear fluid and aqueous humor may be highly valuable for a rapid diagnosis [6, 7]. Currently, PCR analysis is mostly applied for the diagnosis of ocular trachoma and infectious uveitis and is taking a flight for the diagnosis of (mycotic) keratitis and endophthalmitis.

J.D.F. de Groot-Mijnes, PhD
Section Clinical Virology,
Department of Medical Microbiology and
Department of Ophthalmology,
University Medical Center Utrecht,
Heidelberglaan 100, 3584 CX, Utrecht,
The Netherlands
e-mail: j.d.f.degroot@umcutrecht.nl

K. Tabbara et al. (eds.), *Ocular Infections*, Essentials in Ophthalmology,
DOI 10.1007/978-3-662-43981-4_1, © Springer-Verlag Berlin Heidelberg 2014

1.2 Molecular Techniques for the Diagnosis of Ocular Infections

1.2.1 Polymerase Chain Reaction

PCR is a technique whereby with the use of short complementary DNA fragments called primers and DNA polymerase, a single or few copies of a part of the target DNA are amplified across several orders of magnitude, generating millions or more copies of a particular nucleic acid sequence [8]. The introduction of the PCR has greatly improved the detection of infectious agents. Results can be obtained much faster than with culture. Moreover, particular PCR procedures have been designed to be so sensitive as to replace culture in many cases, most notably for viruses and fastidious microorganisms [9, 10].

Next to the basic gel-based PCR method, various more sensitive and specific techniques are available, such as nested PCR and real-time PCR. Nested PCR is a modification of the basic PCR and involves two sets of primers, used in two consecutive amplification runs, the second set intended to amplify a target within the first run product, thereby increasing both sensitivity and specificity [11, 12].

Real-time PCR is also a modification of the basic PCR but adds a fluorescent compound to the reaction allowing for real-time monitoring of the PCR reaction and quantitation of the pathogenic load of the original sample. In case of Taqman real-time PCR, the fluorescent compound constitutes a DNA probe, which in addition to the possibility of quantitation increases the specificity of the reaction.

The introduction of real-time PCR assays in the clinical microbiology laboratory has led to significant improvements in the diagnosis of infectious disease [13, 14]. Contrary to nested PCR assays, real-time methods allow rapid DNA amplification, detection, and quantitation of the pathogenic load. Moreover, as real-time PCR assays are performed in a closed-tube system, the risk of contamination is reduced [15, 16]. However, real-time PCR assays may be less sensitive than nested PCR assays [17, 18].

PCR, most notably real-time PCR, has proven to be valuable for the diagnosis of various intraocular infections, including cytomegalovirus (CMV) retinitis, ocular toxoplasmosis, acute retinal necrosis (ARN), and herpetic anterior uveitis [13, 19–22]. Specific PCR assays are also available for many bacteria, like *Bartonella henselae, Borrelia burgdorferi, Treponema pallidum, Mycobacterium tuberculosis* and Mycobacterium species, and *Coxiella burnetii*, and have been reported to be applicable for the diagnosis of uveitis [23–31]. PCR directed to the 16S rRNA conserved gene sequences of bacteria is applied to detect bacteria that cause endophthalmitis but may also be useful for the diagnosis of uveitis entities [29, 32–35]. The 16S rRNA gene sequences contain hypervariable regions which can provide species-specific sequences which allow for bacterial identification. As a result, 16S rRNA gene sequencing has become prevalent in medical microbiology as a rapid, accurate alternative to phenotypic methods of bacterial identification [36]. Similarly, PCR assays have been developed targeting highly conserved gene sequences in fungi, such as the 18S and 28S rRNA genes. However, one has to be aware of possible contamination with nonpathogenic microorganisms, as these may accidentally be isolated during sampling and surgical procedures [37].

Positive PCR outcomes are directly related to the pathogenic load in the ocular sample. It has therefore been suggested that the probability of detecting viruses by PCR is higher than for bacteria or parasites, because viruses generally produce more progeny [3, 4, 13]. False-positive results for viruses may occur due to contamination of samples, overflow from the peripheral blood into the eye or the (intra)ocular presence of cells infected with infectious agents unrelated to the ocular inflammation [3, 38–40]. Therefore, positive PCR findings do not always prove causality.

False-negative results might occur because of a low inherent (intra)ocular pathogenic load or due to the small volume of ocular fluid available for testing and might also depend on the time interval between the onset of infection and sampling. Therefore, negative PCR results do not entirely exclude the presumed diagnosis and other diagnostic tools should be considered.

1.2.2 Loop-Mediated Isothermal Amplification (LAMP)

Loop-mediated isothermal amplification or LAMP is a novel molecular detection tool capable of amplifying a few copies of DNA to 10^9 in less than 1 h at isothermal conditions [41]. The method uses a set of four primers that produce multiple stem-loop structures resulting in increased amplification of the target DNA as compared to PCR. Moreover, the LAMP primers recognize six distinct regions on the target DNA adding to the specificity. By introducing a reverse transcriptase step to make copy DNA from RNA LAMP can also be used to detect RNA targets [41]. LAMP products can be visualized by agarose gel analysis; however, the high release of pyrophosphate results in a turbidity which is visible by eye. Another improvement is the addition of SYBR green, which induces a clearly visible color change. The LAMP reaction can also be followed in real time by measuring the turbidity in time or by the addition of fluorescent intercalating dyes, reminiscent of real-time PCR methods, allowing for quantitation of pathogenic load of the initial clinical sample.

LAMP is performed isothermally which obviates the need for thermal cyclers, and together with its ruggedness and simplicity, LAMP is highly applicable for laboratories with limited equipment or at the point of care by clinicians. LAMP assays have been developed for the molecular diagnosis of several ocular infections, such as uveitis associated with *Mycobacterium tuberculosis*, herpes simplex virus, Chikungunya virus and West Nile virus, and *Acanthamoeba* keratitis [42–47]. However, so far the sensitivity of the LAMP assays does not exceed that of real-time PCR [42–46].

1.2.3 Restriction Fragment Length Polymorphism, DNA Sequencing, and DNA Microarray

Restriction fragment length polymorphism (RFLP), DNA sequencing, and DNA microarray are molecular assays which are used for pathogen species and strain identification subsequent to PCR analysis. RFLP is a tool by which DNA is cut by sequence-specific restriction enzymes and subsequently analyzed on agarose gel. The resulting fragments are indicative of a particular pathogen species or strain. This method is mostly used for the identification of particular strains, rather than for species identification following broad-range PCR assays for bacteria and fungi. Therefore, RFLP has largely been replaced by DNA sequencing in the diagnostic setting. DNA sequencing involves the actual determination of the genetic code of a particular piece of DNA. Sequencing has been largely automated and may now allow for high-throughput analysis of diagnostic PCR products. DNA sequencing following PCR amplification has become the standard procedure for pathogen species and strain identification and antibiotic resistance profiling.

The DNA microarray technology is a genotyping tool which allows for the simultaneous identification of a wide variety of DNA sequences. An array consists of a large amount of small specific DNA probes spotted onto a matrix. PCR products are then allowed to hybridize to the DNA probes. Due to the introduction of fluorescent identification markers coupled to the PCR products, the arrays are scanned using fluorometry and subsequent data analysis is automated. Like DNA sequencing DNA arrays can be used for species identification and antibiotic resistance profiling [48].

1.3 Molecular Diagnosis of Trachoma

Trachoma is the leading cause of blindness worldwide and is caused by the bacterium *Chlamydia trachomatis*, which is also associated with venereal disease [49]. Different stains, the so-called serovars, have been identified of which only A through C cause trachoma, D through K cause ocular-genital infections, and the L-serovars cause lymphogranuloma venereum (LGV) [50]. Diagnosis of trachoma by clinical appearance is poor and molecular testing is commonly used. Several PCR assays have been developed for the detection of *Chlamydia trachomatis*, most of them were developed for the detection of genital infections. Only two commercial assays have been used to diagnose trachoma, the COBAS® Amplicor CT/NG Test by Roche Diagnostics Solutions (Basel, Switzerland) and the LCx™ by Abbott (Chicago, IL, USA) [51]. More recently, novel molecular diagnostic tools have been developed based on the detection of rRNA targets. The advantage of rRNA amplification over PCR is that these tests are equally specific, but more sensitive due to the high copy number of the rRNAs [52–54]. The new rRNA tests may prove valuable not only in detecting low-level infections but may also contribute to the surveillance of ocular Chlamydia, particularly in areas mass-treated with antibiotics where low-level reinfections are emerging [55, 56, 52].

1.4 Molecular Diagnosis of Microbial Keratitis

Microbial keratitis is an infection and inflammation of the cornea, and due to its progressive and potentially devastating nature, it is considered an ophthalmological emergency. Hence, rapid diagnosis of the causative agent is of the utmost importance. In a recent literature review by Karsten et al., 232 different species were found to be involved in microbial keratitis of which the fungi represent the largest group [57]. The most common causes include herpes simplex virus, varicella zoster virus, the bacteria *Staphylococcus aureus* and *Pseudomonas aeruginosa*, *Acanthamoeba* keratitis, and several fungi among which *Fusarium*, *Aspergillus* species, and *Candida* species [5]. The diagnosis is generally made based on clinical presentation and noninvasive imaging methods, complemented by microbial investigation, such as *in vitro* microscopical examination and culture of corneal scrapings and biopsies. In recent years, PCR analysis of corneal material has become increasingly more popular as it provides a rapid and sensitive tool for the identification of keratitis-causing infectious agents [58]. However, caution should be taken as fluorescein and antibiotics, chemical substances frequently used for the diagnosis and treatment of keratitis, may inhibit the PCR reaction, putatively yielding false-negative PCR outcomes [59].

1.4.1 Viral Keratitis

The most frequent cause of viral keratitis is HSV. In addition to HSV, VZV, adenoviruses and enteroviruses can cause corneal infections [60, 61]. Clinical manifestations of herpes keratitis include epithelial dendritic and stromal keratitis, the latter of which is more prevalent in children [7, 62]. Dendritic keratitis is often diagnosed on clinical presentation. Stromal keratitis on the other hand is clinically more difficult to diagnose. The molecular diagnosis of keratitis involves PCR analysis of corneal swabs or scrapings [7, 63–67]. Due to the location and the nature of the infection, the sensitivity of PCR assay appears to be higher for dendritic keratitis than for stromal keratitis [68]. In case of stromal keratitis or keratouveitis, aqueous humor analysis may add to the diagnosis [69, 68].

A good alternative to corneal scraping and swabs is the collection of tear fluid as this is less damaging to the already fragile cornea [70–76, 68, 60]. However, the sensitivity of the PCR assay on tear fluid may be lower than on corneal scrapings or swabs; Kakimaru-Hasegawa et al. demonstrated by real-time PCR lower copy numbers in tear samples after comparing simultaneously collected tear fluid and corneal scrapings from patients with HSV keratitis [68].

In addition to the diagnosis of keratitis, quantitative PCR analysis of ocular samples can also be used to monitor reaction to treatment and the occurrence of resistance to antivirals [63]. Acyclovir (ACV) resistance of HSV has been described in keratitis, but so far resistance is mostly determined phenotypically, that is, by virus culture in the presence of varying concentrations of ACV [64, 65]. One study described the genotypic identification of ACV resistance in HSV isolates from patients with keratitis [77]. Mutations in the HSV genome associated with ACV resistance have been identified and molecular tests for HSV genotyping are available [78–81]. Genotypic resistance analysis is faster and more sensitive than phenotypic resistance analysis as it obviates the need of cultured virus and may therefore prove valuable for analysis of the small volume ocular samples in the near future.

1.4.2 Nonviral Keratitis

Although in most institutes the diagnosis of nonviral keratitis is still made by more conventional methods, such as clinical presentation and direct staining or culture of ocular material, the molecular diagnosis of bacterial, fungal, and amoebic keratitis is gaining interest fast. Molecular analysis of corneal scrapings and biopsies is fast and sensitive and allows for rapid identification of the infectious species [5, 82–84].

Molecular assays currently described for infectious nonviral keratitis predominantly include broad-range bacterial and fungal PCR assays targeting the 16S rRNA gene and 18S and 28S rRNA genes, respectively [85–88, 37]. Microbial species identification can subsequently be done by sequence analysis of the PCR product or by DNA hybridization procedures [84]. For the identification of *Acanthamoeba* specific PCR assays are available [47, 89, 90].

Due to the high sensitivity and the broad-spectrum nature of the molecular tests for bacteria and fungi, one should be cautious with regard to false-positive results caused by commensal nonpathogenic species [37]. As there appears to be a high concordance between PCR and conventional diagnostic tools, it has been suggested to reserve PCR analysis for those cases where conventional diagnostics yielded negative results or where a rapid definitive diagnosis is crucial [88, 5].

1.5 Molecular Diagnosis of Endophthalmitis

Endophthalmitis is an uncommon but sight-threatening intraocular inflammation and can originate from a trauma or surgical procedure (exogenous endophthalmitis) or from an infection elsewhere in the body through septicemia (endogenous endophthalmitis) [91]. Infectious endophthalmitis can be caused by bacteria, fungi, parasites, and rarely viruses. Bacterial endophthalmitis predominates, with Staphylococci and Streptococci as most common causes, followed by fungal endophthalmitis caused by among others *Candida parapsilosis*, *Aspergillus* ssp, and *Fusarium* ssp. [91]. A rapid diagnosis is often of utmost importance. For the diagnosis of endophthalmitis, investigation of vitreous by direct Gram-staining and/or culture is currently mostly applied. More recently, molecular analysis of ocular fluids is being explored. Large studies comparing PCR to classical diagnostic tools are not available yet, but molecular analysis clearly has its advantages. PCR can be more sensitive than Gram-staining and culture particular in very early stages of the disease, when the causative agent concerns a fastidious pathogen or when the patient has received antimicrobial treatment [92–94]. Also PCR results are acquired faster than culture outcomes. Moreover, with the emergence of antimicrobial resistance, also intraocularly, new PCR assays are being developed which not only identify specific microbes but also determine resistance profiles [95–97].

Molecular assays currently described for infectious endophthalmitis mostly include the broad-range bacterial and fungal PCR assays [94, 98–102]. In addition, Gram-discriminating and microorganism-specific molecular assay are available [103, 104]. Novel explorations include the use of multiplex PCR techniques and DNA microarrays, which may allow for simultaneous detection and identification of a large number of microorganism species and may also include resistance profiling [101, 48].

1.6 Molecular Diagnosis of Infectious Uveitis

As the inner eye is a secluded compartment separated from the periphery by the blood-retina barrier, analysis of peripheral blood is often not informative for the diagnosis of infectious uveitis.

For a definitive diagnosis, the analysis of intraocular fluid is imperative. To obtain intraocular fluid for diagnostic purposes, a vitreous or aqueous tap can be performed [3, 105, 106]. A diagnostic vitrectomy is more aggressive than an aqueous tap but yields a larger amount of ocular fluid (0.5–0.7 mL). Possible complications of vitrectomy are endophthalmitis and retinal detachment; however, their incidence is low [3, 107]. An aqueous tap can be performed in the outpatient setting, providing approximately 0.1–0.2 mL aqueous [108]. This procedure has been shown to be safe in the hands of an experienced ophthalmologist [105, 106]. Various infrequent complications may occur, such as hyphema, occurring mostly in patients with a high intraocular pressure (IOP) at time of paracentesis [106]. To date, no systematic studies have been done to determine whether vitreous or aqueous is superior in ocular fluid analyses nor have investigated whether the choice of aqueous or vitreous aspirate should be dependent on the location of inflammation within the eye. However, it has been reported that aqueous humor analysis provides a safe and useful first laboratory diagnostic tool prior to the more perilous vitrectomy and that subsequent vitreous analysis when the aqueous humor was negative contributes only marginally to the diagnosis of infectious uveitis [108–110].

Polymerase chain reaction (PCR) analysis of intraocular fluids has become an important tool for the diagnosis of infectious uveitis and may yield results close to 100 % for acute retinal necrosis and CMV retinitis [21, 111, 112]. However, in other infectious uveitis entities, PCR yields may be lower. In these cases, analysis of intraocular antibody production by Goldmann-Witmer coefficient (GWC) or Antibody Index (AI) calculation may contribute to the diagnosis of viral and parasitic uveitis entities [13, 113–119]. The GWC or AI is calculated by determining the ratio of pathogen-specific antibody and total antibody, usually immunoglobulin G, in serum and ocular fluid thus allowing for the differentiation between leakage of peripheral antibodies into the intraocular fluid and actual local antibody production.

1.6.1 Diagnosis of Viral Uveitis

The most common viral ocular infections are caused by herpes simplex virus (HSV), varicella zoster virus (VZV), and cytomegalovirus (CMV). However, over the past decade, new viruses have been identified as important etiologies involved in uveitis, such as rubella virus, West Nile virus, dengue virus, and Chikungunya virus [120, 121, 117].

1.6.1.1 Herpetic Uveitis

Herpetic uveitis is an ocular inflammation secondary to viral infection caused by HSV-1 and HSV-2, VZV, or CMV. Intraocular herpetic infections may present as anterior (kerato)-uveitis or as characteristic types of posterior uveitis, such as acute retinal necrosis (ARN), progressive outer retinal necrosis (PORN), and CMV retinitis. More recently, atypical and non-ARN types of posterior ocular infections with HSV and VZV were reported, as well as hypertensive anterior uveitis and Fuchs heterochromic uveitis caused by CMV.[122–128, 112] CMV retinitis and PORN occur predominantly in immunosuppressed patients, whereas the other entities are prevalent mostly in patients with a competent immune system. Peripheral blood analyses for antibodies against HSV, VZV, and CMV are not useful, because the majority of adults are seropositive (up to 90, 100 and 90 % worldwide, respectively) even without a clear clinical history of disease [129–133]. To establish an intraocular herpesviral infection without obvious extraocular signs analysis of aqueous humor or vitreous fluid is required.

PCR on ocular fluids has been widely used to diagnose herpetic posterior and panuveitis [1–4, 13, 129, 108, 19, 134–137, 21, 111, 112]. Particularly in ARN and PORN, PCR analysis has a high success rate. Due to the progressive nature of the infection and the high production of viral progeny, PCR may yield sensitivities up to 100 % [4, 111, 21, 112]. Other HSV- and VZV-induced retinitis entities also benefit from molecular diagnosis albeit with a lower yield [122, 128, 212]. Possibly, because viral replication occurs at a lower level or because the viral load has decreased due to antiviral treatment or due to sampling at a later time point in disease [4, 13, 119, 118]. Atypical presentations of posterior uveitis form a diagnostic challenge, and a delay in treatment can be harmful to vision. Here, the diagnosis may also benefit from quick laboratory testing of aqueous or vitreous specimens.

The diagnosis of CMV retinitis is usually based on the typical ophthalmoscopic picture. However, in an immunosuppressed individual, the introduction of HAART might influence the clinical presentation, rendering the clinical diagnosis more difficult [138–140]. Also for the diagnosis of CMV retinitis, PCR analysis of intraocular fluid may be useful and is highly sensitive particularly in patients with AIDS [141, 108, 134–136, 1, 21, 112, 2].

PCR analysis is also applied for the diagnosis of herpetic anterior uveitis. Sensitivities range between 20 and 80 % and are higher when the analysis includes multiple herpes viruses, such as combined testing for HSV and VZV [136, 112, 127, 142–144]. CMV anterior uveitis is a newly recognized entity and includes a range of ophthalmological manifestations overlapping with HSV, VZV, and rubella virus-induced anterior uveitis [145, 123, 125, 146]. Chee et al. confirmed CMV anterior uveitis by PCR analysis of aqueous humor; however, other groups also diagnosed CMV anterior uveitis by GWC analysis alone, suggesting that the sensitivity of PCR is less than 100 % [124, 126, 147].

In immunocompetent patients, herpes viral nucleic acid can be readily detected in the early stages of the disease, whereas at later stages PCR assays tend to become negative [4, 13, 119, 118]. The most likely explanation is that later in infection, the immune system, whether or not supported by adequate antiviral therapy, has cleared the virus or has reduced the viral load below the detection level. This may explain the high sensitivity of PCR for the diagnosis of ARN, where paracentesis is usually performed very early in the disease [4]. In immunosuppressed individuals, viral replication is hardly or not at all limited in the absence of antiviral therapy explaining the high sensitivity of PCR analysis in CMV retinitis in AIDS patients [134, 2].

In addition to merely diagnosing a viral infection, PCR analysis of sequential ocular samples may be very useful to monitor the efficacy of antiviral therapy particularly when treating devastating entities such as ARN, PORN, and CMV retinitis [141, 148–150]. Moreover, PCR analysis and subsequent sequence or DNA microarray analysis may also be applied to detect antiviral resistance [151].

1.6.1.2 Fuchs Heterochromic Uveitis Syndrome and Rubella Virus-Associated Uveitis

Fuchs heterochromic uveitis syndrome (FHUS) is a chronic low-grade anterior chamber inflammation characterized by typical clinical signs such as fine keratic precipitates, diffuse iris atrophy and/or heterochromia, the development of cataract, and the absence of posterior synechiae prior to surgery. In Europe, FHUS was reported to be highly associated with rubella virus as in almost 100 % of patients intraocular antibody production against rubella virus was demonstrated [117, 152–154, 147]. Moreover, Birnbaum et al. found that the incidence of FHUS was reduced in patients vaccinated against rubella virus, strongly suggesting a causal relationship between FHUS and rubella virus [155]. Additional studies showed that rubella virus-associated uveitis represents a range of clinical manifestations including true FHUS but also FHUS-like entities [156, 146].

Due to the high incidence of natural infection during the pre-vaccination era and recent vaccination programs, the seroprevalence for rubella virus antibodies is very high (94–96 %) [157]. Therefore, serology is not informative for the diagnosis of rubella virus-associated uveitis and intraocular fluid analysis is essential. Several reports showed that intraocular antibody production against Rubella virus is positive in 93–100 % of rubella virus-associated uveitis cases, whereas PCR remains negative in the majority of cases (80–90 %) [117, 152–154]. This may be explained by a persistent low-grade infection resulting in a low viral load in the aqueous humor [117]. However, FHUS representing a chronic autoimmune reaction triggered by the virus also remains a possibility [158]. In short, contrary to herpesviral uveitis, PCR analysis is not recommended as a first diagnostic laboratory tool for rubella virus-associated uveitis, but may be considered when intraocular antibody production is detected against rubella virus.

1.6.1.3 Other Viruses

Other viruses less frequently associated with uveitis can also be identified by PCR analysis such as Chikungunya virus, dengue virus, HIV, human herpes virus 6, and West Nile virus, although information about the sensitivity of the PCR assays is unavailable [120, 39, 159–162, 121]. Epstein-Barr virus can also been identified by PCR in ocular fluids of uveitis patients; however, its role in uveitis remains controversial [39, 163, 112, 164]. A pathognomonic ocular manifestation has not been identified yet. Moreover, intraocular fluids of patients with laboratory-proven *Toxoplasma* chorioretinitis and VZV-induced acute retinal necrosis and of patients without intraocular inflammation have been found PCR-positive for EBV. Therefore, PCR results should be interpreted with caution and preferably performed in combination with other laboratory tests, such as determination of intraocular antibody production [39].

1.6.2 Diagnosis of Parasitic Uveitis

1.6.2.1 Ocular Toxoplasmosis

Ocular toxoplasmosis (OT), caused by the parasite *Toxoplasma gondii*, is the most common identifiable cause of posterior uveitis in many parts of the world and can be acquired either by congenital or postnatal route of infection [165]. Classically, OT presents as a unilateral focal retinochoroidal lesion [166–169]. In immunocompromised patients, OT may exhibit a variety of clinical manifestations, including single foci of retinochoroiditis in one or both eyes, multifocal lesions, or diffuse areas of retinal necrosis, and occasionally as AU [170–172]. *Toxoplasma* infection may also mimic ARN and should be considered when diagnostic testing for HSV, VZV, and CMV is negative [173].

For the diagnosis of OT, detection of anti-*T. gondii* IgG antibodies in peripheral blood is not informative in areas with a medium to high seroprevalence. Detection of serum IgM may be useful, if OT accompanies a recently acquired *Toxoplasma* infection [174, 175]. To confirm the diagnosis of toxoplasmosis, intraocular fluid analysis can be performed to detect *T. gondii* DNA by PCR and/or to establish intraocular antibody production by Goldmann-Witmer coefficient [175]. Immunoblotting has also been described for the detection of serum and intraocular antibody; however, this method is elaborate and quantitation of specific bands is more complicated [22, 176]. Several studies on PCR analysis of *Toxoplasma* in aqueous humor reported positive results ranging from 13 to 36 % [177, 13, 178, 22]. Analysis of intraocular antibody production reportedly yielded positive results up to 93 % and, therefore, appears to play a more decisive role in the diagnosis of intraocular *Toxoplasma* infection [13, 178, 108, 22, 2]. In primary OT, both PCR and GWC analysis contribute equally to the diagnosis of ocular disease [178, 174, 108, 22]. In immunocompromised patients, both assays appear to be valuable; however, PCR was reported to perform best in atypical toxoplasmic chorioretinitis in these patients [178, 2, 174].

Various studies suggest that for the diagnosis of OT, the application of both diagnostic assays is indicated irrespective of the patient's immune status [177, 13, 176, 2].

1.6.3 Diagnosis of Bacterial Uveitis

In uveitis, the bacterial load in ocular fluids is usually too low to be detected by culture. Moreover, the involved bacteria are frequently fastidious or grow obligatory intracellular. PCR analysis may overcome these problems. Several molecular assays exist for the detection of intraocular bacteria. Specific assays are available for *Mycobacterium tuberculosis*, *Treponema pallidum*, and *Tropheryma whipplei* [179–181, 31, 29]. PCR assays are also available for *Borrelia* and *Bartonella*; however, positive results on ocular fluid have sporadically been reported [182, 29]. For the detection of bacteria, the panbacterial 16S rRNA gene-based assay may be used [29]. Identification of the particular bacterial species requires subsequent sequence analysis of the amplification product. The latter method has proven valuable for screening large cohorts of undiagnosed uveitis and endophthalmitis patients but may also be of value for individual ophthalmology patients with a strong suspicion of a bacterial intraocular infection for which a specific PCR assay is not available [35, 29, 99, 183].

1.6.3.1 Ocular Tuberculosis

Ocular tuberculosis may present in many entities including conjunctivitis, keratitis, scleritis, anterior granulomatous inflammation, retinal vasculitis, or chorioretinal lesions similar to serpiginous-like choroiditis. The ability to mimic other infections is in part determined by the variable host response and to the fact that virtually all parts of the eye may be affected [184–186, 83]. This large variation in presentations makes the diagnosis of intraocular tuberculosis difficult. Clinical suspicion is an imperative first step toward the correct diagnosis. Patients suspected of ocular tuberculosis generally undergo a complete physical examination including a Mantoux tuberculin skin test (TST) and chest radiograph. However, the TST test results should be interpreted with care. Vaccination with the bacillus Calmette-Guérin (BCG) vaccine poses a potential source of cross-reactions and may yield false-positive results [184, 187]. Recently, interferon-gamma release assays (IGRAs), such as the QuantiFERON-TB Gold test and the T. Spot-TB® Elispot assay have been added to the diagnostic repertoire [188, 184, 189, 190]. The antigens used in these assays are not shared by the vaccine strain, thus preventing false-positive results in BCG-vaccinated individuals [188, 184]. A positive TST or IGRA only indicates that a person has been exposed to *Mycobacterium tuberculosis*, and does not distinguish between active or latent disease. In fact, in active disease or in AIDS patients with a low CD4 count, both the TST and IGRAs may be negative [191–195].

The diagnosis of ocular tuberculosis is definitive when *M. tuberculosis* is identified in the eye. However, this is rarely achieved, because mycobacterial culture facilities are not readily available and cultures may require several weeks for a positive result [191, 196]. A rapid procedure for diagnosing tuberculosis is the examination of acid-fast (Ziehl-Neelsen) stained smears of infected ocular tissue or fluid. But, as the amount of microorganisms found in intraocular fluids is usually relatively low, direct microscopy of the smears may not be sensitive enough [197, 184]. *M. tuberculosis*-specific molecular tests, mostly PCR assays, are available and have been found useful for the diagnosis of intraocular tuberculosis using several intraocular materials, such as aqueous humor and vitreous fluid, but also chorioretinal biopsies and subretinal fluid [179, 23, 180, 27, 198–200]. Recently, also LAMP assays were developed for *Mycobacterium tuberculosis* [45, 46]. Little information is available on the sensitivity of the molecular tests for the various ocular tuberculosis entities and the ocular material analyzed. However, anecdotal data suggest that these assays are most useful in tuberculosis endemic areas where intraocular bacterial loads may be higher.

1.6.3.2 Ocular Syphilis

The spirochete *Treponema pallidum* is the causative agent of syphilis, a sexually transmitted disease [201]. Uveitis is the most common ocular feature of syphilis and is often associated with neurosyphilis [202]. No pathognomonic features exist for syphilitic uveitis and, hence, the term "great imitator" applies not only to systemic syphilis but also to ocular syphilitic disease. When ocular syphilis is suspected, initially standard syphilis screening assays are performed, such as the *Treponema pallidum* hemagglutination and particle agglutination assays (TPHA and TPPA, respectively), fluorescent treponemal antibody absorption (FTA-ABS) test and the immunoblot on peripheral blood. Enzyme immunoassays are also available and show promising results as screening assays in all stages of syphilis [203, 204]. However, none of these tests discriminate between a previous or active infection.

The non-treponemal Venereal Disease Research Laboratory (VDRL) and the rapid plasma reagin (RPR) tests are applied to determine the activity of disease and can be useful to monitor treatment [201]. Neurosyphilis is confirmed by a positive VDRL in CSF or by the presence of intrathecal antibody production, using the TPHA or TPPA [205–207]. The diagnosis of ocular syphilis is considered proven when ocular disease is present in active syphilis or in combination with proven neurosyphilis. However, in case of severely immunocompromised patients, the possibility of other ocular infections should preferable be excluded. Intraocular fluid analysis is not commonly used for the diagnosis of ocular syphilis. PCR assays are available and have been reported positive for both aqueous and vitreous fluids; however, sensitivity data on the molecular analysis for ocular syphilis are not available [30, 31, 208, 209].

Conclusions

Most molecular assays are expensive and require well-equipped laboratories. Moreover, molecular analysis may not always provide an answer. However, molecular diagnostic tools clearly have their benefits. Particularly PCR analysis of ocular fluids can contribute significantly to the diagnosis of an ocular infection. However, it also has its weaknesses and limitations. A positive PCR result may depend on many factors. Indisputably, it requires the presence of the culprit in the collected ocular sample. Depending on the location and nature of the ocular infection, the pathogenic load in different ocular samples may differ. For instance, in case of herpes keratitis, it was demonstrated that the viral burden is higher in ocular scrapings than in tear fluid [68]. For the same reason, *Chlamydia trachomatis*, an obligate intracellular bacterium, is best detected in conjunctival swabs which contain infected cells. Negative PCR results may also be encountered when a patient has already been treated with antibiotics or antivirals. Furthermore, in subacute or chronic ocular diseases, such as herpetic anterior uveitis and rubella virus-associated uveitis, the pathogenic load may have dropped below the detection level rendering negative PCR results. On the other hand, PCR assays have become so sensitive that occasionally infectious agents are detected that are merely bystanders and do not contribute to the actual disease.

Other diagnostic tools may complement molecular diagnostic tools, not only to confirm a diagnosis in case of a negative PCR result but also to confirm or exclude a diagnosis in case of a putative false-positive PCR result. Antibody detection may provide a valuable addition to the diagnostic repertoire. In keratitis and conjunctivitis, IgA detection in tear fluid can be of help [210, 211]. In infectious uveitis, the detection of intraocular antibody production can play a major role in the diagnosis of herpesviral, rubella viral, and toxoplasmic infections [4, 152, 13, 119, 118, 175, 22].

Compliance with Ethical Requirements

Conflict of Interest The author declares that she has no conflict of interest.

Informed Consent No human studies were carried out by the authors for this article.

Animal Studies No animal studies were carried out by the authors for this article.

References

1. Mitchell SM, Fox JD, Tedder RS, Gazzard BG, Lightman S. Vitreous fluid sampling and viral genome detection for the diagnosis of viral retinitis in patients with AIDS. J Med Virol. 1994;43(4):336–40.
2. Westeneng AC, Rothova A, de Boer JH, de Groot-Mijnes JDF. Infectious uveitis in immunocompromised patients and the diagnostic value of polymerase chain reaction and Goldmann-Witmer coefficient in aqueous analysis. Am J Ophthalmol. 2007;144(5):781–5.
3. Bodaghi B, LeHoang P. Testing ocular fluids in uveitis. Ophthalmol Clin North Am. 2002;15(3):271–9.
4. de Boer JH, Verhagen C, Bruinenberg M, Rothova A, de Jong PT, Baarsma GS, et al. Serologic and polymerase chain reaction analysis of intraocular fluids in the diagnosis of infectious uveitis. Am J Ophthalmol. 1996;121(6):650–8.
5. Thomas PA, Kaliamurthy J. Mycotic keratitis: epidemiology, diagnosis and management. Clin Microbiol Infect. 2013;19(3):210–20.

6. Liu S, Pavan-Langston D, Colby KA. Pediatric herpes simplex of the anterior segment: characteristics, treatment, and outcomes. Ophthalmology. 2012; 119(10):2003–8.
7. Revere K, Davidson SL. Update on management of herpes keratitis in children. Curr Opin Ophthalmol. 2013;24(4):343–7.
8. Saiki RK, Gelfand DH, Stoffel S, Scharf SJ, Higuchi R, Horn GT, et al. Primer-directed enzymatic amplification of DNA with a thermostable DNA polymerase. Science. 1988;239(4839):487–91.
9. Mackay IM, Arden KE, Nitsche A. Real-time PCR in virology. Nucleic Acids Res. 2002;30(6):1292–305.
10. Niesters HG. Clinical virology in real time. J Clin Virol. 2002;25 Suppl 3:S3–12.
11. Dimmock JN, Easton AJ, Leppard KN. Some methods for studying animal viruses. In: Introduction to modern virology. 6th ed. Malden: Blackwell Publishing; 2007. p. 18–29.
12. Persing DH. In vitro nucleic acid amplification techniques. In: Persing DH, Smith TF, Tenover TJ, White TJ, editors. Diagnostic molecular microbiology, principles and applications. Rochester: Mayo Foundation; 1993. p. 51–87.
13. De Groot-Mijnes JDF, Rothova A, Van Loon AM, Schuller M, Ten Dam-Van Loon NH, De Boer JH, et al. Polymerase chain reaction and Goldmann-Witmer coefficient analysis are complimentary for the diagnosis of infectious uveitis. Am J Ophthalmol. 2006;141(2):313–8.
14. Espy MJ, Uhl JR, Sloan LM, Buckwalter SP, Jones MF, Vetter EA, et al. Real-time PCR in clinical microbiology: applications for routine laboratory testing. Clin Microbiol Rev. 2006;19(1):165–256.
15. Costa C, Costa JM, Desterke C, Botterel F, Cordonnier C, Bretagne S. Real-time PCR coupled with automated DNA extraction and detection of galactomannan antigen in serum by enzyme-linked immunosorbent assay for diagnosis of invasive aspergillosis. J Clin Microbiol. 2002;40(6):2224–7.
16. Loeffler J, Henke N, Hebart H, Schmidt D, Hagmeyer L, Schumacher U, et al. Quantification of fungal DNA by using fluorescence resonance energy transfer and the light cycler system. J Clin Microbiol. 2000;38(2):586–90.
17. Buchheidt D, Hummel M, Schleiermacher D, Spiess B, Schwerdtfeger R, Cornely OA, et al. Prospective clinical evaluation of a LightCycler-mediated polymerase chain reaction assay, a nested-PCR assay and a galactomannan enzyme-linked immunosorbent assay for detection of invasive aspergillosis in neutropenic cancer patients and haematological stem cell transplant recipients. Br J Haematol. 2004;125(2):196–202.
18. Spiess B, Buchheidt D, Baust C, Skladny H, Seifarth W, Zeilfelder U, et al. Development of a LightCycler PCR assay for detection and quantification of Aspergillus fumigatus DNA in clinical samples from neutropenic patients. J Clin Microbiol. 2003;41(5):1811–8.
19. Matos K, Muccioli C, Belfort Junior R, Rizzo LV. Correlation between clinical diagnosis and PCR analysis of serum, aqueous, and vitreous samples in patients with inflammatory eye disease. Arq Bras Oftalmol. 2007;70(1):109–14.
20. Fox GM, Crouse CA, Chuang EL, Pflugfelder SC, Cleary TJ, Nelson SJ, et al. Detection of herpesvirus DNA in vitreous and aqueous specimens by the polymerase chain reaction. Arch Ophthalmol. 1991;109(2):266–71.
21. Tran TH, Rozenberg F, Cassoux N, Rao NA, LeHoang P, Bodaghi B. Polymerase chain reaction analysis of aqueous humour samples in necrotising retinitis. Br J Ophthalmol. 2003;87(1):79–83.
22. Villard O, Filisetti D, Roch-Deries F, Garweg J, Flament J, Candolfi E. Comparison of enzyme-linked immunosorbent assay, immunoblotting, and PCR for diagnosis of toxoplasmic chorioretinitis. J Clin Microbiol. 2003;41(8):3537–41.
23. Brisson-Noel A, Gicquel B, Lecossier D, Levy-Frebault V, Nassif X, Hance AJ. Rapid diagnosis of tuberculosis by amplification of mycobacterial DNA in clinical samples. Lancet. 1989;2(8671):1069–71.
24. Gupta V, Arora S, Gupta A, Ram J, Bambery P, Sehgal S. Management of presumed intraocular tuberculosis: possible role of the polymerase chain reaction. Acta Ophthalmol Scand. 1998;76(6):679–82.
25. Hilton E, Smith C, Sood S. Ocular Lyme borreliosis diagnosed by polymerase chain reaction on vitreous fluid. Ann Intern Med. 1996;125(5):424–5.
26. Mikkila H, Karma A, Viljanen M, Seppala I. The laboratory diagnosis of ocular Lyme borreliosis. Graefes Arch Clin Exp Ophthalmol. 1999;237(3):225–30.
27. Ortega-Larrocea G, Bobadilla-del-Valle M, Ponce-de-Leon A, Sifuentes-Osornio J. Nested polymerase chain reaction for Mycobacterium tuberculosis DNA detection in aqueous and vitreous of patients with uveitis. Arch Med Res. 2003;34(2):116–9.
28. Bergmans AM, Groothedde JW, Schellekens JF, van Embden JD, Ossewaarde JM, Schouls LM. Etiology of cat scratch disease: comparison of polymerase chain reaction detection of Bartonella (formerly Rochalimaea) and Afipia felis DNA with serology and skin tests. J Infect Dis. 1995;171(4):916–23.
29. Drancourt M, Berger P, Terrada C, Bodaghi B, Conrath J, Raoult D, et al. High prevalence of fastidious bacteria in 1520 cases of uveitis of unknown etiology. Medicine (Baltimore). 2008;87(3):167–76.
30. Müller M, Ewert I, Hansmann F, Tiemann C, Hagedorn HJ, Solbach W, et al. Detection of Treponema pallidum in the vitreous by PCR. Br J Ophthalmol. 2007;91(5):592–5.
31. Rajan MS, Pantelidis P, Tong CY, French GL, Graham EM, Stanford MR. Diagnosis of Treponema pallidum in vitreous samples using real time polymerase chain reaction. Br J Ophthalmol. 2006;90(5):647–8.
32. Carroll NM, Jaeger EE, Choudhury S, Dunlop AA, Matheson MM, Adamson P, et al. Detection of and discrimination between gram-positive and gram-negative bacteria in intraocular samples by using nested PCR. J Clin Microbiol. 2000;38(5):1753–7.
33. Higashide T, Takahashi M, Kobayashi A, Ohkubo S, Sakurai M, Shirao Y, et al. Endophthalmitis caused by Enterococcus mundtii. J Clin Microbiol. 2005;43(3):1475–6.

34. Kerkhoff FT, van der Zee A, Bergmans AM, Rothova A. Polymerase chain reaction detection of Neisseria meningitidis in the intraocular fluid of a patient with endogenous endophthalmitis but without associated meningitis. Ophthalmology. 2003;110(11):2134–6.
35. Okhravi N, Adamson P, Carroll N, Dunlop A, Matheson MM, Towler HM, et al. PCR-based evidence of bacterial involvement in eyes with suspected intraocular infection. Invest Ophthalmol Vis Sci. 2000;41(11):3474–9.
36. Janda JM, Abbott SL. 16S rRNA gene sequencing for bacterial identification in the diagnostic laboratory: pluses, perils, and pitfalls. J Clin Microbiol. 2007;45(9):2761–4.
37. Kim E, Chidambaram JD, Srinivasan M, Lalitha P, Wee D, Lietman TM, et al. Prospective comparison of microbial culture and polymerase chain reaction in the diagnosis of corneal ulcer. Am J Ophthalmol. 2008;146(5):714–23. 23 e1.
38. Ongkosuwito JV, Feron EJ, van Doornik CE, Van der Lelij A, Hoyng CB, La Heij EC, et al. Analysis of immunoregulatory cytokines in ocular fluid samples from patients with uveitis. Invest Ophthalmol Vis Sci. 1998;39(13):2659–65.
39. de Groot-Mijnes JDF, de Visser L, Zuurveen S, Martinus RA, Volker R, ten Dam-van Loon NH, et al. Identification of new pathogens in the intraocular fluid of patients with uveitis. Am J Ophthalmol. 2010;150(5):628–36.
40. Bijlsma WR, Kalmann R, Dekkers J, Paridaens D, Mourits MP, Kloos R, et al. Identification of infectious entities in idiopathic orbital inflammation biopsies. Br J Ophthalmol. 2013;97(5):664–5.
41. Notomi T, Okayama H, Masubuchi H, Yonekawa T, Watanabe K, Amino N, et al. Loop-mediated isothermal amplification of DNA. Nucleic Acids Res. 2000;28(12):E63.
42. Kaneko H, Iida T, Aoki K, Ohno S, Suzutani T. Sensitive and rapid detection of herpes simplex virus and varicella-zoster virus DNA by loop-mediated isothermal amplification. J Clin Microbiol. 2005;43(7):3290–6.
43. Mohan A, Kiran DH, Manohar IC, Kumar DP. Epidemiology, clinical manifestations, and diagnosis of Chikungunya fever: lessons learned from the re-emerging epidemic. Indian J Dermatol. 2010;55(1):54–63.
44. Shukla J, Saxena D, Rathinam S, Lalitha P, Joseph CR, Sharma S, et al. Molecular detection and characterization of West Nile virus associated with multifocal retinitis in patients from southern India. Int J Infect Dis. 2012;16(1):e53–9.
45. Iwamoto T, Sonobe T, Hayashi K. Loop-mediated isothermal amplification for direct detection of Mycobacterium tuberculosis complex, M. avium, and M. intracellulare in sputum samples. J Clin Microbiol. 2003;41(6):2616–22.
46. Mitarai S, Okumura M, Toyota E, Yoshiyama T, Aono A, Sejimo A, et al. Evaluation of a simple loop-mediated isothermal amplification test kit for the diagnosis of tuberculosis. Int J Tuberc Lung Dis. 2011;15(9):1211–7. i.
47. Ge Z, Qing Y, Zicheng S, Shiying S. Rapid and sensitive diagnosis of Acanthamoeba keratitis by loop-mediated isothermal amplification. Clin Microbiol Infect. 2013;19:1042–8.
48. Sakai T, Kohzaki K, Watanabe A, Tsuneoka H, Shimadzu M. Use of DNA microarray analysis in diagnosis of bacterial and fungal endophthalmitis. Clin Ophthalmol. 2013;6:321–6.
49. Bhosai SJ, Bailey RL, Gaynor BD, Lietman TM. Trachoma: an update on prevention, diagnosis, and treatment. Curr Opin Ophthalmol. 2012; 23(4):288–95.
50. Schaeffer A, Henrich B. Rapid detection of Chlamydia trachomatis and typing of the Lymphogranuloma venereum associated L-Serovars by TaqMan PCR. BMC Infect Dis. 2008;8:56.
51. Mabey D, Solomon AW. Application of molecular tools in the control of blinding trachoma. Am J Trop Med Hyg. 2003;69(5 Suppl):11–7.
52. Yang JL, Hong KC, Schachter J, Moncada J, Lekew T, House JI, et al. Detection of Chlamydia trachomatis ocular infection in trachoma-endemic communities by rRNA amplification. Invest Ophthalmol Vis Sci. 2009;50(1):90–4.
53. Burton MJ, Holland MJ, Jeffries D, Mabey DC, Bailey RL. Conjunctival chlamydial 16S ribosomal RNA expression in trachoma: is chlamydial metabolic activity required for disease to develop? Clin Infect Dis. 2006;42(4):463–70.
54. Yang JL, Schachter J, Moncada J, Habte D, Zerihun M, House JI, et al. Comparison of an rRNA-based and DNA-based nucleic acid amplification test for the detection of Chlamydia trachomatis in trachoma. Br J Ophthalmol. 2007;91(3):293–5.
55. West SK, Munoz B, Mkocha H, Holland MJ, Aguirre A, Solomon AW, et al. Infection with Chlamydia trachomatis after mass treatment of a trachoma hyperendemic community in Tanzania: a longitudinal study. Lancet. 2005;366(9493):1296–300.
56. Burton MJ, Holland MJ, Makalo P, Aryee EA, Alexander ND, Sillah A, et al. Re-emergence of Chlamydia trachomatis infection after mass antibiotic treatment of a trachoma-endemic Gambian community: a longitudinal study. Lancet. 2005;365(9467):1321–8.
57. Karsten E, Watson SL, Foster LJ. Diversity of microbial species implicated in keratitis: a review. Open Ophthalmol J. 2012;6:110–24.
58. Thompson PP, Kowalski RP. A 13-year retrospective review of polymerase chain reaction testing for infectious agents from ocular samples. Ophthalmology. 2011;118(7):1449–53.
59. Goldschmidt P, Rostane H, Saint-Jean C, Batellier L, Alouch C, Zito E, et al. Effects of topical anaesthetics and fluorescein on the real-time PCR used for the diagnosis of Herpesviruses and Acanthamoeba keratitis. Br J Ophthalmol. 2006;90(11):1354–6.
60. Miyakoshi A, Takemoto M, Shiraki K, Hayashi A. Varicella-zoster virus keratitis with asymptomatic

conjunctival viral shedding in the contralateral eye. Case Rep Ophthalmol. 2012;3(3):343–8.
61. Banik U, Adhikary AK, Suzuki E, Inada T, Okabe N. Multiplex PCR assay for rapid identification of oculopathogenic adenoviruses by amplification of the fiber and hexon genes. J Clin Microbiol. 2005;43(3):1064–8.
62. Rowe AM, St Leger AJ, Jeon S, Dhaliwal DK, Knickelbein JE, Hendricks RL. Herpes keratitis. Prog Retin Eye Res. 2013;32:88–101.
63. Hlinomazova Z, Loukotova V, Horackova M, Sery O. The treatment of HSV1 ocular infections using quantitative real-time PCR results. Acta Ophthalmol. 2012;90(5):456–60.
64. Choong K, Walker NJ, Apel AJ, Whitby M. Aciclovir-resistant herpes keratitis. Clin Experiment Ophthalmol. 2010;38(3):309–13.
65. Turner LD, Beckingsale P. Acyclovir-resistant herpetic keratitis in a solid-organ transplant recipient on systemic immunosuppression. Clin Ophthalmol. 2013;7:229–32.
66. Praidou A, Androudi S, Kanonidou E, Konidaris V, Alexandridis A, Brazitikos P. Bilateral herpes simplex keratitis presenting as peripheral ulcerative keratitis. Cornea. 2012;31(5):570–1.
67. Tsagkataki M, Trainor E, Kaye LC, Hopkins MJ, Kaye SB. Adenoviral keratoconjunctivitis associated with stromal oedema and keratic precipitates. Clin Exp Ophthalmol. 2013;41:715–6.
68. Kakimaru-Hasegawa A, Kuo CH, Komatsu N, Komatsu K, Miyazaki D, Inoue Y. Clinical application of real-time polymerase chain reaction for diagnosis of herpetic diseases of the anterior segment of the eye. Jpn J Ophthalmol. 2008;52(1):24–31.
69. Usui M, Usui N, Goto H, Minoda H, Rai T. Polymerase chain reaction for diagnosis of herpetic intraocular inflammation. Ocul Immunol Inflamm. 1993;1(1–2):105–12.
70. Hidalgo F, Melon S, de Ona M, Do Santos V, Martinez A, Cimadevilla R, et al. Diagnosis of herpetic keratoconjunctivitis by nested polymerase chain reaction in human tear film. Eur J Clin Microbiol Infect Dis. 1998;17(2):120–3.
71. Koizumi N, Nishida K, Adachi W, Tei M, Honma Y, Dota A, et al. Detection of herpes simplex virus DNA in atypical epithelial keratitis using polymerase chain reaction. Br J Ophthalmol. 1999;83(8):957–60.
72. Kudo E, Shiota H, Kinouchi Y, Mimura Y, Itakura M. Detection of herpes simplex virus DNA in tear fluid of stromal herpetic keratitis patients by nested polymerase chain reaction. Jpn J Ophthalmol. 1996;40(3):390–6.
73. Tei M, Nishida K, Kinoshita S. Polymerase chain reaction detection of herpes simplex virus in tear fluid from atypical herpetic epithelial keratitis after penetrating keratoplasty. Am J Ophthalmol. 1996;122(5):732–5.
74. Robert PY, Traccard I, Adenis JP, Denis F, Ranger-Rogez S. Multiplex detection of herpesviruses in tear fluid using the "stair primers" PCR method: prospective study of 93 patients. J Med Virol. 2002;66(4):506–11.
75. Fukuda M, Deai T, Hibino T, Higaki S, Hayashi K, Shimomura Y. Quantitative analysis of herpes simplex virus genome in tears from patients with herpetic keratitis. Cornea. 2003;22(7 Suppl):S55–60.
76. Khodadoost MA, Sabahi F, Behroz MJ, Roustai MH, Saderi H, Amini-Bavil-Olyaee S, et al. Study of a polymerase chain reaction-based method for detection of herpes simplex virus type 1 DNA among Iranian patients with ocular herpetic keratitis infection. Jpn J Ophthalmol. 2004;48(4):328–32.
77. Duan R, de Vries RD, Osterhaus AD, Remeijer L, Verjans GM. Acyclovir-resistant corneal HSV-1 isolates from patients with herpetic keratitis. J Infect Dis. 2008;198(5):659–63.
78. Andrei G, Fiten P, De Clercq E, Snoeck R, Opdenakker G. Evaluating phenotype and genotype of drug-resistant strains in herpesviruses. Mol Biotechnol. 2001;18(2):155–67.
79. Frobert E, Cortay JC, Ooka T, Najioullah F, Thouvenot D, Lina B, et al. Genotypic detection of acyclovir-resistant HSV-1: characterization of 67 ACV-sensitive and 14 ACV-resistant viruses. Antiviral Res. 2008;79(1):28–36.
80. Malartre N, Boulieu R, Falah N, Cortay JC, Lina B, Morfin F, et al. Effects of mutations on herpes simplex virus 1 thymidine kinase functionality: an in vitro assay based on detection of monophosphate forms of acyclovir and thymidine using HPLC/DAD. Antiviral Res. 2012;95(3):224–8.
81. Venard V, Dauendorffer JN, Carret AS, Corsaro D, Edert D, Bordigoni P, et al. Investigation of aciclovir-resistant herpes simplex virus I infection in a bone marrow transplantation unit: genotyping shows that different strains are involved. J Hosp Infect. 2001;47(3):181–7.
82. Thomas PA, A Teresa P, Theodore J, Geraldine P. PCR for the molecular diagnosis of mycotic keratitis. Expert Rev Mol Diagn. 2012;12(7):703–18.
83. Tabbara KF. Tuberculosis. Curr Opin Ophthalmol. 2007;18(6):493–501.
84. Kuo MT, Chang HC, Cheng CK, Chien CC, Fang PC, Chang TC. A highly sensitive method for molecular diagnosis of fungal keratitis: a dot hybridization assay. Ophthalmology. 2012;119(12):2434–42.
85. Ferrer C, Colom F, Frases S, Mulet E, Abad JL, Alio JL. Detection and identification of fungal pathogens by PCR and by ITS2 and 5.8S ribosomal DNA typing in ocular infections. J Clin Microbiol. 2001;39(8):2873–9.
86. Bharathi MJ, Ramakrishnan R, Meenakshi R, Mittal S, Shivakumar C, Srinivasan M. Microbiological diagnosis of infective keratitis: comparative evaluation of direct microscopy and culture results. Br J Ophthalmol. 2006;90(10):1271–6.
87. Eleinen KG, Mohalhal AA, Elmekawy HE, Abdulbaki AM, Sherif AM, El-Sherif RH, et al. Polymerase chain reaction-guided diagnosis of

infective keratitis – a hospital-based study. Curr Eye Res. 2012;37(11):1005–11.
88. Embong Z, Wan Hitam WH, Yean CY, Rashid NH, Kamarudin B, Abidin SK, et al. Specific detection of fungal pathogens by 18S rRNA gene PCR in microbial keratitis. BMC Ophthalmol. 2008;8:7.
89. Yang HW, Lee YR, Inoue N, Jha BK, Danne DB, Kim HK, et al. Loop-mediated isothermal amplification targeting 18S ribosomal DNA for rapid detection of Acanthamoeba. Korean J Parasitol. 2013;51(3):269–77.
90. Laummaunwai P, Ruangjirachuporn W, Boonmars T. A simple PCR condition for detection of a single cyst of Acanthamoeba species. Parasitol Res. 2012;110(4):1569–72.
91. Safneck JR. Endophthalmitis: a review of recent trends. Saudi J Ophthalmol. 2012;26(2):181–9.
92. Lohmann CP, Linde HJ, Reischl U. Improved detection of microorganisms by polymerase chain reaction in delayed endophthalmitis after cataract surgery. Ophthalmology. 2000;107(6):1047–51; discussion 51–2.
93. Okhravi N, Adamson P, Lightman S. Use of PCR in endophthalmitis. Ocul Immunol Inflamm. 2000;8(3):189–200.
94. Chiquet C, Cornut PL, Benito Y, Thuret G, Maurin M, Lafontaine PO, et al. Eubacterial PCR for bacterial detection and identification in 100 acute post-cataract surgery endophthalmitis. Invest Ophthalmol Vis Sci. 2008;49(5):1971–8.
95. Rossney AS, Herra CM, Brennan GI, Morgan PM, O'Connell B. Evaluation of the Xpert methicillin-resistant Staphylococcus aureus (MRSA) assay using the GeneXpert real-time PCR platform for rapid detection of MRSA from screening specimens. J Clin Microbiol. 2008;46(10):3285–90.
96. Boehme CC, Nabeta P, Hillemann D, Nicol MP, Shenai S, Krapp F, et al. Rapid molecular detection of tuberculosis and rifampin resistance. N Engl J Med. 2010;363(11):1005–15.
97. Melo GB, Bispo PJ, Yu MC, Pignatari AC, Hofling-Lima AL. Microbial profile and antibiotic susceptibility of culture-positive bacterial endophthalmitis. Eye (Lond). 2011;25(3):382–7; quiz 8.
98. Sugita S, Kamoi K, Ogawa M, Watanabe K, Shimizu N, Mochizuki M. Detection of Candida and Aspergillus species DNA using broad-range real-time PCR for fungal endophthalmitis. Graefes Arch Clin Exp Ophthalmol. 2012;250(3):391–8.
99. Sugita S, Shimizu N, Watanabe K, Katayama M, Horie S, Ogawa M, et al. Diagnosis of bacterial endophthalmitis by broad-range quantitative PCR. Br J Ophthalmol. 2011;95(3):345–9.
100. Ogawa M, Sugita S, Watanabe K, Shimizu N, Mochizuki M. Novel diagnosis of fungal endophthalmitis by broad-range real-time PCR detection of fungal 28S ribosomal DNA. Graefes Arch Clin Exp Ophthalmol. 2012;250(12):1877–83.
101. Bharathi MJ, Rameshkumar G, Ramakrishnan R, Venugopal Reddy YC, Shivkumar C, Ramesh S. Comparative evaluation of uniplex, nested, semi-nested, multiplex and nested multiplex PCR methods in the identification of microbial etiology of clinically suspected infectious endophthalmitis. Curr Eye Res. 2013;38(5):550–62.
102. Cornut PL, el Youssef B, Bron A, Thuret G, Gain P, Burillon C, et al. A multicentre prospective study of post-traumatic endophthalmitis. Acta Ophthalmol. 2013;91(5):475–82.
103. Melo GB, Bispo PJ, Campos Pignatari AC, Hofling-Lima AL. Real-time polymerase chain reaction test to discriminate between contamination and intraocular infection after cataract surgery. J Cataract Refract Surg. 2011;37(7):1244–50.
104. Smith WM, Fahle G, Nussenblatt RB, Sen HN. A rare case of endogenous Aspergillus conicus endophthalmitis in an immunocompromised patient. J Ophthalmic Inflamm Infect. 2013;3(1):37.
105. Cheung CM, Durrani OM, Murray PI. The safety of anterior chamber paracentesis in patients with uveitis. Br J Ophthalmol. 2004;88(4):582–3.
106. Van der Lelij A, Rothova A. Diagnostic anterior chamber paracentesis in uveitis: a safe procedure? Br J Ophthalmol. 1997;81(11):976–9.
107. Davis JL, Miller DM, Ruiz P. Diagnostic testing of vitrectomy specimens. Am J Ophthalmol. 2005; 140(5):822–9.
108. Rothova A, de Boer JH, Ten Dam-van Loon NH, Postma G, de Visser L, Zuurveen SJ, et al. Usefulness of aqueous humor analysis for the diagnosis of posterior uveitis. Ophthalmology. 2008; 115(2):306–11.
109. Harper TW, Miller D, Schiffman JC, Davis JL. Polymerase chain reaction analysis of aqueous and vitreous specimens in the diagnosis of posterior segment infectious uveitis. Am J Ophthalmol. 2009;147(1):140–7 e2.
110. Oahalou A, Schellekens PA, De Groot-Mijnes JD, Rothova A. Diagnostic pars plana vitrectomy and aqueous analyses in patients with uveitis of unknown cause. Retina. 2014;34:108–14.
111. Gargiulo F, De Francesco MA, Nascimbeni G, Turano R, Perandin F, Gandolfo E, et al. Polymerase chain reaction as a rapid diagnostic tool for therapy of acute retinal necrosis syndrome. J Med Virol. 2003;69(3):397–400.
112. Sugita S, Shimizu N, Watanabe K, Mizukami M, Morio T, Sugamoto Y, et al. Use of multiplex PCR and real-time PCR to detect human herpes virus genome in ocular fluids of patients with uveitis. Br J Ophthalmol. 2008;92(7):928–32.
113. Goldmann H, Witmer R. Antikörper im Kammerwasser. Ophthalmologica. 1954;127(4–5):323–30.
114. Desmonts G. Definitive serological diagnosis of ocular toxoplasmosis. Arch Ophthalmol. 1966; 76(6):839–51.
115. Dussaix E, Cerqueti PM, Pontet F, Bloch-Michel E. New approaches to the detection of locally produced antiviral antibodies in the aqueous of patients

with endogenous uveitis. Ophthalmologica. 1987;194(2–3):145–9.
116. Garweg JG, Jacquier P, Boehnke M. Early aqueous humor analysis in patients with human ocular toxoplasmosis. J Clin Microbiol. 2000;38(3):996–1001.
117. Quentin CD, Reiber H. Fuchs heterochromic cyclitis: rubella virus antibodies and genome in aqueous humor. Am J Ophthalmol. 2004;138(1):46–54.
118. Errera MH, Goldschmidt P, Batellier L, Degorge S, Heron E, Laroche L, et al. Findings in detection of Herpesviridae by polymerase chain reaction and intraocular antibody production in a case series of anterior uveitis. Ocul Immunol Inflamm. 2013;21(1):61–8.
119. Errera MH, Goldschmidt P, Batellier L, Degorge S, Heron E, Laroche L, et al. Real-time polymerase chain reaction and intraocular antibody production for the diagnosis of viral versus toxoplasmic infectious posterior uveitis. Graefes Arch Clin Exp Ophthalmol. 2011;249(12):1837–46.
120. Khairallah M, Chee SP, Rathinam SR, Attia S, Nadella V. Novel infectious agents causing uveitis. Int Ophthalmol. 2010;30(5):465–83.
121. Khairallah M, Kahloun R, Ben Yahia S, Jelliti B, Messaoud R. New infectious etiologies for posterior uveitis. Ophthalmic Res. 2013;49(2):66–72.
122. Bodaghi B, Rozenberg F, Cassoux N, Fardeau C, LeHoang P. Nonnecrotizing herpetic retinopathies masquerading as severe posterior uveitis. Ophthalmology. 2003;110(9):1737–43.
123. Chee SP, Jap A. Presumed fuchs heterochromic iridocyclitis and Posner-Schlossman syndrome: comparison of cytomegalovirus-positive and negative eyes. Am J Ophthalmol. 2008;146(6):883–9 e1.
124. de Schryver I, Rozenberg F, Cassoux N, Michelson S, Kestelyn P, Lehoang P, et al. Diagnosis and treatment of cytomegalovirus iridocyclitis without retinal necrosis. Br J Ophthalmol. 2006;90(7):852–5.
125. Markomichelakis NN, Canakis C, Zafirakis P, Marakis T, Mallias I, Theodossiadis G. Cytomegalovirus as a cause of anterior uveitis with sectoral iris atrophy. Ophthalmology. 2002;109(5):879–82.
126. van Boxtel LA, van der Lelij A, van der Meer J, Los LI. Cytomegalovirus as a cause of anterior uveitis in immunocompetent patients. Ophthalmology. 2007;114(7):1358–62.
127. Van der Lelij A, Ooijman FM, Kijlstra A, Rothova A. Anterior uveitis with sectoral iris atrophy in the absence of keratitis: a distinct clinical entity among herpetic eye diseases. Ophthalmology. 2000;107(6):1164–70.
128. Wensing B, de Groot-Mijnes JDF, Rothova A. Necrotizing and nonnecrotizing variants of herpetic uveitis with posterior segment involvement. Arch Ophthalmol. 2011;129(4):403–8.
129. Gaynor BD, Margolis TP, Cunningham Jr ET. Advances in diagnosis and management of herpetic uveitis. Int Ophthalmol Clin. 2000;40(2):85–109.
130. Kramer MA, Uitenbroek DG, Ujcic-Voortman JK, Pfrommer C, Spaargaren J, Coutinho RA, et al. Ethnic differences in HSV1 and HSV2 seroprevalence in Amsterdam, the Netherlands. Euro Surveill. 2008;13(24):1–5.
131. McCrary ML, Severson J, Tyring SK. Varicella zoster virus. J Am Acad Dermatol. 1999;41(1):1–14.
132. Wharton M. The epidemiology of varicella-zoster virus infections. Infect Dis Clin North Am. 1996;10(3):571–81.
133. Staras SA, Dollard SC, Radford KW, Flanders WD, Pass RF, Cannon MJ. Seroprevalence of cytomegalovirus infection in the United States, 1988–1994. Clin Infect Dis. 2006;43(9):1143–51.
134. Doornenbal P, Seerp Baarsma G, Quint WG, Kijlstra A, Rothbarth PH, Niesters HG. Diagnostic assays in cytomegalovirus retinitis: detection of herpesvirus by simultaneous application of the polymerase chain reaction and local antibody analysis on ocular fluid. Br J Ophthalmol. 1996;80(3):235–40.
135. Knox CM, Chandler D, Short GA, Margolis TP. Polymerase chain reaction-based assays of vitreous samples for the diagnosis of viral retinitis. Use in diagnostic dilemmas. Ophthalmology. 1998;105(1):37–44.
136. Yamamoto S, Pavan-Langston D, Kinoshita S, Nishida K, Shimomura Y, Tano Y. Detecting herpesvirus DNA in uveitis using the polymerase chain reaction. Br J Ophthalmol. 1996;80(5):465–8.
137. Silverstein BE, Conrad D, Margolis TP, Wong IG. Cytomegalovirus-associated acute retinal necrosis syndrome. Am J Ophthalmol. 1997;123(2):257–8.
138. Heiligenhaus A, Helbig H, Fiedler M. Herpesviruses. In: Foster CS, Vitale AT, editors. Diagnosis and treatment of uveitis. Philadelphia: W.B. Saunders Company; 2002. p. 315–32.
139. Sobrin L, Foster CS. Cytomegalovirus retinitis after one decade of HAART. Int Ophthalmol Clin. 2007;47(2):155–64.
140. Goldberg DE, Smithen LM, Angelilli A, Freeman WR. HIV-associated retinopathy in the HAART era. Retina. 2005;25(5):633–49.
141. Fenner TE, Garweg J, Hufert FT, Boehnke M, Schmitz H. Diagnosis of human cytomegalovirus-induced retinitis in human immunodeficiency virus type 1-infected subjects by using the polymerase chain reaction. J Clin Microbiol. 1991;29(11):2621–2.
142. Schacher S, Garweg JG, Russ C, Bohnke M. Die Diagnostik der herpetischen Uveitis und Keratouveitis. Klin Monatsbl Augenheilkd. 1998;212(5):359–62.
143. Siverio Junior CD, Imai Y, Cunningham Jr ET. Diagnosis and management of herpetic anterior uveitis. Int Ophthalmol Clin. 2002;42(1):43–8.
144. Miyanaga M, Sugita S, Shimizu N, Morio T, Miyata K, Maruyama K, et al. A significant association of viral loads with corneal endothelial cell damage in

cytomegalovirus anterior uveitis. Br J Ophthalmol. 2010;94(3):336–40.
145. Chee SP, Bacsal K, Jap A, Se-Thoe SY, Cheng CL, Tan BH. Clinical features of cytomegalovirus anterior uveitis in immunocompetent patients. Am J Ophthalmol. 2008;145(5):834–40.
146. Wensing B, Relvas LM, Caspers LE, Valentincic NV, Stunf S, de Groot-Mijnes JD, et al. Comparison of rubella virus- and herpes virus-associated anterior uveitis: clinical manifestations and visual prognosis. Ophthalmology. 2011;118(10):1905–10.
147. Kongyai N, Sirirungsi W, Pathanapitoon K, Tananuvat N, Kunavisarut P, Leechanachai P, et al. Viral causes of unexplained anterior uveitis in Thailand. Eye (Lond). 2012;26(4):529–34.
148. Asano S, Yoshikawa T, Kimura H, Enomoto Y, Ohashi M, Terasaki H, et al. Monitoring herpesvirus DNA in three cases of acute retinal necrosis by real-time PCR. J Clin Virol. 2004;29(3):206–9.
149. Cottet L, Kaiser L, Hirsch HH, Baglivo E. HSV2 acute retinal necrosis: diagnosis and monitoring with quantitative polymerase chain reaction. Int Ophthalmol. 2009;29(3):199–201.
150. Yin PD, Kurup SK, Fischer SH, Rhee HH, Byrnes GA, Levy-Clarke GA, et al. Progressive outer retinal necrosis in the era of highly active antiretroviral therapy: successful management with intravitreal injections and monitoring with quantitative PCR. J Clin Virol. 2007;38(3):254–9.
151. van Velzen M, Missotten T, van Loenen FB, Meesters RJ, Luider TM, Baarsma GS, et al. Acyclovir-resistant herpes simplex virus type 1 in intra-ocular fluid samples of herpetic uveitis patients. J Clin Virol. 2013;57(3):215–21.
152. de Groot-Mijnes JDF, de Visser L, Rothova A, Schuller M, van Loon AM, Weersink AJ. Rubella virus is associated with fuchs heterochromic iridocyclitis. Am J Ophthalmol. 2006;141(1):212–4.
153. Ruokonen PC, Metzner S, Ucer A, Torun N, Hofmann J, Pleyer U. Intraocular antibody synthesis against rubella virus and other microorganisms in Fuchs' heterochromic cyclitis. Graefes Arch Clin Exp Ophthalmol. 2009;248(4):565–71.
154. Suzuki J, Goto H, Komase K, Abo H, Fujii K, Otsuki N, et al. Rubella virus as a possible etiological agent of Fuchs heterochromic iridocyclitis. Graefes Arch Clin Exp Ophthalmol. 2010;248(10):1487–91.
155. Birnbaum AD, Tessler HH, Schultz KL, Farber MD, Gao W, Lin P, et al. Epidemiologic relationship between fuchs heterochromic iridocyclitis and the United States rubella vaccination program. Am J Ophthalmol. 2007;144(3):424–8.
156. de Visser L, Braakenburg A, Rothova A, de Boer JH. Rubella virus-associated uveitis: clinical manifestations and visual prognosis. Am J Ophthalmol. 2008;146(2):292–7.
157. de Melker HE, van den Hof S, Berbers GA, Conyn-van Spaendonck MA. Evaluation of the national immunisation programme in the Netherlands: immunity to diphtheria, tetanus, poliomyelitis, measles, mumps, rubella and Haemophilus influenzae type b. Vaccine. 2003;21(7–8):716–20.
158. Rothova A. The riddle of fuchs heterochromic uveitis. Am J Ophthalmol. 2007;144(3):447–8.
159. Mahendradas P, Shetty R, Malathi J, Madhavan HN. Chikungunya virus iridocyclitis in Fuchs' heterochromic iridocyclitis. Indian J Ophthalmol. 2010;58(6):545–7.
160. Babu K, Murthy GJ. Chikungunya virus iridocyclitis in Fuchs' heterochromic iridocyclitis. Indian J Ophthalmol. 2012;60(1):73–4.
161. Rothova A, Schneider M, de Groot-Mijnes JDF. Human immunodeficiency virus-induced uveitis: intraocular and plasma human immunodeficiency virus-1 RNA loads. Ophthalmology. 2008;115(11):2062–4.
162. Sugita S, Shimizu N, Kawaguchi T, Akao N, Morio T, Mochizuki M. Identification of human herpesvirus 6 in a patient with severe unilateral panuveitis. Arch Ophthalmol. 2007;125(10):1426–7.
163. Ongkosuwito JV, Van der Lelij A, Bruinenberg M, Wienesen-van Doorn M, Feron EJ, Hoyng CB, et al. Increased presence of Epstein-Barr virus DNA in ocular fluid samples from HIV negative immunocompromised patients with uveitis. Br J Ophthalmol. 1998;82(3):245–51.
164. Yamamoto S, Sugita S, Sugamoto Y, Shimizu N, Morio T, Mochizuki M. Quantitative PCR for the detection of genomic DNA of Epstein-Barr virus in ocular fluids of patients with uveitis. Jpn J Ophthalmol. 2008;52(6):463–7.
165. Holland GN. Ocular toxoplasmosis: a global reassessment. J Ophthalmol. 2003;136(6):973–88.
166. Antoniazzi E, Guagliano R, Meroni V, Pezzotta S, Bianchi PE. Ocular impairment of toxoplasmosis. Parassitologia. 2008;50(1–2):35–6.
167. Holland GN. Ocular toxoplasmosis: a global reassessment. Part II: disease manifestations and management. Am J Ophthalmol. 2004;137(1):1–17.
168. Pereira Da Mata A, Oréfice F. Toxoplasmosis. In: Foster CS, Vitale AT, editors. Diagnosis and treatment of uveitis. Philadelphia: W.B. Saunders Company; 2002. p. 385–410.
169. Nussenblatt RB. Ocular toxoplasmosis. In: Nussenblatt RB, Whitcup SM, editors. Uveitis. Fundamentals and clinical practice. 3rd ed. Philadelphia: Mosby; 2004. p. 214–34.
170. Cano-Parra JL, Diaz LML, Cordoba JL, Gobernado ML, Navea AL, Menezo JL. Acute iridocyclitis in a patient with AIDS diagnosed as toxoplasmosis by PCR. Ocul Immunol Inflamm. 2000;8(2):127–30.
171. Holland GN. Ocular toxoplasmosis in the immunocompromised host. Int Ophthalmol. 1989;13(6):399–402.
172. Rehder JR, Burnier Jr MB, Pavesio CE, Kim MK, Rigueiro M, Petrilli AM, et al. Acute unilateral toxoplasmic iridocyclitis in an AIDS patient. Am J Ophthalmol. 1988;106(6):740–1.
173. Balansard B, Bodaghi B, Cassoux N, Fardeau C, Romand S, Rozenberg F, et al. Necrotising

retinopathies simulating acute retinal necrosis syndrome. Br J Ophthalmol. 2005;89(1):96–101.
174. Ongkosuwito JV, Bosch-Driessen EH, Kijlstra A, Rothova A. Serologic evaluation of patients with primary and recurrent ocular toxoplasmosis for evidence of recent infection. Am J Ophthalmol. 1999;128(4):407–12.
175. Garweg JG, de Groot-Mijnes JD, Montoya JG. Diagnostic approach to ocular toxoplasmosis. Ocul Immunol Inflamm. 2011;19(4):255–61.
176. Fekkar A, Bodaghi B, Touafek F, Le Hoang P, Mazier D, Paris L. Comparison of immunoblotting, calculation of the Goldmann-Witmer coefficient, and real-time PCR using aqueous humor samples for diagnosis of ocular toxoplasmosis. J Clin Microbiol. 2008;46(6):1965–7.
177. Aouizerate F, Cazenave J, Poirier L, Verin P, Cheyrou A, Begueret J, et al. Detection of Toxoplasma gondii in aqueous humour by the polymerase chain reaction. Br J Ophthalmol. 1993;77(2):107–9.
178. Fardeau C, Romand S, Rao NA, Cassoux N, Bettembourg O, Thulliez P, et al. Diagnosis of toxoplasmic retinochoroiditis with atypical clinical features. Am J Ophthalmol. 2002;134(2):196–203.
179. Bowyer JD, Gormley PD, Seth R, Downes RN, Lowe J. Choroidal tuberculosis diagnosed by polymerase chain reaction. A clinicopathologic case report. Ophthalmology. 1999;106(2):290–4.
180. Gupta V, Gupta A, Arora S, Bambery P, Dogra MR, Agarwal A. Presumed tubercular serpiginouslike choroiditis: clinical presentations and management. Ophthalmology. 2003;110(9):1744–9.
181. Touitou V, Fenollar F, Cassoux N, Merle-Beral H, LeHoang P, Amoura Z, et al. Ocular Whipple's disease: therapeutic strategy and long-term follow-up. Ophthalmology. 2012;119(7):1465–9.
182. Kerkhoff FT, Bergmans AM, van Der Zee A, Rothova A. Demonstration of Bartonella grahamii DNA in ocular fluids of a patient with neuroretinitis. J Clin Microbiol. 1999;37(12):4034–8.
183. Sugita S, Ogawa M, Shimizu N, Morio T, Ohguro N, Nakai K, et al. Use of a comprehensive polymerase chain reaction system for diagnosis of ocular infectious diseases. Ophthalmology. 2013;120(9):1761–8.
184. Gupta V, Gupta A, Rao NA. Intraocular tuberculosis – an update. Surv Ophthalmol. 2007;52(6):561–87.
185. Bodaghi B, LeHoang P. Ocular tuberculosis. Curr Opin Ophthalmol. 2000;11(6):443–8.
186. Yeh S, Sen HN, Colyer M, Zapor M, Wroblewski K. Update on ocular tuberculosis. Curr Opin Ophthalmol. 2012;23(6):551–6.
187. Nienhaus A, Schablon A, Diel R. Interferon-gamma release assay for the diagnosis of latent TB infection – analysis of discordant results, when compared to the tuberculin skin test. PLoS One. 2008;3(7):e2665.
188. Andersen P, Munk ME, Pollock JM, Doherty TM. Specific immune-based diagnosis of tuberculosis. Lancet. 2000;356(9235):1099–104.
189. Kurup SK, Buggage RR, Clarke GL, Ursea R, Lim WK, Nussenblatt RB. Gamma interferon assay as an alternative to PPD skin testing in selected patients with granulomatous intraocular inflammatory disease. Can J Ophthalmol. 2006;41(6):737–40.
190. Mackensen F, Becker MD, Wiehler U, Max R, Dalpke A, Zimmermann S. QuantiFERON TB-Gold – a new test strengthening long-suspected tuberculous involvement in serpiginous-like choroiditis. Am J Ophthalmol. 2008;146(5):761–6.
191. Bramante CT, Talbot EA, Rathinam SR, Stevens R, Zegans ME. Diagnosis of ocular tuberculosis: a role for new testing modalities? Int Ophthalmol Clin. 2007;47(3):45–62.
192. Winqvist N, Bjorkman P, Noren A, Miorner H. Use of a T cell interferon gamma release assay in the investigation for suspected active tuberculosis in a low prevalence area. BMC Infect Dis. 2009;9:105.
193. Ang M, Htoon HM, Chee SP. Diagnosis of tuberculous uveitis: clinical application of an interferon-gamma release assay. Ophthalmology. 2009; 116(7):1391–6.
194. Lütkemeyer AF, Charlebois ED, Flores LL, Bangsberg DR, Deeks SG, Martin JN, et al. Comparison of an interferon-gamma release assay with tuberculin skin testing in HIV-infected individuals. Am J Respir Crit Care Med. 2007; 175(7):737–42.
195. Stephan C, Wolf T, Goetsch U, Bellinger O, Nisius G, Oremek G, et al. Comparing QuantiFERON-tuberculosis gold, T-SPOT tuberculosis and tuberculin skin test in HIV-infected individuals from a low prevalence tuberculosis country. AIDS. 2008;22(18):2471–9.
196. Thompson MJ, Albert DM. Ocular tuberculosis. Arch Ophthalmol. 2005;123(6):844–9.
197. Biswas J, Badrinath SS. Ocular morbidity in patients with active systemic tuberculosis. Int Ophthalmol. 1995;19(5):293–8.
198. Arora SK, Gupta V, Gupta A, Bambery P, Kapoor GS, Sehgal S. Diagnostic efficacy of polymerase chain reaction in granulomatous uveitis. Tuber Lung Dis. 1999;79(4):229–33.
199. Salman A, Parmar P, Rajamohan M, Thomas PA, Jesudasan N. Subretinal fluid analysis in the diagnosis of choroidal tuberculosis. Retina. 2003;23(6): 796–9.
200. Shanmugam M. Subretinal fluid analysis in the diagnosis of choroidal tuberculosis. Retina. 2004;24(4):659.
201. Aldave AJ, King JA, Cunningham Jr ET. Ocular syphilis. Curr Opin Ophthalmol. 2001;12(6):433–41.
202. Chao JR, Khurana RN, Fawzi AA, Reddy HS, Rao NA. Syphilis: reemergence of an old adversary. Ophthalmology. 2006;113(11):2074–9.
203. Sambri V, Marangoni A, Simone MA, D'Antuono A, Negosanti M, Cevenini R. Evaluation of recomWell Treponema, a novel recombinant antigen-based enzyme-linked immunosorbent assay for the diagnosis of syphilis. Clin Microbiol Infect. 2001;7(4):200–5.
204. Schmidt BL, Edjlalipour M, Luger A. Comparative evaluation of nine different enzyme-linked

immunosorbent assays for determination of antibodies against Treponema pallidum in patients with primary syphilis. J Clin Microbiol. 2000;38(3):1279–82.
205. Clyne B, Jerrard DA. Syphilis testing. J Emerg Med. 2000;18(3):361–7.
206. Luger AF, Schmidt BL, Kaulich M. Significance of laboratory findings for the diagnosis of neurosyphilis. Int J STD AIDS. 2000;11(4):224–34.
207. Marra CA. Neurosyphilis: a guide for clinicians. Infect Dis Clin Pract. 1996;5:33–41.
208. Cornut PL, Sobas CR, Perard L, De Bats F, Salord H, Manificat HJ, et al. Detection of Treponema pallidum in aqueous humor by real-time polymerase chain reaction. Ocul Immunol Inflamm. 2011; 19(2):127–8.
209. Troutbeck R, Chhabra R, Jones NP. Polymerase chain reaction testing of vitreous in atypical ocular syphilis. Ocul Immunol Inflamm. 2013;21(3):227–30.
210. Friedman MG. Antibodies in human tears during and after infection. Surv Ophthalmol. 1990; 35(2):151–7.
211. Pramod NP, Dhevahi E, Sudhamathi K, Kannan K, Thyagarajan SP. Tear secretory IgA: evaluation of usefulness as a diagnostic marker in herpetic keratitis. Ocul Immunol Inflamm. 1999;7(2):61–7.
212. Knox CM, Chandler D, Short GA, Margolis TP. Polymerase chain reaction-based assays of vitreous samples for the diagnosis of viral retinitis. Use in diagnostic dilemmas. Ophthalmology 1998;105:37–44.

2 Antimicrobial Agents in Ophthalmology

Khalid F. Tabbara

2.1 Introduction

The US Food and Drug Administration has approved more new antibiotics in the past 20 years than all antibiotics discovered in the twentieth century. The recent proliferation of new antibiotics has made the selection more difficult [1–5]. The selection of an antibiotic depends on the clinical findings, the most likely causative organism, the laboratory confirmation, and the pharmacokinetics of the drug.

The purpose of this chapter is to put in the hands of the ophthalmologist a concise approach to the selection of topical or systemic antimicrobial agents in the management of infections of the eye. This would provide practical, concise, and objective information on antimicrobial agents used in the treatment of infections of the eye. The information is useful as a rapid reference for the eye care practitioner. The use of antibiotics in ocular infection can be preventive, preemptive, curative, or prophylaxis. The guidelines for the proper use of antimicrobial agents in ophthalmology are outlined (Table 2.1).

The dramatic decrease in the incidence of classic infectious diseases is due largely to, first, mass vaccination, which has eradicated certain infectious disease such as smallpox; second, the implementation of rigorous public health measures by many countries; and, third, the introduction of newly discovered antimicrobial agents. In the first decade of the twenty-first century, infectious diseases continue to be a serious cause of visual loss, mortality, and morbidity. We should not rest on the laurels we have won for overcoming the classic infections, but we should, rather, prepare ourselves to confront the microorganisms emerging from the degradation of our ecosystem as well as those bacteria that are becoming increasingly antibiotic resistant. Several new infectious agents have been recently identified as a cause of disease in man (Table 2.2).

Chemicals were used as early as the seventeenth century to treat infectious disease. Quinine was used for malaria, and emetine was used for amebiasis. Antibiotics, however, can cause harm as well as good. Erlich, in 1900 in Germany, introduced the concept of selective toxicity of chemicals, showing that it is possible to use an antibiotic that is toxic to the microorganism but does not harm the host. In 1929, Fleming recorded his observation that agar plates in his laboratory contaminated with *Penicillium* spp. were free of other bacteria such as staphylococci and went to discover penicillin. In 1935 in Germany, Domagk

K.F. Tabbara, MD, ABO, FRCOphth
Department of Ophthalmology,
The Eye Center and The Eye Foundation
for Research in Ophthalmology, Riyadh, Saudi Arabia

Department of Ophthalmology,
College of Medicine, King Saud University,
Riyadh, Saudi Arabia

The Wilmer Ophthalmological Institute,
The Johns Hopkins University School of Medicine,
Baltimore, MD, USA
e-mail: kftabbara@yahoo.com

K. Tabbara et al. (eds.), *Ocular Infections*, Essentials in Ophthalmology,
DOI 10.1007/978-3-662-43981-4_2,

Table 2.1 Guidelines for the proper use of antibiotics for ocular infections

1. The use of antibiotics for treatment of ocular infections should be initiated whenever a patient has an infection which is microbial in nature and the organism is susceptible to the antibiotic prescribed
2. The patient's history and eye examination should be consistent with the diagnosis of microbial infection
3. Ocular specimens for stain, cultures, or molecular diagnosis (e.g., PCR) should be obtained before the initiation of therapy and sent immediately to the laboratory. The etiologic organism causing the infection should be identified
4. In serious infections, treatment may be started empirically before laboratory results are obtained
5. The selection of the antibiotic should be based on the susceptibility of the organisms, adverse effects, penetration into the affected tissue, and cost
6. Discrepancies between the results of the laboratory sensitivity tests and the patient clinical response should be carefully evaluated
7. Adverse effects from the use of the antibiotic (allergic or toxic) should be taken into account in the selection and administration of antibiotic agents' autotoxicity, nephrotoxicity, or hepatotoxicity. The antibiotic should be discontinued if an allergic or serious adverse reaction occurs after its use
8. Blood level monitoring of systemic antibiotics should be assessed whenever indicated
9. Duration of therapy is dependent on the nature of the infection and site of the infection but should not be less than 1 week
10. The route of antibiotics should be given at a dosage level that will allow penetration of the antibiotic into the desirable infected site within the safe margin and for the shortest period of time to eradicate the offending agent
11. The possibility of a superinfection should always be kept in mind when antibiotics are used for a prolonged period of time
12. The use of antibiotic combinations should be avoided unless the organism has not been cultured and the findings are highly suggestive of infectious etiology
13. Antibiotic prophylaxis in surgery should be used very carefully; the antibiotic used should cover both Gram-negative and Gram-positive organisms and be started just before surgery and discontinued immediately following surgery
14. Long-term use of antibiotics should be avoided

described sulfonamide, not only winning the Nobel Prize in 1939 but also launching a new era of antimicrobial agents. It was not until 1940, however, when Chain and Florey used penicillin in the treatment of *Streptococcus pneumoniae* infections, and that was the turning point in the management of infectious diseases.

Table 2.2 Newly discovered microbial pathogens

Disease	Cause
Cat scratch disease	*Bartonella henselae*
Pneumonia	Hanta virus
Kaposi's sarcoma	Human herpes simplex virus type 6
Autoimmune deficiency syndrome (AIDS)	Human immunodeficiency virus type 1 and type 2
T cell lymphoma	Human T cell lymphoma virus
Lyme disease	*Borrelia burgdorferi*
Whipple's disease	*Treponema whippelii*
Severe acute respiratory syndrome (SARS)	Corona virus
Middle East Respiratory Syndrome (MERS)	Corona virus
Avian influenza	H_5N_1 virus

Streptomycin was described in the late 1940s; tetracyclines were launched in the early 1950s, followed by chloramphenicol and later followed by lincomycin in the 1960s. Lincomycin was described from the systematic analysis of soil samples in Lincoln, Nebraska, in the United States and was named after the state's capital city, Lincoln. It was produced by a strain of *Streptomyces lincolnensis.* After this discovery, extensive soil sampling was conducted worldwide to isolate and identify antibiotic-producing organisms.

There are so many different types and generations of antibiotics. It is important, therefore, to identify those which are useful in ophthalmology and those that are not. It is of paramount importance to select the right antibiotic to treat ocular infection; fundamental to this is the identification of the organism responsible for the infection.

The initial selection of antibiotics for the treatment of ocular infections is based on the most frequently encountered organism, pharmacokinetics of the antibiotic, dosage, and cost.

The great stumbling blocks to safe and effective antibiotic therapy are resistance and toxicity, two factors which must always be taken into account when choosing an antibiotic. Cost is another factor and one that is often overlooked. It is important to be aware of the fact that some antibiotics are expensive. There have been instances of patients receiving very expensive therapy when in fact the organism responsible for their infection was sensitive to much cheaper antibiotics. The combination of antibiotic agents may be used simultaneously in the following conditions:

(a) In a severe devastating vision-threatening ocular infection of unknown etiology and after lab tests have been initiated to determine a specific etiologic agent
(b) If an infection is caused by more than one organism
(c) The emergence of resistant strains of bacteria during the treatment
(d) In case of infections caused by organisms that are known to respond better to simultaneous use of more than one antibiotic such as *Toxoplasma* and *Acanthamoeba*
(e) Organisms not cultured and the clinical findings are highly suggestive of infectious etiology

2.2 Mechanism of Action

Although antibiotics can be described as being either bacteriostatic or bactericidal, this is a less useful classification than the one which is based on the drug mechanism of action, namely, how and where they affect the target organism. Under this system of classification, the first group of antibiotics inhibits synthesis of the cell wall, the second group inhibits the cell membrane, the third group affects ribosomal function and protein synthesis, and the fourth group affects nucleic acid synthesis.

Topical antimicrobial agents used in ocular infections are listed in Table 2.3. The antimicrobial agents that can be compounded for the treatment of ocular infections for topical, subconjunctival, intravitreal, and intravenous are summarized in Table 2.4. Antibiotics that are used for bacterial (Table 2.5), fungal (Table 2.6), viral infections (Table 2.7) are also listed.

Table 2.3 Commercially available topical ophthalmic antibacterial agents

		Concentration	
Generic name	Trade name	Ophthalmic solution	Ophthalmic ointment
Individual agents			
Bacitrin		Not available	500 units/g
Besifloxacin	Besivance	0.6 %	Not available
Ciprofloxacin hydrochloride	Ciloxan	0.3 %	0.3 %
Erythromycin		Not available	0.5 %
Gatifloxacin	Zymar, Tymer	0.3 %	Not available
Gentamicin sulfate	Genoptic, Garamycin	0.3 %	0.3 %
Lomefloxacin	Okacin		
Levofloxacin	Iquix	1.5 %	Not available
	Quixin	0.5 %	Not available
Moxifloxacin	Vigamox	0.5 %	Not available
Ofloxacin	Oflox, Optiflox	0.3 %	Not available
Sulfacetamide	Bleph-10	10 %	Not available
	Sulf-10 (15 mL) or preservative-free	10 %	Not available
	Generic	10 %	10 %
Tobramycin sulfate	Tobrex	0.3 %	0.3 %
	Generic	0.3 %	Not available
Tosufloxacin	Ozex	0.3 %	Not available
Mixtures			
Chloramphenicol eyedrops and ointment	Generic	0.5 %	
Polymyxin B/bacitracin zinc	AK-Poly-Bac Polysporin Polycin-B Generic	Not available	10,000 units – 500 units/g

(continued)

Table 2.3 (continued)

Generic name	Trade name	Concentration	
		Ophthalmic solution	Ophthalmic ointment
Polymyxin B/neomycin/bacitracin	Neosporin Generic	Not available	10,000 units – 3.5 mg – 400 units/g
Polymyxin B/neomycin/gramicidin	Neosporin Generic	10,000 units – 1.75 mg – 0.025 mg/mL	Not available
Polymyxin B/trimethoprim	Polytrim Generic	10,000 units – 1 mg/mL	Not available

Table 2.4 Compounding of major antibiotics for the treatment of ocular infections

		Route of administration		
Drug name[a]	Topical	Subconjunctival	Intravitreal	Intravenous[b]
Amikacin sulfate	10 mg/mL	25 mg	400 μgm	15 mg/kg daily in 2–3 doses
Ampicillin sodium	50 mg/mL	50–150 mg	5 mg	4–12 g daily in 4 doses
Bacitracin zinc	10,000 units/mL	5,000 units	–	–
Cefazolin sodium	50 mg/mL	100 mg	2,250 μgm	2–4 g daily in 3–4 doses
Ceftazidime	50 mg/mL	100 mg	2,000 μgm	1 g daily in 2–3 doses
Ceftriaxone	50 mg/mL	–	–	1–4 g daily in 1–2 doses
Clindamycin	50 mg/mL	15–50 mg	1,000 μgm	900–1,800 mg daily in 2–3 doses
Colistimethate sodium	10 mg/mL	15–25 mg	100 μgm	2.5–5 mg/kg daily in 2–4 doses
Erythromycin	50 mg/ml	100 mg	500 μgm	–
Gentamicin sulfate	8–15 mg/ml	10–20 mg	100–200 μgm	3–5 mg/kg daily in 2–3 doses
Imipenem/cilastatin sodium	5 mg/ml	–	–	2 g daily in 3–4 doses
Kanamycin sulfate	30–50 mg/ml	30 mg	500 mg	–
Neomycin sulfate	5–8 mg/ml	125–250 mg	–	–
Penicillin G	100,000 units/mL	0.5–1.0 million units	300 units	12–24 million units daily in 4–6 doses
Piperacillin	12.5 mg/mL	100 mg	–	–
Polymyxin B sulfate	10,000 units/mL	100,000 units	–	–
Ticarcillin disodium	6 mg/mL	100 mg	–	200–300 mg/kg daily 3 × in 4–6 doses
Tobramycin sulfate	8–15 mg/mL	10–20 mg	100–200 μgm	3–5 mg/kg daily in 2–3 doses
Vancomycin hydrochloride[c]	20–25 mg/mL	25 mg	1,000 μgm	15–30 mg/kg daily in 1–2 doses

[a]Most penicillins and cephalosporins are physically incompatible when combined in the same bottle with aminoglycosides such as amikacin, gentamicin, or tobramycin
[b]Adult doses
[c]Usage discouraged by CDC because of increased resistant organisms

2.3 Antibiotics That Inhibit Cell Wall Synthesis

Several antibiotics affect the cell wall of organisms including penicillins, cephalosporins, gramicidin, and bacitracin [6–17]. Bacterial survival can be compromised without a cell wall. The cell wall protects bacteria from the environmental noxious agents and maintains the intracellular milieu. The thickness of bacterial cell walls varies: Gram-positive bacteria have thick cell walls, and Gram-negative bacteria have thin cell walls. The internal osmotic pressure of Gram-positive organisms is higher than that in Gram-negative

Table 2.5 Bacterial keratitis therapy (initial therapy for bacterial keratitis)

Organism	Antibiotic	Topical dose	Subconjunctival dose
Gram(+) cocci	Cefazolin	50 mg/mL	100 mg in 0.5 mL
	Vancomycin[a]	50 mg/mL	25 mg in 0.5 ML
Gram(−) rods	Tobramycin	9–14 mg/mL	20 mg in 0.5 mL
	Ceftazidime	50 mg/mL	100 mg in 0.5 mL
	Fluoroquinolones	3 mg/mL	Not available
No organism or multiple types of organisms	Cefazolin	50 mg/mL	100 mg in 0.5 mL
	with		
	Tobramycin	9–14 mg/mL	20 mg in 0.5 mL
	or		
	Fluoroquinolones	3 mg/mL	Not available
Gram(−) cocci	Ceftriaxone	50 mg/mL	100 mg in 0.5 mL
	Ceftazidime	50 mg/mL	
Mycobacteria	Amikacin	20 mg/mL	20 mg in 0.5 mL
	Azithromycin	1.5 mg/ml (0.15 %)	

[a]For resistant *Staphylococcus* species

Table 2.6 Antimicrobial agents for fungal keratitis

Generic (trade) name	Route	Dosage
Amphotericin B (Fungizone®)	Topical	0.1–0.5 % solution (most commonly 0.15 %); dilute with water for injection or dextrose 5 % in water
	Subconj.	0.8–1.0 mg
	Intravitreal	5 mcg
Liposomal amphotericin B	Intravenous	
Fluconazole (Diflucan®)	Oral	200 mg on day 1, then 100 mg daily in divided doses
		400 mg on day 1, then 200 mg daily in divided doses
Intravenous	IV	200–400 mg
Flucytosine (Ancobon®)	Oral	50–150 mg/kg daily 4 divided doses
Itraconazole (Sporanox®)	Oral	200–400 mg/kg daily
	Intravenous	200 mg IV twice a day for 4 doses, then 200 mg IV daily for 14 days
Ketoconazole (Nizoral®)	Oral	200–400 mg daily
Natamycin (Natacyn®)	Topical	5 % suspension
Voriconazole (Vfend®)	Oral	200 mg twice a day
	Intravenous	3–6 mg/kg every 12 h
	Intracorneal	25 µgm
	Topical	1 % eyedrops

Table 2.7 Antimicrobial agents for viral ocular infections

Generic (trade) name	Topical conc.	Intravit. dose	Systemic dosage
Trifluridine (Viroptic®)	1.0 %	–	–
Acyclovir sodium	–	24,000 µgm	Oral – *herpes simplex* keratitis: 200 mg 5 times daily for 7–10 days
			Oral – *herpes zoster ophthalmicus*: 600–800 mg 5 times daily for 10 days; IV therapy
Cidofovir (Vistide®)	–	–	IV – induction: 5 mg/kg constant infusion over 1 h administered once weekly for 2 consecutive weeks
			Maintenance: 5 mg/kg constant infusion over 1 h administered once every 2 weeks

(continued)

Table 2.7 (continued)

Generic (trade) name	Topical conc.	Intravit. dose	Systemic dosage
Famciclovir (Famvir®)	–	–	Oral – *herpes zoster ophthalmicus* 500 mg 3 times daily for 7 days
Fomivirsen (Vitravene®)	–	330 μgm	Every other week for 4 doses, then every 4 weeks. Contains 6.6 mg/mL, in a 0.25-ml vial
Foscarnet sodium (Foscavir®)	–	1 mg	IV – by controlled infusion only, either by central vein or by peripheral vein induction: 60 mg/kg (adjusted for renal function) given over 1 h every 8 h for 14–21 days Maintenance: 90–120 mg/kg given over 2 h once daily
Ganciclovir (gel) (Zirgan®, Virgan)	0.15 %		
Ganciclovir sodium (Cytovene®)	–	0.2 mg	IV – induction: 5 mg/kg every 12 h for 14–21 days Maintenance: 5 mg/kg daily for 7 days or 6 mg once daily for 5 days/week Oral – after IV induction: 1,000 mg 3 times daily with food or 500 mg 6 times daily every 3 h
Ganciclovir sodium (Vitrasert®)[a]	–	4.5 mg	
Valacyclovir (Valtrex®)	–	–	Oral – *herpes zoster ophthalmicus*: 1 g 3 times daily for 7 days Herpes simplex virus (types 1 & II): 1 g 2 times daily

[a]Sterile intravitreal insert designed to release the drug over a 5–8-month period

organisms. A Gram-positive organism, in particular, is under considerable risk of death when the cell wall is compromised.

Bacterial cell wall contains peptidoglycans and ligands of alternating pyranoside residues of two amino sugars, *N*-acetylglucosamine and *N*-acetylmuramic acid (the latter is not found in mammalian cells), and is cross-linked by pentapeptide chains. Pentapeptide cross-linking gives the cell wall its rigidity; consequently, the introduction of antimicrobial agents or antibiotics that interfere with cross-linking causes the cell wall to weaken and the organism to die.

Unlike bacteria, mammalian cells do not have cell walls a selective target and an example of selective toxicity.

2.3.1 Penicillins

Penicillins are beta-lactam antibiotics. There are four generations of penicillins. The first three are important in the treatment of ocular infections. The first-generation penicillins are penicillin G and penicillinase-resistant penicillins, of which there are two types, methicillin and nafcillin. Methicillin was used to treat beta-lactamase-producing organisms. Methicillin can cause interstitial nephritis and is no longer used in most centers. The penicillins are used specifically to treat ocular infections caused by *Streptococcus*, *Neisseria*, *Clostridium* spp., syphilis, and *Actinomyces*.

The second-generation penicillins include ampicillin and amoxicillin. These antibiotics have a slightly broader spectrum than those of the first generation. The second-generation penicillins are used to treat ocular infections caused by *Haemophilus* species and enterococci.

The third-generation penicillins are carbenicillin and ticarcillin. Ticarcillin has been combined with clavulanic acid as a suicide inhibitor of beta-lactamase. These antibiotics occupy receptor sites on Gram-negative bacteria making them more active against Gram-negative bacteria. Until recently, carbenicillin was used to treat *Pseudomonas* infections. Ticarcillin has replaced carbenicillin and may be used in combination with aminoglycosides. The fourth group of penicillins comprises of mezlocillin, piperacillin and azlocillin which are derivatives of ampicillin and are similar to carbenicillin and ticarcillin. These antibiotics are also effective against Gram-negative organisms because they have a greater affinity to cell wall receptor sites in Gram-negative organisms than in Gram-positive organisms. The fourth-generation penicillins have limited role in ophthalmology. New generations of antibiotics are not necessarily better or more effective than earlier generations. Each generation of antibiotics plays a specific role and has specific indication and advantages in the treatment of infections caused by susceptible organisms.

Organisms become resistant by producing beta-lactamase. The enzyme disrupts the beta-lactam ring, rendering it ineffective. In order to counteract this, an antibiotic called clavulanic acid, produced by *Streptomyces* spp., has been introduced. Clavulanic acid has a very weak antibiotic effect and binds to beta-lactamase and inhibits its effects, "suicide inhibition." Clavulanic acid has unique affinity to beta-lactamase and leads to its deactivation. The combination of clavulanic acid to existing antibiotics does not constitute a new generation of antibiotics but is a new therapeutic strategy to improve the effectiveness of existing antibiotics.

A combination of 500 mg amoxicillin and 250 mg clavulanic acid (Augmentin®) is effective against beta-lactamase-producing organisms such as *Haemophilus* and streptococci. The drug is used for the treatment of preseptal cellulitis in young children where *Haemophilus* is a common cause. Similarly, a combination of ticarcillin and clavulanic acid (Timentin®).

Cloxacillin is similar to clavulanic acid (Timentin®) in that it has strong affinity for beta-lactamase and neutralizes its effects.

2.3.2 Monobactam Antibiotics

Several examples of monobactam antibiotics are available which are Impenem meropenen, ectapenem which have wide antimicrobial activity. Impenen is effective against anaerobes, Gram-positive and Gram-negative organisms, *Streptococcus pneumoniae*, *Streptococcus* Group A, *Staphylococcus aureus*, *Streptococcus faecalis*, and *Haemophilus influenzae*. The minimum inhibitory concentration of imipenem to *Haemophilus influenzae* and *Neisseria* spp. is less than 0.6 μg/ml. Imipenem is also effective against *Enterobacteriaceae*, *Pseudomonas*, and *Acinetobacter calcoaceticus*. Imipenem has been marketed in combination with silastin. Silastin inhibits hydropeptidase, an enzyme released by the brush border of the kidney which destroys imipenem. Consequently, cilastatin prolongs the half-life of imipenem and increases the concentration of imipenem in the urine. Imipenem should not be used in conjunction with cephalosporin because of potential antagonism.

2.3.3 Cephalosporins

Cephalosporins are an important group accounting for some 50 % of all antibiotics prescribed in hospitals (Tables 2.8a and 2.8b). Over 25 cephalosporins are available, and many more are under investigation. The advantages of cephalosporins include a broad-spectrum bactericidal with selective toxicity. Cephalosporins (first generation) are effective against penicillinase-producing *Staphylococcus aureus*. The disadvantages of cephalosporins include low CSF level, and therefore the agents are not recommended to treat meningitis. They have limited effects against enterococci, and they may potentiate nephrotoxicity if they are used intravenously in combination with aminoglycosides.

The first generation of cephalosporins was introduced in the 1970s. One of the antibiotics in this generation is cefazolin. As with other groups of antibiotics, each generation of cephalosporins has its own spectrum: the first-generation cephalosporins are more effective against Gram-positive cocci than the third- or fourth-generation cephalosporins.

The second-generation cephalosporins include cefuroxime and cefonicid. Cefuroxime

Table 2.8a The major cephalosporins

First generation	Second generation	Third generation
Parenteral	*Parenteral*	*Parenteral*
Cephalothin (Keflin)	Cefamandole (Mandol)	Cefotaxime (Claforan)
Cefazolin (Ancef, Kefzol)	Cefoxitin (Mefoxin)	Cefoperazone (Cefobid)
Cephapirin (Cefadyl)	Cefuroxime (Zinacef)	Ceftizoxime (Cefizox)
Cephradine (Velosef)	Cefotetan (Cefotan)	Ceftriaxone (Rocephin)
		Ceftazidime (Fortaz, Tazidime, or Tazicef)
		Cefepime (Maxipime)
Oral	*Oral*	*Oral*
Cephalexin (Keflex)	Cefuroxime axetil (Ceftin)	Cefixime (Suprax)
Cephradine (Velosef, Anspor)	Cefprozil (Cefzil)	Cefpodoxime (Vantin)
	Loracarbef (Lorabid)	Ceftibuten (Cedax)
Cefadroxil (Duricef)	Cefaclor (Ceclor)	Cefdinir (Omnicef)

Table 2.8b Selective oral cephalosporins for ocular and adnexal infections

Agent	Indication
First generation	
Cephalexin (Keflex) or	Eyelid minor soft tissue infections due to methicillin susceptible *S. aureus* and/or *S. pyogenes*
Cephradine (Anspor, Velosef)	Alternative in streptococcal pharyngitis
Second generation	
Cefuroxime (Ceftin), or	Alternative therapy in orbital cellulitis, otitis media, sinusitis, bronchitis
Cefprozil (Cefzil), or	Cefuroxime axetil has been used in Lyme disease
Loracarbef (Lorabid)	Alternate therapy in early selected cases of community-acquired pneumonia (CAP)
Cefaclor (Ceclor)	
Third generation	
Cefixime (Suprax)	Alternate therapy for *H. influenza* and *M. catarrhalis*
	Alternate for uncomplicated gonorrheal conjunctivitis
Ceftibuten (Cedax)	No unique role, possible alternative
Cefdinir (Omnicef)	No unique role
Ceftriaxone (Rocephin)	Lyme disease, leptospirosis, syphilis, gonorrheal conjunctivitis
Ceftazidime (Fortaz)	Endophthalmitis combined with vancomycin

is the treatment of choice for sinus infections. It has been used intracamerally in phacoemulsification for the prevention of postoperative endophthalmitis. Unfortunately, it has no effects against *Pseudomonas* or other enteric Gram-negative organisms. It is a good single drug for the treatment of patients with sinusitis or orbital cellulitis as it covers most of the Gram-positive cocci (staphylococci, streptococci) as well as non-enteric Gram-negative organisms; it is also effective against *Haemophilus*. In addition, cefuroxime has a long half-life and can be administered intravenously twice daily. Unlike cefamandole, cefuroxime does not cause bleeding tendencies and is well tolerated. The disadvantages of cefuroxime are as follows: (1) it is not active against *Pseudomonas* spp., enterococci, or *B. fragilis*, and (2) the drug is relatively expensive. Cefaclor is for oral administration.

The third-generation cephalosporins include ceftazidime, cefotaxime, and ceftriaxone. Ceftriaxone is the drug of choice for treating *Neisseria gonorrhoeae*. Most current strains of *N. gonorrhoeae* are resistant to penicillins, and many of them are resistant to other antimicrobial agents as well. Ceftriaxone is effective against infections caused by *Neisseria meningitidis*. Ceftriaxone is used for the treatment of ocular infections caused by *Borrelia*, *Leptospira*, and *Treponema* and infections caused by *Haemophilus* and beta-lactamase-producing organisms. Other advantages of ceftriaxone include its long half-life and, therefore, can be used once or twice daily (unlike other cephalosporins which have to be administered three or four times daily) which makes it cost-effective. Ceftriaxone has certain disadvantages including its limited value in the treatment of infections caused by *Pseudomonas* spp. except when combined with aminoglycosides and has little or no effect against *Staphylococcus aureus* and may prolong the bleeding time.

The fourth and fifth generations of cephalosporins have so far limited use in ocular infections.

Teicoplanin (Targocid®, Sanofi Aventis Ltd.) is a glycopeptide antibiotic similar to vancomycin and is effective against Gram-positive cocci including methicillin-resistant staphylococci (MRSA) [18, 19]. The drug affects the cell wall synthesis of Gram-positive bacteria. Experience in ophthalmic infections is limited. Oral teicoplanin has been shown to be effective in the treatment of *Clostridium difficile*-associated pseudomembranous colitis [20].

Fumagillin is used for the treatment of corneal microsporidiosis [21]. It is compounded as eyedrops at a concentration level of 0.113 mg/ml (Leiter's Pharmacy Inc., 1700 Park Ave #30, San Jose CA, USA, Telephone No.: 800-292-6773). It has also been shown to inhibit angiogenesis.

2.4 Antibiotics That Inhibit Cell Membrane Function

Antibiotics that inhibit cell membrane function include polymyxin B, amphotericin B, colistin, imidazoles, and polyenes. Some of these antibiotics, such as amphotericin B and the polyenes, act against fungi and do not affect bacterial cell membranes.

Polyenes bind to ergosterol, a sterol moiety in the cell membrane of fungi. Ergosterol is not present in mammalian or bacterial cell membranes.

The imidazoles act against fungi but have different modes of action from the polyenes. Imidazoles act by inhibiting ergosterol synthesis leading to disruption of cell membrane function. In addition, imidazoles inhibit cytochrome C and peroxidase and allow the intracellular accumulation of hydrogen peroxidase leading to death of the fungus. Since ergosterol is the binding site for amphotericin B, the use of imidazoles may render amphotericin B less effective by competing ergosterol in the fungal cell membrane. Polymyxins bind to phosphatidylethanolamine-rich membranes, particularly in Gram-negative organisms. They have a detergent-like effect which disrupts the cell membrane, eventually causing death of the organism.

Polymyxins are effective in treating infections caused by species of *Pseudomonas* as well as certain other Gram-negative organisms. Polymyxins cannot be given systemically because of nephrotoxicity [22–26].

Daptomycin is a new lipopeptide antibiotic used for the treatment of resistant Gram-positive organisms. It is produced by the fungus *Streptomyces roseosporus*. The trade name is Cubicin®.

It binds to the bacterial cell membrane leading to depolarization and loss of membrane function. Daptomycin may also act by inhibiting protein synthesis.

Daptomycin is effective against Gram-positive cocci and shows significant corneal penetration following 1 % topical eyedrops in rabbits [27]. Daptomycin appears to be safe and effective when given intravitreally [28].

2.5 Antibiotics That Inhibit Protein Synthesis

The third group of antibiotics consists of compounds which inhibit protein synthesis and include chloramphenicol, tetracycline, lincomycin, clindamycin, aminoglycosides, and macrolides. They are used extensively in ocular infections [22]. Binding to bacterial ribosomes by erythromycin leads to inhibition of protein synthesis. Inhibition of protein synthesis is also achieved when tetracyclines and aminoglycosides bind to 30S portion of the bacterial ribosome, while the chloramphenicols, lincomycins, and erythromycin bind to the 50S portion of the bacterial ribosome. The selectivity is partial and these antibiotics may have some toxic effect on human cells. Topical chloramphenicol, is widely used to treat ocular surface infections. There have been several reports of fatal aplastic anemia following topical administration of chloramphenicol. The incidence of idiosyncracy to chloramphenicol is not high; nonetheless, if large numbers of patients are given topical chloramphenicol, cases of fatal aplastic anemia will occur.

In other situations, the use of certain antibiotics is neither ideal nor appropriate. Approximately 30 % of staphylococci isolated from ocular infections are resistant to erythromycin. Erythromycin cannot be considered the drug of choice for the treatment of infections caused by these organisms. Fusidic acid is another antibiotic in this group and is helpful in the treatment of staphylococcal blepharitis [29, 30].

We recovered 163 staphylococcal isolates from ocular infection sites and assessed their sensitivity to different antibiotics [29]. Vancomycin was found to be the most effective antibiotic against all types of staphylococci, including *Staphylococcus epidermidis* and *Staphylococcus aureus*. The results showed that while 95 % of strains of *S. epidermidis* were sensitive to fusidic acid and 84 % were sensitive to bacitracin, only 45 % were sensitive to methicillin, 53 % to gentamicin, 56 % to erythromycin, and 33 % to chloramphenicol [29]. Unfortunately, resistant strains *of* staphylococci to fusidic acid started to appear. Currently, close to 52 % of ocular isolates of staphylococci are sensitive to fusidic acid. The topical use of antibiotics such as chloramphenicol is less effective and carries risks of systemic adverse effects. Chloramphenicol is an antibiotic which is considered to have a very narrow spectrum, with many organisms resistant to it, and carries the risk of aplastic anemia. It is vital that chloramphenicol be prescribed only when absolutely necessary, for example, treating strains of *Haemophilus* that are resistant to other antibiotics.

Vancomycin is a valuable antibiotic that should be used carefully. Wide or inappropriate use may lead to emergence of resistant strains. In addition, nephrotoxicity is likely to increase when systemic vancomycin is combined with gentamicin.

There is antagonism when tetracycline is used in combination with quinolone, erythromycin, and all the beta-lactam antibiotics. A beta-lactam antibiotic should not be used in combination with tetracyclines, erythromycin, or chloramphenicol; since the latter inhibit ribosomal function, they will interfere with the effects of beta-lactam antibiotics.

Azithromycin is a macrolide antibiotics belonging to the azalide group. It has been shown to be highly effective against chlamydial infections as well as against Gram-positive bacteria [31–33]. Azithromycin has a long elimination life reaching 68 h. Azithromycin has been found to be effective in the treatment of genital *Chlamydia*. A single, 1-g dose is sufficient to eradicate it. Azithromycin is also effective in the treatment of trachoma [34]. A 1-week course or repeated 3-day courses of azithromycin are required in chronic active cases of trachoma. The drug has high intracellular concentration in the macrophages and polymorphonuclear cells. Following a single oral dose of azithromycin, the drug remains in the conjunctiva above the minimum inhibitory concentration (MIC) of *Chlamydia* for up to 2 weeks [31]. The drug is currently available as eyedrops at a concentration of 1.5 % as Azyter® (Laboratoires Theá, Clermont-Ferrand, France) and 1.0 % concentration as Azasite (Inspire Pharmaceuticals Inc, NC, USA). The tear concentration of topical azithromycin was studied following topical administration of a single dose of azithromycin 1.0 and 1.5 % in healthy volunteers [32]. This study was a prospective, randomized double-masked study. A total of 91 healthy volunteers with normal tear functions were included. Twenty-three subjects received azithromycin 0.5 % eyedrops, 58 subjects received azithromycin 1.0 % eyedrops, and 38 subjects received azithromycin 1.5 % eyedrops. Tears were collected from each subject at seven time points over a 24-h period using the Schirmer strips that were weighed before and after tear sampling. The tear samples were analyzed for azithromycin by high-performance liquid chromatography mass spectrometry (HPLC-MS). The peak of azithromycin was noted 10 min after instillation and the mean concentration remained above 7 mg/l for 24 h. A late-onset increase in the tear concentration of azithromycin was noted at 8–12 h and may be explained by the known azithromycin release from the tissues after storage in the cells [31, 35, 36].

In another study, Kuehne and coworkers [33] measured the concentration of azithromycin and clarithromycin in rabbit corneal tissue following topical application of 2 mg/ml (0.2 %) of azithromycin and 10 mg/ml (0.1 %) of clarithromycin. It was shown that topical azithromycin concentrations were higher in the corneal tissue than clarithromycin. Azithromycin is used for the treatment of chlamydial conjunctivitis, trachoma, keratitis due to *Mycobacterium chelonae*, and chronic blepharitis [31, 36–38].Topical azithromycin is used for the treatment of blepharitis [36–38]. Corneas exposed to desiccation showed significant increase in the azithromycin tissue level compared to normal eyes following topical application of azithromycin 1.5 % eyedrops [39]. It appears that dryness may increase the tissue absorption of the cornea [39].

Linezolid (Zyvox®) is a synthetic antibiotic, is a member of the oxazolidinones used for the treatment of serious infections caused by Gram-positive bacteria [40]. Linezolid inhibits protein synthesis and appears to work by disrupting the translation of messenger RNA into proteins in the ribosomes. Linezolid binds to 50S subunit of the ribosome. It has been shown that linezolid is most active against Gram-positive bacteria including streptococci, vancomycin-resistant-enterococci, and methicillin-resistant-*Staphylococcus aureus* (MRSA). The main indications of linezolid are infections of the skin and soft tissues and pneumonia. The drug is available in the United States and the United Kingdom under the name of Zyvox® and in European countries under the name of Zyvoxid®. On the other hand, in Canada and Mexico, the drug is known as Zyvixam®. Generics of these drugs are available in India under the name of Linospan by Cipla.

Linezolid is an oxazolidinone antibiotic which is a protein synthesis inhibitor. Resistance to linezolid by bacteria has remained low. Linezolid has proven to be safe and effective in infections due to susceptible organisms. The US Food and Drug Association approved linezolid in April 2000. It is considered a bacteriostatic agent, and the main indication of linezolid is the treatment of severe infections caused by Gram-positive bacteria that are resistant to other antibiotics. It has a narrow spectrum and, therefore, remains a reserved antibiotic for cases with severe infections due to resistant bacteria. Linezolid has been associated with *Clostridium difficile*-associated diarrhea and pseudomembranous colitis. The long-term use of linezolid may lead to bone marrow suppression and thrombocytopenia.

2.6 Antibiotics That Inhibit Nucleic Acid Synthesis

The fourth group of antibiotics, the quinolones, comprises antibiotics which inhibit nucleic acid synthesis [5, 41–66].

Pyrimethamine interferes with the synthesis of the hydrofolate which is an important building block of bacterial DNA. The drug is used for the treatment of *Toxoplasma*. Rifamycin interferes with nucleic acid synthesis by the inhibition of RNA-dependent DNA polymerase. Sulfonamides are synergistic with trimethoprim and, have been combined for systemic use.

Fluoroquinolones have a fluorine substitution at position 6 of the quinolone molecule. Additional substitutions at position 1 and position 7 markedly affect antimicrobial efficacy as well as penetration. These alterations have substantially improved the antimicrobial effects against Gram-positive as well as Gram-negative organisms in addition to improving solubility in ophthalmic solutions. Norfloxacin was the first fluoroquinolone to be used topically for ocular infections. It has primarily Gram-negative activity, including antipseudomonal activity as well as limited Gram-positive activity.

The regulation of DNA supercoiling is essential to DNA transcription and replication. In supercoiling, the DNA molecule coils up and shortens the molecule. The DNA helix must unwind to permit the proper function of the enzymatic machinery involved in these processes. Topoisomerases serve to maintain both the transcription and replication of DNA. Type I and type II topoisomerases cut one strand or two strands of DNA, respectively.

The underlying mechanism of action is reversible trapping of DNA gyrase (topoisomerase II) and topoisomerase IV-DNA complexes. Complex formation is followed by reversible inhibition of DNA synthesis. As fluoroquinolone concentrations increase, cell death occurs as double-stranded DNA breaks releasing trapped gyrase and/or topoisomerase IV complexes. In many Gram-negative bacteria, resistance arises primarily from mutation of the gyrase A protein, while in some Gram-positive bacteria, primary resistance occurs via mutation in topoisomerase IV. In addition, efflux pumps that actively pump antibiotics out of the bacteria confer multidrug resistance via these membrane-associated efflux pumps. Gatifloxacin and moxifloxacin are more resistant to these efflux pumps. This change additionally confers added anaerobic activity. Gram-negative organisms may also exhibit decreased levels of outer membrane proteins that facilitate diffusion into the bacterial cell of drug, thereby conferring additional resistance, which can work in concert with the efflux pumps. These last two mechanisms confer a form of resistance and can be overwhelmed by higher concentrations of drug [65].

Fluoroquinolones include moxifloxacin, gatifloxacin, besifloxacin, ciprofloxacin, fleroxacin, lomefloxacin, norfloxacin, ofloxacin, perfloxacin, and temfloxacin, all of which are C-7 1-piperazinyl and C-7 fluoro-substituted quinolones. The drugs are more potent than the original nalidixic acid structure. Several quinolones are available in topical eyedrop form. These drugs have good in vitro actions against many Gram-negative and Gram-positive bacteria, while action against anaerobic bacteria remains poor. The mechanism of action of the quinolones is through inhibition of DNA gyrase. Lomefloxacin is effective against most Gram-negative and Gram-positive organisms. Studies on *Chlamydia trachomatis* show that this organism is moderately susceptible to lomefloxacin.

These susceptibilities are in contrast to the aminoglycosides and β-lactam antibiotics which have activity against bacterial cells in the growth phase, whereas fluoroquinolones are rapidly bactericidal in vitro and in vivo in both growth phase and secondary phase of cell growth.

Studies carried out on the rabbit model have revealed that lomefloxacin readily penetrates the cornea, iris, and ciliary body of the eye and reaches an appreciable concentration in the aqueous. Penetration occurs after both local and systemic administration and penetration have been shown to be increased in the presence of melanin.

The fluoroquinolones have two pKa values on each side of physiological pH with an isoelectric point at pH 7.4. Unionized fluoroquinolones are considered to be very lipophilic, a factor that is thought to influence considerably the mechanism by which these compounds penetrate bacterial cell membranes. Fluoroquinolones are approximately 20–30 % protein bound. This value has been found to be independent of the drug concentration. Following oral administration of lomefloxacin, 10 % of the drug is protein bound in the serum. Evidence from animal studies suggests that lomefloxacin is excreted unchanged by the kidney, although small concentrations of 5 metabolites have been described. The most notable drug interaction occurring is the effect of fluoroquinolones on the clearance of theophylline. Plasma concentrations of theophylline are raised by approximately 19 % during coadministration with perfloxacin as compared to 111 % for enoxacin and 23 % for ciprofloxacin. Ofloxacin and nalidixic acid do not increase the apparent plasma level of theophylline. The interaction is supposed to rise, not through the parent fluoroquinolone but through their 4-oxo metabolites. This interaction is produced through the effect on hepatic p450-related isoenzymes resulting in reduced capacity of *N*-demethylation of theophylline. No oxo-metabolite is produced in the metabolic elimination of lomefloxacin, and the drug is extensively excreted. Theophylline adjustment does not seem to be necessary in patients receiving concomitant lomefloxacin.

Quinolones are interesting in ophthalmology because several of them are available in topical forms. Levofloxacin, lomefloxacin, ciprofloxacin, ofloxacin, norfloxacin, moxifloxacin, gatifloxacin, besifloxacin, and temefloxacin are available for topical use. They are effective against Gram-negative organisms, and in topical form ciprofloxacin has a useful role in the treatment of bacterial keratitis caused by *Pseudomonas.* Certain fourth-generation quinolones, however, have limited efficacy against Gram-positive cocci.

Quinolones are highly effective against Gram-negative organisms and have intermediate activity against staphylococci. They are effective against group B streptococci but not useful against group A streptococci, *Streptococcus pneumonia*, and anaerobes. Clearly, these antibiotics have selective effects against microorganisms, making them unsuitable for "blind shot blanket" therapy. In addition, systemic fluoroquinolones may cause cartilage erosion in children. They should not be used in children or pregnant women. As the case with tetracyclines, antacids may decrease absorption of oral quinolones.

The antibiotics of choice for common ocular pathogens are shown in Table 2.9. The compounding dosages for intravitreal injections of antimicrobial agents are shown in Table 2.10. The antimicrobial therapy for tuberculosis (Table 2.11) and for ocular toxoplasmosis is also listed (Table 2.12).

Compliance with Ethical Requirements

Conflict of Interest The author declares that he has no conflict of interest.

Informed Consent No human studies were carried out by the authors for this article.

Animal Studies No animal studies were carried out by the authors for this article.

Table 2.9 Antibiotics of choice for common ocular pathogens

Pathogen	Antibiotic of first choice	Alternative agents
Viridans group		
S. pneumoniae	Penicillin G (with or without gentamicin)	Cefazolin, vancomycin
	Penicillin G	Cefazolin, vancomycin
Gram-negative cocci		
Neisseria gonorrhoeae	Ceftriaxone or cefixime or ofloxacin	Cefotaxime, spectinomycin, cefoxitin
N. meningitides	Penicillin G	Third-generation cephalosporin, chloramphenicol
Moraxella (Branhamella) catarrhalis	Trimethoprim-sulfamethoxazole	Amoxicillin-clavulanic acid, erythromycin, clarithromycin, azithromycin, cefixime, third-generation cephalosporin, tetracycline
Gram-positive bacilli		
Clostridium perfringens and *Clostridium* spp.	Penicillin G	Metronidazole, clindamycin, imipenem, meropenem, chloramphenicol
Listeria monocytogenes	Ampicillin with gentamicin	Trimethoprim-sulfamethoxazole (TMP-SMX)
Gram-negative bacilli		
Acinetobacter	Imipenem or meropenem	Tobramycin, gentamicin, or amikacin, usually with (or similar agent); TMP-SMX*; a ciprofloxacin
Enterobacter spp.	Imipenem or meropenem	An aminoglycoside and piperacillin or ticarcillin or mezlocillin; a third-generation cephalosporin; TMP-SMX*
		Aztreonam
		Ciprofloxacin

(continued)

Table 2.9 (continued)

Pathogen	Antibiotic of first choice	Alternative agents
Escherichia coli	TMP-SMX* or ciprofloxacin	A cephalosporin or a fluoroquinolones
Haemophilus influenzae	Cefotaxime or ceftriaxone	Chloramphenicol; cefuroxime, gatifloxacin, moxifloxacin, azithromycin
Gram-negative bacilli		
Klebsiella pneumoniae	Ceftriaxone or cefotaxime	Aminoglycoside, imipenem, or meropenem, TMP-SMX*, ticarcillin-clavulanic acid, ampicillin-sulbactam, piperacillin-tazobactam; aztreonam; a fluoroquinolone; amoxicillin-clavulanic acid
Proteus spp.		
Indole positive	Cefotaxime, ceftizoxime, ceftriaxone of cefepime	Aminoglycoside; ticarcillin or piperacillin or mezlocillin; TMP-SMX*; amoxicillin-clavulanic acid; ticarcillin-clavulanic acid, ampicillin-sulbactam, piperacillin-tazobactam; a fluoroquinolone; aztreonam; imipenem
Pseudomonas aeruginosa	Gentamicin or tobramycin or amikacin (combined with ticarcillin, piperacillin, etc., for serious infections)	Aminoglycoside and ceftazidime; imipenem or meropenem, or aztreonam plus an aminoglycoside; ciprofloxacin; trovafloxacin
	Ciprofloxacin, polymyxin B	Ticarcillin piperacillin, or ceftazidime; imipenem or meropenem; aztreonam, an aminoglycoside; cefepime
Gram-negative bacilli		
Serratia	Cefotaxime, ceftizoxime, or ceftriaxone	Gentamicin or amikacin; imipenem; TMP-SMX*; ticarcillin, piperacillin, or mezlocillin, which can be combined with an aminoglycoside; aztreonam; afluoroquinolones
Nocardia spp.	TMP-SMX* Amikacin Rifampin	Tetracycline
Acanthamoeba	Propamidine (0.1 %) Chlorhexidine (0.02 %) Aminoglycoside Voriconazole (1 %)	Polyhexamethylene biguanide
Microsporidia	Fumagillin 0.113 mg/ml Voriconazole 1 % Fluconazole 2 mg/ml	Ketaconazole Itraconazole Albendazole

**TMP-SMX* Trimethoprim-sulfamethazazole

Table 2.10 Intravitreal injections of antimicrobial agents

Acyclovir	2.4 mg/0.1 ml
Amikacin sulfate	0.4 mg/0.1 ml
Ampicillin sodium	5 mg
Cefazolin sodium	2,250 μgm
Ceftazidime	2.25 mg/0.1 ml
Ceftriaxone	2 mg/0.1 ml
Clindamycin	1,000 μgm
Daptomycin	0.2 mg/.05 ml
Dexamethasone	0.4 mg/0.1 ml

Table 2.10 (continued)

Erythromycin	500 μgm
Foscarnet	2.4 mg/0.1 ml
Ganciclovir	0.2 mg/0.05 ml
Gentamicin sulfate	100–200 μgm
Tobramycin sulfate	100–200 μgm
Triamcinolone acetonide	4 mg/0.1 ml
Vancomycin hydrochloride	1 mg/0.1 ml
Voriconazole	0.2 mg/0.1 ml

Table 2.11 Antimicrobial therapy for tuberculosis (adult) [67]

Drug	Daily dose (mg)	Duration (months)	Adverse effects
Isoniazid	300	6	Peripheral neuropathy, hepatotoxicity
Rifampin	600	6	Hepatotoxicity, pink urine
Pyrazinamide	1,500–2,000	6	Liver toxicity, hyperuricemia
Ethambutol	800	2	Optic neuropathy, retinal ganglion cell loss

Table 2.12 Antimicrobial therapy for ocular toxoplasmosis

Treatment regimen (adult)
Pyrimethamine 200 mg orally on day 1, followed by 50 mg orally daily for 4 weeks
Sulfadiazine 2 g orally as a loading dose followed by 1 g orally 4 times daily for 4 weeks
Folinic acid 15 mg orally every other day twice a week
Force fluids and give sodium bicarbonate
Alternate regimen (adult)
Azithromycin, 500 mg orally twice daily for 4 weeks, or clindamycin 300–450 mg orally q 6 h for 4 weeks
Trimethoprim, 160 mg/sulfamethoxazole 800 mg twice daily for 4 weeks
Vision-threatening lesions
Corticosteroids to be used only when vision is threatened: prednisone, 1 mg to 1.5 mg/kg/day, gradually tapered over a period of 4 weeks, or periocular injection of triamcinolone acetonide 40 mg once
Give corticosteroids 3 days after initiation of antimicrobial agents
Congenital toxoplasmosis
Pyrimethamine, 1 mg/kg/day orally once every 3 days, and sulfadiazine, 50 mg to 100 mg/kg/day orally in two divided doses for 3 weeks
Corticosteroids for vision-threatening lesions: 1 mg/kg/day orally in two divided doses. The dosage should be tapered progressively and later discontinued
Folinic acid, 3 mg twice weekly during treatment with pyrimethamine

Adapted and modified from [1, 68]

References

1. Karlowsky JA, Thornsberry C, Jones ME, Evangelista AT, Critchley IA, Sahm DF. TRUST surveillance program. Factors associated with relative rates of antimicrobial resistance among streptococcus pneumoniae in the United States: Results from the TRUST Surveillance Program 1998–2002. Clin Infect Dis. 2003;36(8):963–70.
2. Alfonso E, Crider J. Ophthalmic infections and their anti-infective challenges. Surv Ophthalmol. 2005;50 Suppl 1:S1–6.
3. Tabbara KF. The new era of infections [editorial]. Arch Soc Esp Oftalmol. 1996;70:527–8.
4. Tabbara KF. Antibiotics in ophthalmology [editorial]. Saudi J Ophthalmol. 1999;13(1):1–2.
5. Ayaki M, Iwasawa A, Niwano Y. In vitro assessment of the cytotoxicity of six topical antibiotics to four cultured ocular surface cell lines. Biocontrol Sci. 2012;17(2):93–9.
6. Hong J, Chen J, Sun X, Deng SX, Chen L, Cao W, Yu X, Xu J. Pediatric bacterial keratitis cases in Shanghai: microbiological profile, antibiotic susceptibility and visual outcome. Eye (Lond). 2012;26(12):1571–8. doi:10.1038/eye.2012.210.
7. Barreau G, Mounier M, Marin B, Adenis JP, Robert PY. Intracameral cefuroxime injection at the end of cataract surgery to reduce the incidence of endophthalmitis: French study. J Cataract Refract Surg. 2012;38(8):1370–5.
8. Robert MC, Moussally K, Harissi-Dagher M. Review of endophthalmitis following Boston Keratoprosthesis type 1. Br J Ophthalmol. 2012;96(6):776–80.
9. Cheung CS, Wong AW, Lui A, Kertes PJ, Devenyi RG, Lam WC. Incidence of endophthalmitis and use of antibiotic prophylaxis after intravitreal injections. Ophthalmology. 2012;119(8):1609–14.
10. Mathias MT, Horsley MB, Mawn LA, Laquis SJ, Cahill KV, Foster J, Amato MM, Durairaj VD. Atypical presentations of orbital cellulitis caused by methicillin-resistant Staphylococcus aureus. Ophthalmology. 2012;119(6):1238–43.
11. Scott WJ, Eck CD. Povidone-iodine and ophthalmia neonatorum. Ophthalmology. 2012;119(3):653–4; author reply 654.
12. Emmett Hurley P, Harris GJ. Subperiosteal abscess of the orbit: duration of intravenous antibiotic therapy in

nonsurgical cases. Ophthal Plast Reconstr Surg. 2012;28(1):22–6.
13. Gupta M, Durand ML, Sobrin L. Vancomycin resistance in ocular infections. Int Ophthalmol Clin. 2011;51(4):167–81. Review.
14. Yiu G, Young L, Gilmore M, Chodosh J. Prophylaxis against postoperative endophthalmitis in cataract surgery. Int Ophthalmol Clin. 2011;51(4):67–83. Review.
15. Mataftsi A, Tsinopoulos IT, Tsaousis KT, Dimitrakos SA. Perioperative antibiotic prophylaxis during cataract surgery in Greece. J Cataract Refract Surg. 2011;37(9):1732–3.
16. Jayahar BM, Ramakrishnan R, Ramesh S, Murugan N. Extended-spectrum beta-lactamase resistance among bacterial isolates recovered from ocular infections. Ophthalmic Res. 2012;47(1):52–6.
17. Burton MJ, Pithuwa J, Okello E, Afwamba I, Onyango JJ, Oates F, Chevallier C, Hall AB. Microbial keratitis in East Africa: why are the outcomes so poor? Ophthalmic Epidemiol. 2011;18(4):158–63.
18. Hadatsch B, Butz D, Schmiederer T, Steudle J, Wohlleben W, Süssmuth R, Stegmann E. The biosynthesis of teicoplanin-type glycopeptide antibiotics: assignment of p450 mono-oxygenases to side chain cyclizations of glycopeptide a47934. Chem Biol. 2007;14(9):1078–89.
19. Ho JY, Huang YT, Wu CJ, Li YS, Tsai MD, Li TL. Glycopeptide biosynthesis: Dbv21/Orf2 from dbv/tcp gene clusters are N-Ac-Glm teicoplanin pseudoaglycone deacetylases and Orf15 from cep gene cluster is a Glc-1-P thymidyltransferase. J Am Chem Soc. 2006;128(42):13694–5.
20. de Lalla F, Nicolin R, Rinaldi E, Scarpellini P, Rigoli R, Manfrin V, Tramarin A. Prospective study of oral Teicoplanin versus oral vancomycin for therapy of pseudomembranous colitis and *Clostridium difficile* associated diarrhea. Antimicrob Agents Chemother. 1992;36:2192–6.
21. Molina JM, Tourneur M, Sarfati C, Chevret S, de Gouvello A, Gobert JG, Balkan S, Derouin F, Agence Nationale de Recherches sur le SIDA 090 Study Group . Fumagillin treatment of intestinal microsporidiosis. N Engl J Med. 2002;346(25):1963–9.
22. Tabbara KF, Hyndiuk RA, editors. Infections of the eye. Boston: Little, Brown and Company Publishers; 1996.
23. Tabbara KF, Al-Jabarti A. Hospital construction-associated outbreak of ocular aspergillosis after cataract surgery. Ophthalmology. 1998;105(3):522–6.
24. Parchand S, Gupta A, Ram J, Gupta N, Chakrabarty A. Voriconazole for fungal corneal ulcers. Ophthalmology. 2012;119(5):1083.
25. Prokosch V, Gatzioufas Z, Thanos S, Stupp T. Microbiological findings and predisposing risk factors in corneal ulcers. Graefes Arch Clin Exp Ophthalmol. 2012;250(3):369–74.
26. Oldenburg CE, Acharya NR, Tu EY, Zegans ME, Mannis MJ, Gaynor BD, Whitcher JP, Lietman TM, Keenan JD. Practice patterns and opinions in the treatment of acanthamoeba keratitis. Cornea. 2011;30(12):1363–8.
27. Sakarya R, Sakarya Y, Ozcimen M, Kesli R, Alpfidan I, Kara SJ. Ocular penetration of topically applied 1% daptomycin in a rabbit model. J Ocul Pharmacol Ther. 2013;29(1):75–8. doi:10.1089/jop.2012.0111.
28. Comer GM, Miller JB, Schneider EW, Khan NW, Reed DM, Elner VM, Zacks DN. Intravitreal daptomycin: a safety and efficacy study. Retina. 2011;31(6):1199–206.
29. Tabbara KF, Antonios S, Alvarez H. Effects of fusidic acid on staphylococcal keratitis. Br J Ophthalmol. 1989;73(2):136–9.
30. Taylor PB, Burd EM, Tabbara KF. Corneal and intraocular penetration of topical and subconjunctival fusidic acid. Br J Ophthalmol. 1987;1(8):598–601.
31. Tabbara KF, Al Kharashi SA, Al-Mansouri SM, Al-Omar OM, Cooper H, Abu El-Asrar AM, Foulds G. Ocular levels of azithromycin. Arch Ophthalmol. 1998;116:1625–8.
32. Chiambaretta F, Garraffo R, Elena PP, Pouliquen P, Delval L, Rigal D, Dubray C, Goldschmidt P, Tabbara K, Cochereau I. Tear concentrations of azithromycin following topical administration of a single dose of azithromycin 0.5%, 1.0%, and 1.5% eyedrops (T1225) in healthy volunteers. Eur J Ophthalmol. 2008;18(1):13–20.
33. Kuehne JJ, Yu AL, Holland GN, et al. Corneal pharmacokinetics of topically applied azithromycin and clarithromycin. Am J Ophthalmol. 2004;138(4):547–53.
34. Tabbara KF, Abu El-Asrar AM, Al-Omar OM, Choudhury AH, Al-Faisal ZK. Single-dose Azithromycin in the treatment of trachoma: a randomized, controlled study. Ophthalmology. 1996;103(5):842–6.
35. Abshire R, Cockrum P, Crider J, Schlech B. Topical antibacterial therapy for mycobacterial keratitis: potential for surgical prophylaxis and treatment. Clin Ther. 2004;26(2):191–6.
36. Luchs J. Efficacy of tropical azithromycin ophthalmic solution 1% in the treatment of posterior blepharitis. Adv Ther. 2008;25(9):855–70.
37. Igami TZ, Holzchuh R, Osaki TH, Santo RM, Kara-Jose N, Hida RY. Oral azithromycin for treatment of posterior blepharitis. Cornea. 2011;30(10):1145–9.
38. Veldman P, Colby K. Current evidence for topical azithromycin 1% ophthalmic solution in the treatment of blepharitis and blepharitis-associated ocular dryness. Int Ophthalmol Clin. 2011;51(4):43–52. Review.
39. Tabbara KF, Kotb AK, Hammouda EF, Elkum N. Effects of dehydration on corneal tissue absorption of topical azithromycin in rabbits. Curr Eye Res. 2005;30:915–8.
40. Tascini C, Gemignani G, Doria R, Biancofiore G, Urbani L, Mosca C, Malacarne P, Papineschi F, Passaglia C, Dal Canto L, Procaccini M, Furneri G, Didoni G, Filipponi F, Menichetti F. Linezolid treatment for gram positive infections: a retrospective comparison with teicoplanin. J Chemother. 2009;21(3):311–6.
41. Blondeau JM. Fluoroquinolones: mechanism of action, classification, and development of resistance. Surv Ophthalmol. 2004;49 Suppl 2:S73–8.

42. Tabbara KF, El-Sheikh HF, Islam SMM, Hammouda E. Treatment of acute bacterial conjunctivitis with topical Lomefloxacin 0.3% compared to topical Ofloxacin 0.3%. Eur J Ophthalmol. 1999;4(4):269–75.
43. Alexandrakis G, Alfonso EC, Miller D. Shifting trends in bacterial keratitis in South Florida and emerging resistance to fluoroquinolones. Ophthalmology. 2000;107:1497–502.
44. Chaudhry NA, Flynn Jr HW, Murray TG, Tabandeh H, Mello Jr MO, Miller D. Emerging ciprofloxacin-resistant Pseudomonas aeruginosa. Am J Ophthalmol. 1999;128(4):509–10.
45. Goldstein MH, Kowalski RP, Gordon YJ. Emerging fluoroquinolone resistance in bacterial keratitis: a 5-year review. Ophthalmology. 1999;106:131–8.
46. Aliprandis E, Ciralsky J, Lai H, Herling I, Katz HR. Comparative efficacy of topical moxifloxacin versus ciprofloxacin and vancomycin in the treatment of P. aeruginosa and ciprofloxacin-resistant MRSA keratitis in rabbits. Cornea. 2005;24(2):201–5.
47. Caballero AR, Marquart ME, O'Callaghan RJ, Thibodeaux BA, Johnston KH, Dajcs JJ. Effectiveness of fluoroquinolones against Mycobacterium abscessus in vivo. Curr Eye Res. 2006;31(1):23–9.
48. Callegan MC, Ramirez R, Kane ST, Cochran DC, Jensen H. Antibacterial activity of the fourth-generation fluoroquinolones gatifloxacin and moxifloxacin against ocular pathogens. Adv Ther. 2003;20(5):246–52.
49. Dajcs JJ, Thibodeaux BA, Marquart ME, Girgis DO, Traidej M, O'Callaghan RJ. Effectiveness of ciprofloxacin, levofloxacin or moxifloxacin for treatment of experimental Staphylococcus aureus keratitis. Antimicrob Agents Chemother. 2004;48(6):1948–52.
50. El-Sheikh HF, Tabbara KF, Islam SMM, Hammouda E. Susceptibility of clinically significant ocular isolates to Lomefloxacin 0.3%. Saudi J Ophthalmol. 1999;13(1):31–6.
51. Herrygers LA, Noecker RJ, Lane LC, Levine JM. Comparison of corneal surface effects of gatifloxacin and moxifloxacin using intensive and prolonged dosing protocols. Cornea. 2005;24(1):66–71.
52. Hofling-Lima AL, de Freitas D, Sampaio JL, Leao SC, Contarini P. In vitro activity of fluoroquinolones against Mycobacterium abscessus and Mycobacterium chelonae causing infectious keratitis after LASIK in Brazil. Cornea. 2005;24(6):730–4.
53. Lee SB, Oliver KM, Strube YN, Mohan SK, Slomovic AR. Fourth-generation fluoroquinolones in the treatment of mycobacterial infectious keratitis after laser-assisted in situ keratomileusis surgery. Can J Ophthalmol. 2005;40(6):750–3.
54. Levine JM, Noecker RJ, Lane LC, Herrygers L, Nix D, Snyder RW. Comparative penetration of moxifloxacin and gatifloxacin in rabbit aqueous humor after topical dosing. J Cataract Refract Surg. 2004;30(10):2177–82.
55. Moshirfar M, Mirzaian G, Feiz V, Kang PC. Fourth-generation fluoroquinolone-resistant bacterial keratitis after refractive surgery. J Cataract Refract Surg. 2006;32(3):515–8.
56. Patel NR, Reidy JJ, Gonzalez-Fernandez F. Nocardia keratitis after laser in situ keratomileusis: clinicopathologic correlation. J Cataract Refract Surg. 2005;31(10):2012–5.
57. Price MO, Price Jr FW, Maclellan D. Effect of gatifloxacin 0.3% and moxifloxacin 0.5% ophthalmic solutions on human corneal epithelium following 2 dosing regimens. J Cataract Refract Surg. 2005;31(11):2137–41.
58. Rhee MK, Kowalski RP, Romanowski EG, Mah FS, Ritterband DC, Gordon YJ. A laboratory evaluation of antibiotic therapy for ciprofloxacin-resistant Pseudomonas aeruginosa. Am J Ophthalmol. 2004;138(2):226–30.
59. Robertson SM, Curtis MA, Schlech BA, Rusinko A, Owen GR, Dembinska O, Liao J, Dahlin DC. Ocular pharmacokinetics of moxifloxacin after topical treatment of animals and humans. Surv Ophthalmol. 2005;50 Suppl 1:S32–45.
60. Tabbara KF, Cooper H, Shareef AH. Decrease in tear bioavailability of ciprofloxacin in eyes with carbon containing eyeliners. Saudi Med J. 1999;20(9):717–8.
61. Thibodeaux RA, Dajcs JJ, Caballero AR, Marquart ME, Girgis DO, O'Callaghan RJ. Quantitative comparison of fluoroquinolone therapies of experimental gram-negative bacterial keratitis. Curr Eye Res. 2004;28(5):337–42.
62. Malhotra R, Gira J, Berdy GJ, Brusatti R. Safety of besifloxacin ophthalmic suspension 0.6% as a prophylactic antibiotic following routine cataract surgery: results of a prospective, parallel-group, investigator-masked study. Clin Ophthalmol. 2012;6:855–63.
63. Fukuda M, Yamada M, Kinoshita S, Inatomi T, Ohashi Y, Uno T, Shimazaki J, Satake Y, Maeda N, Hori Y, Nishida K, Kubota A, Nakazawa T, Shimomura Y. Comparison of corneal and aqueous humor penetration of moxifloxacin, gatifloxacin and levofloxacin during keratoplasty. Adv Ther. 2012;29(4):339–49.
64. Miyake T, Ito N, Tajima K, Goto H, Furukawa T. Comparison of moxifloxacin and levofloxacin in an epithelial disorder model using cultured rabbit corneal epithelial cell sheets. Graefes Arch Clin Exp Ophthalmol. 2012;250(7):1035–41.
65. Shalchi Z, Gurbaxani A, Baker M, Nash J. Antibiotic resistance in microbial keratitis: ten-year experience of corneal scrapes in the United Kingdom. Ophthalmology. 2011;118(11):2161–5.
66. Cervantes LJ, Mah FS. Clinical use of gatifloxacin ophthalmic solution for treatment of bacterial conjunctivitis. Clin Ophthalmol. 2011;5:495–502.
67. Tabbara KF. Tuberculosis. Curr Opin Ophthalmol. 2007;18(6):493–501.
68. Tabbara KF. Ocular toxoplasmosis. In: Tasman W, Jaeger EA, editors. Duane's clinical ophthalmology, vol. Uvea section. Baltimore: Lippincott Williams & Wilkins; 2008.

Infections of the Orbit

3

Moncef Khairallah and Sonia Attia

3.1 Introduction

The term "orbital infections" refers to an invasive bacterial or nonbacterial infection of periorbital and orbital structures. Although less common since the advent of antibiotics, this ophthalmic infectious condition still accounts for 60 % of primary orbital disease processes. Orbital infection is usually due to adjacent paranasal sinusitis, but numerous other local or systemic conditions should be considered in the differential diagnosis (Table 3.1) [1]. All age groups may be affected, but the condition is more prevalent in children and young individuals [2, 3].

Diagnosis and characterization of orbital infection as preseptal infection or postseptal infection (orbital cellulitis) are primarily based on clinical findings, and imaging is very helpful in confirming the diagnosis and evaluating the extension of the infectious process. Early diagnosis and prompt, proper management of orbital infection is essential to prevent sight-threatening, as well as life-threatening, complications.

M. Khairallah, MD (✉) • S. Attia, MD
Department of Ophthalmology, Fattouma Bourguiba University Hospital, Monastir, Tunisia

Faculty of Medicine, University of Monastir, Monastir, Tunisia
e-mail: moncef.khairallah@rns.tn

3.2 Pathophysiology

Orbital infections can develop by extension of infection from adjacent paranasal sinuses or upper respiratory infection, ocular and adnexal structures, direct inoculation as a result of trauma or surgery, or hematogenous spread in the setting of bacteremia [4–7]. The pathophysiology of orbital infection is related to local anatomical structures, especially the orbital septum and the lamina papyracea. According to a classification system proposed by Chandler in 1970 (Fig. 3.1), the orbital septum delineates orbital infections into preseptal (type 1) and retroseptal (type 2) cellulitis [5, 8]. The lamina papyracea, which is the medial orbital wall, is the thinnest bone separating the orbit from the sinuses and has numerous natural dehiscences as well as being perforated by numerous vessels and nerves [9]. This may explain why sinusitis and upper respiratory tract infection are the most common causes of orbital infection and why the ethmoid sinus is the most frequent orbital infection source [2, 10–12]. Natural defects on the lamina papyracea also facilitate communication between the ethmoid air cells and the subperiosteal space on the medial wall of the orbit leading to subperiosteal abscess (type 3 cellulitis). Moreover, the lack of lymphatic channels promotes the spread of infection from superficial tissues into the orbit. Orbital veins lack valves, so passage of infectious processes in both anterograde and retrograde directions is possible. Following

K. Tabbara et al. (eds.), *Ocular Infections*, Essentials in Ophthalmology,
DOI 10.1007/978-3-662-43981-4_3, © Springer-Verlag Berlin Heidelberg 2014

Table 3.1 Main causes of orbital infections

Etiologies of preseptal cellulitis
Infection of ocular adnexa: *conjunctivitis, chalazia, hordeola, blepharitis, dacryocystitis, trauma with or without foreign body, insect bites, skin face wound, dacryoadenitis, impetigo*
Hematogenous spread
Acute ethmoid or maxillary sinusitis
Etiologies of retroseptal cellulitis
Acute sinusitis
Trauma with or without foreign body
Progression of preseptal cellulitis
Hematogenous spread
Ophthalmic surgery: *anterior segment surgery, eyelid surgery, strabismus surgery, peribulbar injection, orbital implants*
Dental abscess
Otitis media
Endophthalmitis
Inhaled cocaine abuse

progressive preseptal or orbital cellulitis, the inflammatory process may progress to abscess formation occurring inside or outside the muscle cone leading to an orbital abscess (type 4 cellulitis). Additionally, valveless orbital veins allow for the intracranial retrograde spread of infection to the cavernous sinus causing infectious cavernous sinus thrombosis (CST) (type 5 cellulitis). Sources of orbital infections other than paranasal sinusitis and upper respiratory infection include orbital trauma, with or without foreign body, dacryocystitis, ruptured dacryocele or dermoid cyst, dental infections, otitis media, endogenous endophthalmitis, ophthalmic surgery, eyelid lesions (chalazia, hordeola), insect bites, and impetigo (Table 3.1) [2, 10, 13–22]. Risk factors for orbital infection include diabetic ketoacidosis, history of HIV or immunosuppressive therapy, hematological malignancies, and renal transplant.

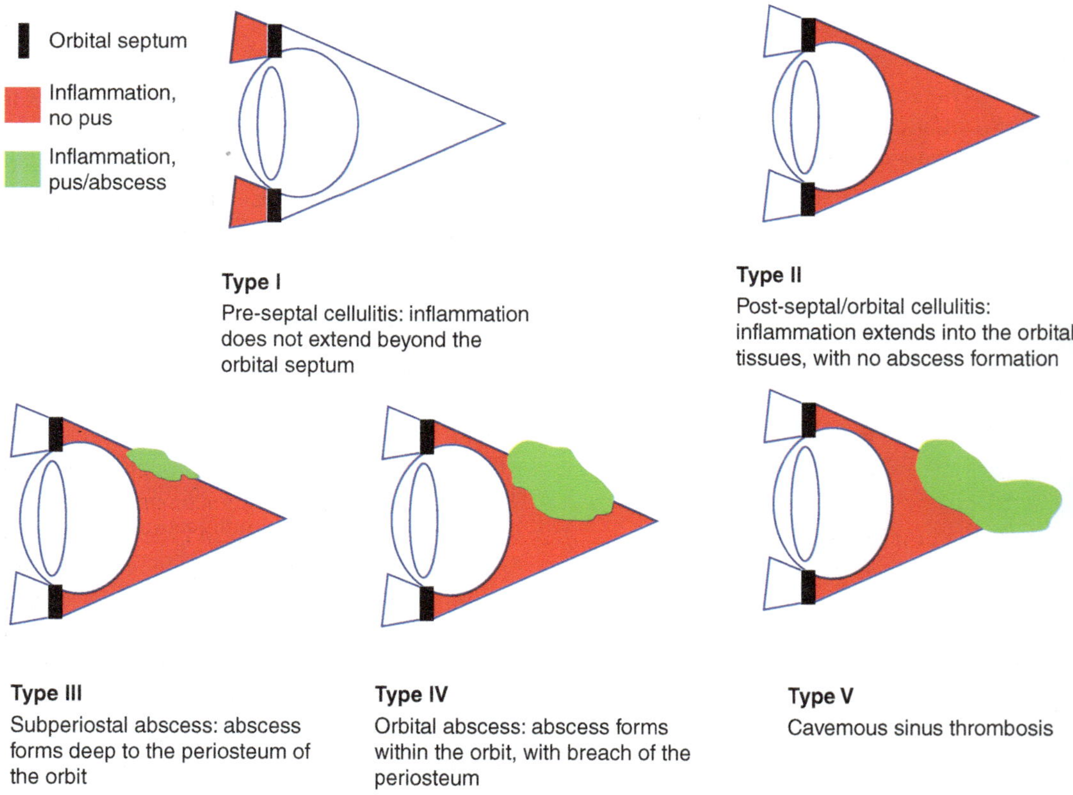

Fig. 3.1 Chandler classification of orbital infections (Adapted from Buchanam et al. [8])

3.3 Symptoms and Signs

A patient with orbital infection usually presents with unilateral painful eyelid edema and erythema (Figs. 3.2 and 3.3). There may be a history of acute sinusitis or upper respiratory tract infection. Past medical history significant for HIV, diabetes, immunosuppression, steroid use, hematological malignancies, or renal disease is important to consider [23]. Early diagnosis and characterization of orbital cellulitis as preseptal or retroseptal infection are primarily based on clinical findings, and this is of utmost importance for prompt initiation of appropriate therapy to prevent ocular and systemic morbidity.

Patients with preseptal cellulitis (type1) will present with preserved visual function, without proptosis, and full ocular motility without painful movement, as the extent of infection is superficial and does not extend posteriorly into the orbit (Table 3.2). Preseptal cellulitis may extend posteriorly, owing to the valveless communication of the facial and ophthalmic veins to the cavernous sinus, to cause one of the retroseptal infections (types 2–5) [24, 25]. Retroseptal septal infection (orbital cellulitis) is characterized by the presence of orbital signs including chemosis, proptosis, resistance to retropulsion of the eye, and extraocular muscle motility disturbance, with the potential for severe vision loss and life-threatening complications [13, 26, 27].

Search for abnormal vital signs (e.g., tachycardia, hyperpyrexia) is recommended. However, normal temperature or vital signs should not rule out postseptal infection. Orbital cellulitis may or may not progress to a significant subperiosteal abscess (Fig. 3.3b), orbital abscess, or cavernous sinus thrombosis. When a fluctuant mass is palpable along the orbital rim with local tenderness, a subperiosteal abscess (type 3) should be considered. If a patient presents with decreased visual acuity, afferent pupillary defect, retinal venous dilatation, optic disk swelling, ptosis, severe directional proptosis, and ophthalmoplegia, an orbital abscess (type 4) should be suspected. Extension of orbital infection posteriorly into the cavernous sinus leads to cavernous sinus thrombosis (CST) (type 5). This serious complication is clinically characterized by headache, generalized sepsis, nausea, vomiting, high fever, periorbital edema, increasing proptosis, chemosis, afferent pupillary defect, and paralysis of eye movements. Infectious CST may cause meningitis with signs of meningeal irritation and loss of consciousness.

Orbital infections should be differentiated from nonspecific orbital inflammation, which usually presents with eyelid swelling/mass, less ocular pain than orbital infection, and no identifiable associated local or systemic causes. Other diseases that may mimic orbital infections include thyroid ophthalmopathy, which is typically bilateral and

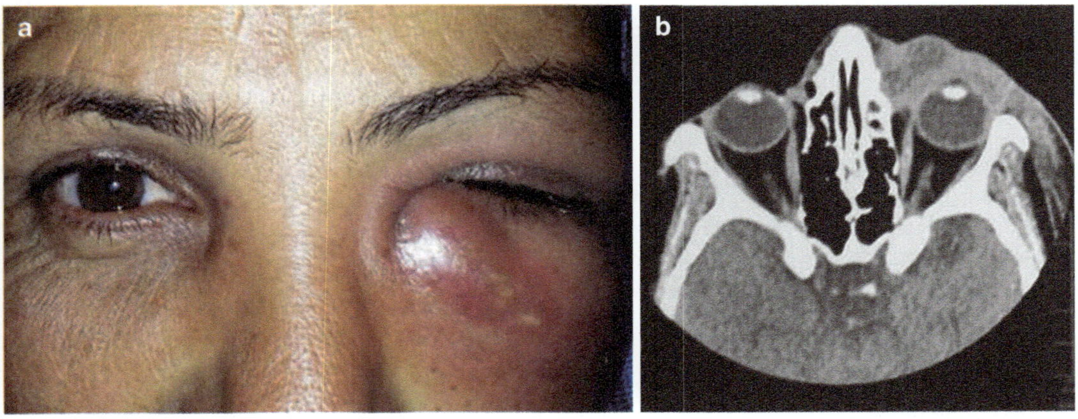

Fig. 3.2 (**a**) Photograph of a 38-year-old woman with 1-week history of acute dacryocystitis shows left inferior eyelid edema and erythema. (**b**) Axial CT scan shows left eyelid swelling and extent of preseptal inflammatory swelling in periorbital tissues consistent with preseptal cellulitis

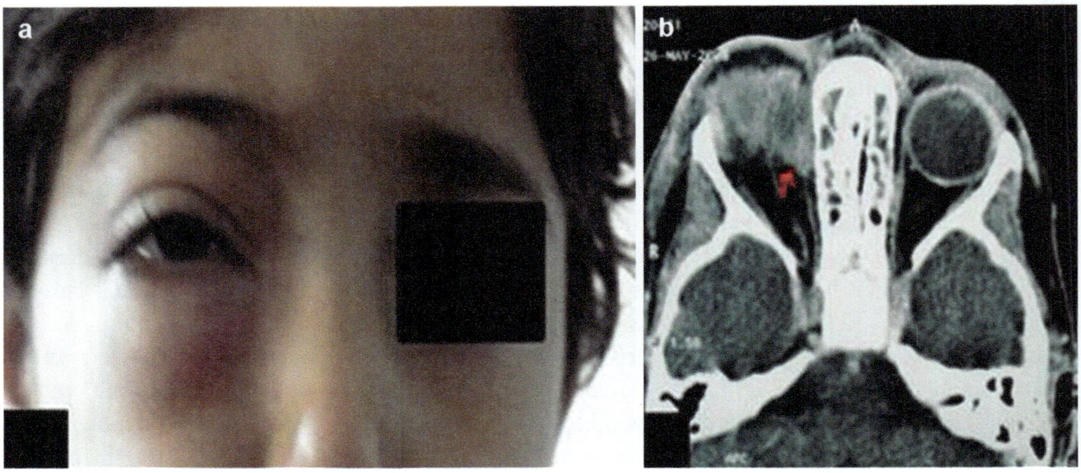

Fig. 3.3 (**a**) Photograph of an 8-year-old girl shows palpebral swelling with erythema and mild proptosis. (**b**) Axial CT scan shows subperiosteal abscess (type 3 orbital infection, *red arrow*) adjacent to the medial rectus and ethmoid sinusitis

Table 3.2 Clinical signs of orbital infections

Type	Diagnosis	Clinical signs
I	Periorbital (preseptal) cellulitis	Upper eyelid swelling causing ptosis without extraocular or visual changes
II	Orbital (postseptal) cellulitis	Eyelid swelling, periorbital swelling, ptosis, proptosis, chemosis, limited or no impairment of extraocular movement
III	Subperiosteal abscess	Displacement of the globe downward and laterally, impairment of extraocular movement with diplopia, decreased VA (later finding), RAPD
IV	Orbital abscess	Severe proptosis, complete ophthalmoplegia, decreased VA that can progress to irreversible blindness, RAPD
V	Cavernous sinus thrombosis	Orbital pain, chemosis, proptosis, sepsis, ophthalmoplegia. Can progress to the other eye

VA visual acuity, *RAPD* relative afferent pupillary defect

painless; orbital myositis, which may produce mild vascular congestion and proptosis; rhabdomyosarcoma; and metastatic orbital tumor, especially from breast carcinoma. Magnetic resonance imaging (MRI) may be helpful in the differential diagnosis of orbital infection.

Vision loss in patients with orbital infection can occur due to corneal damage secondary to proptosis or neurotrophic keratitis, persistent raised intraocular pressure, central retinal artery occlusion, or septic, inflammatory, or ischemic optic neuropathy [10, 28].

3.4 Laboratory Tests and Imaging

Blood testing may show high white cell count, particularly in children with orbital cellulitis [29]. Blood cultures may be positive in children [30], but they are usually negative in adults [6, 10, 31]. Abscess and sinus aspiration remain invasive surgical procedures and should be performed only in case of clinical worsening despite a broad-spectrum antibiotic therapy. Surgical specimens are more likely than swabbing nasal mucosa or conjunctiva to provide positive results [6, 10, 30–32].

Orbital infections have been associated with a wide range of organisms. *Staphylococcus*, followed by *Streptococcus species*, are the most common pathogens, particularly in pediatric population, and methicillin-resistant *S. aureus* accounts for more than 70 % of *S. aureus* isolates [12, 32–34]. The incidence of *Haemophilus influenza* has declined due to the wide use and introduction of *Haemophilus influenza* type B vaccine [35]. Polymicrobial infections with aerobic and anaerobic bacteria are more common in patients aged 16 years or older [12, 32, 36]. *Escherichia coli*, *Enterobacter* species, *Actinobacter* species, and *Proteus mirabilis* can rarely be responsible for orbital infection secondary to hematogenous spread, especially in elderly or immunocompromised patients [10, 16, 37]. Fungal infection (mucormycosis or *Aspergillosis* species) usually occurs in association with diabetic ketoacidosis or immunosuppression, leading to a high mortality rate [38].

Cranio-orbital high-resolution contrast-enhanced computed tomography (CT) scanning remains the gold standard investigation in the diagnosis and management of orbital infections. It should be performed within 24 h in all patients with signs and symptoms suggestive of postseptal infections. It is useful to classify the postseptal infection according to Chandler classification into type 2–5, and may recognize the origin of the sinus infection or a foreign body when it is present in a patient with a history of trauma [39–43].

In patients with preseptal infections, CT imaging should be performed in cases failing to improve following 48 h of IV antibiotic therapy. Axial contrast-enhanced CT scan shows lid swelling and extent of preseptal inflammatory swelling in periorbital tissues (Fig. 3.2b), and even preseptal abscesses.

Signs consistent with postseptal cellulitis revealed by axial contrast-enhanced CT scan include preseptal soft tissue thickening, proptosis, rectus muscle enlargement, soft tissue swelling, and retrobulbar fat stranding. Intraorbital fluid collection with displacement of the globe consistent with orbital abscess may also be observed.

CT images may provide diagnosis of sinusitis showing mucosal thickening of the paranasal sinuses. Both in children and in adults, there is a predilection for the anterior ethmoid and the maxillary sinus [9, 10, 44].

Axial CT scan views should include low narrow cuts of the frontal lobes to rule out peridural and parenchymal brain abscess. However, MRI is superior to CT for the identification of intracranial involvement.

3.5 Management

Patients with orbital infection should be managed promptly in close collaboration with otorhinolaryngologist and infectious disease specialist. Nearly all patients with preseptal cellulitis are managed with oral antibiotics, but they should as well be informed to maintain vigilance and go back for evaluation if there is evidence of clinical worsening. Most cases of postseptal cellulitis are managed with intravenous antibiotics [45]. However, hospital admission with intravenous antibiotics is recommended in patients with preseptal cellulitis in the following situations: children less than 1 year of age, immunosuppressed patients, those who lack immunization against *H. influenzae*, and those with severe systemic infection [9]. Given the origin of orbital infection, antibiotic selection is directed toward causative agents of upper respiratory infections and sinusitis, particularly *Staphylococcus* and *Streptococcus* species [26, 31]. But the initial antibiotic regimen should be changed if the response is insufficient or if the cultures dictate otherwise. Consultation by an infectious disease specialist can be helpful in the selection of appropriate antimicrobial therapy. The most common antibiotic regimen includes cephalosporins or amoxicillin/clavulanic acid combined with other antibiotics. Depending on the source of infection, these antibiotics may include flucloxacillin, vancomycin, and/or fosfomycin [9]. The use of clindamycin is recommended in the presence of infections that involve the bone with osteomyelitis or those individuals who are allergic to cephalosporins or to penicillin. Metronidazole is used in orbital cellulitis to cover anaerobic bacteria [10]. In case of fungal infection, antifungal drug such as amphotericin B or voriconazole is required. Intravenous antimicrobial treatment in patients with orbital cellulitis is continued until there is apparent clinical improvement; after which, continued recovery should be assessed on oral antibiotics on an outpatient basis for additional 7–10 days.

Corticosteroids may be helpful, but they should be initiated 2–3 days after appropriate antibiotics and if clinical improvement is noted. Nasal decongestants are recommended in those cases with acute sinusitis. Ocular antihypertensive therapy should be promptly initiated in case of secondary glaucoma. Tetanus prophylaxis should be given according to standard protocol in cases of posttraumatic orbital cellulitis.

Surgical therapy should be considered in patients with type 3–5 postseptal cellulitis, especially in the presence of a CT scan evidence of suppuration, associated visual loss, immunosuppression, or disease progression despite antibiotic therapy [36, 46]. Surgical intervention consists mostly with combined endoscopic sinus surgery with transnasal orbital abscess drainage [10]. Medial subperiosteal abscesses are usually drained endoscopically, whereas lateral or intraconal abscesses require an open procedure [45]. Concomitant treatment of sinusitis needs to be continued if present. Finally, there is no foolproof method for the prevention of orbital infection, but appropriate treatment of conditions that may lead to this disease (e.g., sinusitis, dacryocystitis, dental disease) is the best way.

Compliance with Ethical Requirements

Conflict of Interest The authors declare that they have no conflict of interest.

Informed Consent No human studies were carried out by the authors for this article.

Animal Studies No animal studies were carried out by the authors for this article.

References

1. Som PM, Curtin HD, editors. Head and neck imaging. St Louis: Mosby; 1996. p. 1090–5.
2. Bagheri A, Tavakoli M, Aletaha M, Salour H, Ghaderpanah M. Orbital and preseptal cellulitis: a 10-year survey of hospitalized patients in a tertiary eye hospital in Iran. Int Ophthalmol. 2012;32(4):361–7.
3. Connell B, Kamal Z, McNab AA. Fulminant orbital cellulitis with complete loss of vision. Clin Exp Ophthalmol. 2001;29:260–1.
4. Harris GJ. Subperiosteal abscess of the orbit. Arch Ophthalmol. 1983;101:751–7.
5. Chandler JR, Langenbrunner DJ, Stevens ER. The pathogenesis of orbital complications in acute sinusitis. Laryngoscope. 1970;80(9):1414–28.
6. Oxford LE, McClay J. Complications of acute sinusitis in children. Otolaryngol Head Neck Surg. 2005;133(1):32–7.
7. Kikkawa DO, Heinz GW, Martin RT, Nunery WN, Eiseman AS. Orbital cellulitis and abscess secondary to dacryocystitis. Arch Ophthalmol. 2002;120(8):1096–9.
8. Buchanan MA, Muen W, Heinz P. Management of periorbital and orbital cellulitis: review article. Paediatr Child Health. 2012;22(2):72–7.
9. Lee S, Yen MT. Management of preseptal and orbital cellulitis. Saudi J Ophthalmol. 2011;25:21–9.
10. Chaudhry IA, Shamsi FA. Outcome of treated orbital cellulitis in a tertiary eye care center in the middle East. Ophthalmology. 2007;114(2):345–54.
11. Sultész M, Csákányi Z, Majoros T, et al. Acute bacterial rhinosinusitis and its complications in our pediatric otolaryngological department between 1997 and 2006. Int J Pediatr Otorhinolaryngol. 2009;73(11):1507–12.
12. Ho CF, Huang YC, Wang CJ, et al. Clinical analysis of computed tomography-staged orbital cellulitis in children. J Microbiol Immunol Infect. 2007;40(6):518–24.
13. Schmitt NJ, Beatty RL, Kennerdell JS. Superior ophthalmic vein thrombosis in a patient with dacryocystitis-induced orbital cellulitis. Ophthal Plast Reconstr Surg. 2005;21(5):387–9.
14. Maheshwari R, Maheshwari S, Shah T. Acute dacryocystitis causing orbital cellulitis and abscess. Orbit. 2009;28(2–3):196–9.
15. Akhaddar A, Elasri F, Elouennass M, et al. Orbital abscess associated with sinusitis from odontogenic origin. Intern Med. 2010;49(5):523–4.
16. Argelicha R, Ibáñez-Floresb N, Bardaviob J, et al. Orbital cellulitis and endogenous endophthalmitis secondary to Proteus mirabilis cholecystitis. Diagn Microbiol Infect Dis. 2009;64(4):442–4.
17. Armesto A, Ugrin MC. Orbital cellulitis after faden operation on the medial rectus. Strabismus. 2007;15(4):215–9.
18. McLeod SD, Flowers CW, Lopez PF, Marx J, McDonnell PJ. Endophthalmitis and orbital cellulitis after radial keratotomy. Ophthalmology. 1995;102(12):1902–7.
19. Hofbauer JD, Gordon LK, Palmer J. Acute orbital cellulitis after peribulbar injection. Am J Ophthalmol. 1994;118(3):391–2.
20. Cox NH, Knowles MA, Porteus ID. Pre-septal cellulitis and facial erysipelas due to Moraxella species. Clin Exp Dermatol. 1994;19(4):321–3.
21. Molarte AB, Isenberg SJ. Periorbital cellulitis in infancy. J Pediatr Ophthalmol Strabismus. 1989;26(5):232–4.

22. Smith TF, O'Day D, Wright PF. Clinical implications of preseptal (periorbital) cellulitis in childhood. Pediatrics. 1978;62(6):1006–9.
23. Rumelt S, Rubin PA. Potential sources for orbital cellulitis. Int Ophthalmol Clin. 1996;36(3):207–21.
24. Howe L, Jones NS. Guidelines for the management of periorbital cellulitis/abscess. Clin Otolaryngol. 2004; 29(6):725–8.
25. Jones DB, Steinkuller PG. Strategies for the initial management of acute preseptal and orbital cellulitis. Trans Am Ophthalmol Soc. 1988;86:94–108.
26. Lessner A, Stern GA. Preseptal and orbital cellulitis. Infect Dis Clin North Am. 1992;6(4):933–52.
27. Yeh CH, Chen WC, Lin MS, Huang HT, Chao SC, Lo YC. Intracranial brain abscess preceded by orbital cellulitis and sinusitis. J Craniofac Surg. 2010;21(3):934–6.
28. Ferguson MP, McNab AA. Current treatment and outcome in orbital cellulitis. Aust N Z J Ophthalmol. 1999;27(6):375–9.
29. Weiss A, Friendly D, Eglin K, Chang M, Gold B. Bacterial periorbital and orbital cellulitis in childhood. Ophthalmology. 1983;90(3):195–203.
30. Robinson A, Beech T, McDermott AL, Sinha A. Investigation and management of adult periorbital and orbital cellulitis. J Laryngol Otol. 2007;121(6):545–7.
31. Uzcátegui N, Warman R, Smith A, Howard CW. Clinical practice guidelines for the management of orbital cellulitis. J Pediatr Ophthalmol Strabismus. 1998;35(2):73–9.
32. McKinley SH, Yen MT, Miller AM, Yen KG. Microbiology of pediatric orbital cellulitis. Am J Ophthalmol. 2007;144(4):497–501.
33. Seltz LB, Smith J, Durairaj VD, Enzenauer R, Todd J. Microbiology and antibiotic management of orbital cellulitis. Pediatrics. 2011;127(3):566–72.
34. Fanella S, Singer A, Embree J. Presentation and management of pediatric orbital cellulitis. Can J Infect Dis Med Microbiol. 2011;22(3):97–100.
35. Ambati BK, Ambati J, Azar N, Stratton L, Schmidt EV. Periorbital and orbital cellulitis before and after the advent of Haemophilus influenzae type B vaccination. Ophthalmology. 2000;107(8):1450–3.
36. Patt BS, Manning SC. Blindness resulting from orbital complications of sinusitis. Otolaryngol Head Neck Surg. 1991;104(6):789–95.
37. Suneetha N, Battu RR, Thomas RK, Bosco A. Orbital abscess: management and outcome. Indian J Ophthalmol. 2000;48(2):129–34.
38. Toumi A, Larbi Ammari F, Loussaief C, Hadhri R, Ben Brahim H, Harrathi K, Ben Romdhane F, Koubaa J, Chakroun M. Rhino-orbito-cerebral mucormycosis: five cases. Med Mal Infect. 2012; 42(12):591–8.
39. O'Ryan F, Diloreto D, Barber HD, Bruckner R. Orbital infections: clinical and radiographic diagnosis and surgical treatment. J Oral Maxillofac Surg. 1988;46(11):991–7.
40. Hornblass A, Herschorn BJ, Stern K, Grimes C. Orbital abscess. Surv Ophthalmol. 1984;29(3): 169–78.
41. Harris GJ. Subperiosteal abscess of the orbit. Age as a factor in the bacteriology and response to treatment. Ophthalmology. 1994;101(3):585–95.
42. Harris GJ. Subperiosteal abscess of the orbit: computed tomography and the clinical course. Ophthal Plast Reconstr Surg. 1996;12(1):1–8.
43. Harris GJ. Subperiosteal abscess of the orbit: older children and adults require aggressive treatment. Ophthal Plast Reconstr Surg. 2001;17(6):395–7.
44. Botting AM, McIntosh D, Mahadevan M. Paediatric pre- and post-septal peri-orbital infections are different diseases. A retrospective review of 262 cases. Int J Pediatr Otorhinolaryngol. 2008;72(3): 377–83.
45. Bedwell J, Bauman NM. Management of pediatric orbital cellulitis and abscess. Curr Opin Otolaryngol Head Neck Surg. 2011;19(6):467–73.
46. Yang M, Quah BL, Seah LL, Looi A. Orbital cellulitis in children-medical treatment versus surgical management. Orbit. 2009;28(2–3):124–36.

4 Infections of the Lacrimal System

Khalid F. Tabbara

4.1 Introduction

The lacrimal apparatus consists of the lacrimal gland and the nasolacrimal drainage system. The accessory lacrimal glands include the glands of Krause and Wölfring; a mucinous layer is secreted by the conjunctival goblet cells and oily secretions by the meibomian glands. The lacrimal gland is oval in shape and has two portions: the palpebral portion and the orbital portion divided anteriorly in two by the lateral horn of the levator aponeurosis. For this reason, inflammations of the lacrimal gland may lead to temporal ptosis. The palpebral portion of the lacrimal gland may be seen in the upper lid in the superior lateral conjunctival fornix. The lacrimal gland has pink-gray color with lobulation which makes it different from the yellowish orbital fat. There are approximately 12–14 lacrimal ductules from each lacrimal gland that produce tears into the superior temporal conjunctival fornix. The tears enter the ocular surface and are secreted via the puncta through the lacrimal canaliculi where the two canaliculi join beneath the anterior crest of the medial canthal ligament to form a common canaliculus before entering the lacrimal sac. The common canaliculus opens in the lacrimal sac and is protected by mucosal fold that prevents the reflux of tears into the conjunctiva. In patients with nasolacrimal duct obstruction, the lacrimal sac can swell because of the mucosal valve over the common canaliculus. The lacrimal sac is found in the bony fossa of the anterior medial orbital wall adjacent to the middle nasal bone of the nose. Anterior ethmoid cells may be found between the lacrimal sac and the nasal mucosa.

4.2 Canaliculitis

Canaliculitis is a condition characterized by infection of the upper or lower canaliculus. It is associated with obstruction of the outflow of the lacrimal secretion, and patients develop epiphora. The causes of canaliculitis include bacteria, fungi, viruses, and *Chlamydia* [1–5]. The most common cause of canaliculitis is *Actinomyces israelii* [6]. The diagnosis is commonly missed and is usually unilateral. Punctal plugs and stents may be complicated by bacterial or fungal canaliculitis [4, 7–9].

4.2.1 Clinical Findings

Patients with canaliculitis present with history of epiphora and unilateral mucopurulent conjunctivitis.

K.F. Tabbara, MD, ABO, FRCOphth
Department of Ophthalmology, The Eye Center and The Eye Foundation for Research in Ophthalmology, Riyadh, Saudi Arabia

Department of Ophthalmology, College of Medicine, King Saud University, Riyadh, Saudi Arabia

The Wilmer Ophthalmological Institute of The Johns Hopkins University School of Medicine, Baltimore, MD, USA
e-mail: kftabbara@yahoo.com

K. Tabbara et al. (eds.), *Ocular Infections*, Essentials in Ophthalmology,
DOI 10.1007/978-3-662-43981-4_4, © Springer-Verlag Berlin Heidelberg 2014

The clinical findings consist of swelling of the lid margin with erythema of the skin, injection of the conjunctiva, and edema and pounding of the punctum with thick tenacious mucopurulent exudates extruding from the punctum. The diagnosis is usually delayed because of the paucity of signs.

4.2.2 Laboratory Diagnosis

The diagnosis of canaliculitis is made clinically. Excretion from the canaliculus can be done, and exudates are subjected to Gram stain, Giemsa stain, and cultures on blood agar, chocolate agar, and thioglycolate. Pressure should be applied over the canaliculus with cotton-tip swabs. In patients with canaliculitis, there is no distention or swelling of the lacrimal sac. The inner part of the eyelid may be tender, and pressure on the canaliculus may cause reflux exudates to come through the punctum. It is believed that patients with canaliculitis have internal diverticula that allow anaerobic growth of *Actinomyces israelii*. Gram and Giemsa stains help to identify the causative organism. Filamentous, non-branching Gram-positive organisms are found in infection caused by *Actinomyces* species. Irrigation may allow reflux of cheesy excretions to come out, and this can be stained on slides for the diagnosis of *Actinomyces* species. *Candida* infection can be detected by demonstrating budding yeasts, and *Aspergillus* can be diagnosed by typical dichotomous branching of the hyphae. Concomitant skin lesions are seen in patients with viral infections due to herpes simplex.

4.2.3 Treatment

Patients with *Actinomyces* canaliculitis may be treated with punctal dilation and curretting of cheesy material and secretions from the canaliculus. Patients usually have cheesy white concretions. Diverticula may be found in the canaliculus. Canaliculotomy may be indicated. The probe may be used to express the cheesy material from the canaliculus and to remove the exudates following the curettage of the canaliculus. Antibiotics consisting of ampicillin 100 mg/ml may be used to irrigate the canaliculus. Therapy of *Actinomyces* canaliculitis require long term oral and topical antibiotics for a period of 3 to 6 months. Patients are treated with compounded penicillin G eye drops or ampicillin eye drops. Systemic oral therapy with ampicillin. Alternative drugs include doxycycline and azithromycin. *Candida* canaliculitis and *Aspergillus* canaliculitis may be treated with voriconazole 2 % eye drops topically every 2 h and oral voriconazole (VFend®) 450 mg orally twice a day for a period of 2 weeks. In patients with active trachoma, canaliculitis may be treated with azithromycin 500 mg orally daily for a period of 6 days. Valacyclovir 500 mg orally twice daily may be given for herpetic canaliculitis and dermatitis.

4.3 Dacryocystitis

Dacryocystitis is an infection of the nasolacrimal sac which can be acute or chronic. It is the most common infection of the lacrimal apparatus. The infection is usually preceded by obstruction of the nasolacrimal duct and may occur at any age. Persistent congenital obstruction of the nasolacrimal duct is due to chronic inflammation of the ductal mucosa which may lead to scarring and fibrosis. Chlamydial infections of the lacrimal sac cause scarring of the mucosa and obstruction of the nasolacrimal duct. Follicles may be seen in the mucus membrane of the nasolacrimal duct in patients with active trachoma. Follicles may undergo necrosis leading of scarring and obstruction. Tumors and mucosal hypertrophy of the nasal mucosa may also lead to obstruction of the nasolacrimal duct. Stenosis following the nasolacrimal duct obstruction can lead to accumulation of tears, mucus secretions, and inflammatory cells. The presence of lacrimal tubes (stents) may predispose to dacryocystitis. Infections may lead to mucocele or mucopyocele. The causes of acute dacryocystitis include *Streptococcus pneumoniae*, *Haemophilus influenzae*, *Staphylococcus aureus*, *and Pseudomonas aeruginosa and Proteus* species. In chronic dacryocystitis, mixed bacterial isolates may occur and most commonly

Streptococcus pneumoniae and *Staphylococcus* species. *Mycobacterium tuberculosis* is a rare cause of infection of the lacrimal sac [10]. Fungal infections of the nasolacrimal system are rare but may be caused by *Candida* species or *Aspergillus* species. *Chlamydia trachomatis* may cause clinical dacryocystitis leading to mucosal fibrosis and obstruction of the nasolacrimal duct.

4.3.1 Clinical Findings

Acute dacryoadenitis occurs more commonly in adults than in children. The disease is characterized by an acute onset of swelling, redness, and pain over the area of the nasolacrimal sac. There is swelling and epiphora with discharge. On the other hand, chronic dacryocystitis may be asymptomatic. Patients may complain of epiphora, but in patients with dry eye syndrome and tear deficiency, epiphora may not be appreciated. In such patients, there is increased risk of bacterial corneal ulcers especially due to *Streptococcus pneumoniae*. Patients with chronic dacryocystitis should not undergo intraocular procedures until the dacryocystitis is resolved and dacryocystorhinostomy (DCR) is performed. Pressure over the lacrimal sac may express mucus or purulent discharge. Swelling of the valve over the common canaliculus (Rosenmüller's valve) may lead to distention swelling of the lacrimal sac with severe pain over the lacrimal sac area. Percutaneous aspiration of the lacrimal sac with needle may be indicated for relieving the pain and obtaining purulent discharge for Gram stain and culture.

Complications of bacterial dacryocystitis include facial cellulitis, lacrimal sac abscess and cutaneous fistula. Mucocele and mucopyocele may precede the fistulization. Dacryocystography is also helpful in the diagnosis of localized tumors or dacryolith. Acquired obstruction of the nasolacrimal duct may occur more frequently in females than males in the fifth decade. Malignancy should be suspected in patients with blood-tinged tears.

Certain drugs such as docetaxel (Taxotere®) used for chemotherapy in cases of cancer of the breast may cause acquired nasolacrimal duct (NLD) obstruction. Other causes of iatrogenic NLD obstruction include topical antiglaucoma eyedrops, radiation, and use of 5-Fluorouracil.

4.3.2 Laboratory Diagnosis

Purulent discharge of pus is subjected to Gram stain and cultures on blood agar, chocolate agar, thioglycolate, and Sabouraud's agar.

A computed tomography (CT) scan is done to assess the sinuses and to help in identifying causes of obstruction such as dacryocystitis, tumors, or bone defects. Nasal endoscopy should be done to assess the inferior turbinate and the opening of the nasolacrimal duct. In cases of tumors of the nasolacrimal sac, biopsy specimens should be obtained.

4.3.3 Treatment

4.3.3.1 Congenital Nasolacrimal Duct (NLD) Obstruction

In over 90 % of the cases with congenital nasolacrimal duct obstruction will become patent at 1 year of age. Conservative management includes lacrimal sac massage and topical antibiotics. A course of azithromycin (Azyter®, Laboratoires Théa, Clermont-Ferrand, Cedex, France) 1.5 % eye drops twice daily for 3 weeks is given for infections caused by Gram-positive organisms, or tobramycin 0.3 % eye drops for Gram-negative organisms. If the epiphora persists beyond 1 year of age, probing of the NLD may be indicated.

4.3.3.2 Acute Dacryocystitis

The treatment of acute dacryocystitis in an adult depends on the causative agent. Initial empiric therapy with Augmentin® (amoxicillin-potassium-clavulanate) can be initiated and later guided by the results of the culture. Decompression of the nasolacrimal sac and aspiration of the pus may be done transcutaneously by a 22 g needle. Special care should be exercised to avoid the angular vein.

4.3.3.3 Chronic Dacryocystitis

The infection of the nasolacrimal sac may be treated with systemic antibiotics. The definitive therapy for chronic dacryocystitis with nasolacrimal duct obstruction is dacryocystorhinostomy (DCR). The procedure may be done transcutaneously or endoscopically through the nasal mucosa.

4.3.3.4 Prophylaxis

Povidone-iodine 2.5 % eye drops may be given at birth. Prophylaxis for ophthalmic neonatorum consists of $AgNO_3$ 1 % or erythromycin ointment [11].

4.4 Dacryoadenitis

4.4.1 Clinical Findings

The lacrimal gland may be the target of insult brought by a variety of infectious and noninfectious disorders [12–19]. Infectious causes of the lacrimal gland may be secondary to hematogenous seeding of the gland or by microorganisms ascending through the ductules. Causes of infectious dacryoadenitis include viruses, bacteria, fungi, and parasites. Table 4.1 shows the causes of infectious dacryoadenitis.

Acute dacryoadenitis is an infection of the lacrimal gland characterized by pain, tenderness, and swelling of the lacrimal gland. The disease is usually unilateral associated with eyelid swelling, ptosis, and erythema. The lacrimal gland palpebral or orbital portion may be involved. Patients may have conjunctival injection and chemosis with watery mucoid discharge in patients with bacterial dacryoadenitis. On the other hand, patients with viral dacryoadenitis such as mumps have no discharge and are associated with swelling of the parotid glands. The most commonly encountered organisms in bacterial dacryoadenitis include *Staphylococcus* species, *Streptococcus* species, *Haemophilus influenzae, and Neisseria gonorrhoeae*. In patients with *N. gonorrhoeae*, the purulent discharge is profuse. Localized abscess of the lacrimal gland may be seen. In cases of involvement of the orbital lobe of the lacrimal gland, there is slight proptosis with inferomedial displacement of the globe. Patients may have diplopia and compromised extraocular motility. Preauricular lymphadenopathy and facial cellulitis may occur. Patients may develop fever or malaise. In patients with dacryoadenitis caused by *Vaircella zoster virus*, the skin lesions may show evidence of cutaneous vesicular eruptions along the lacrimal nerve, a branch of the first division of the trigeminal nerve.

Table 4.1 Causes of infectious dacryoadenitis

I.	Viruses	Mumps, measles, influenza, Epstein-Barr virus, herpes zoster, herpes simplex
II.	Bacteria	Staphylococci, streptococci, *Neisseria gonorrhoeae, Mycobacterium tuberculosis, Mycobacterium leprae, Treponema pallidum, Chlamydia trachomatis, Lymphogranuloma venereum*
III.	Fungi	Phycomycetes
IV.	Parasites	*Schistosoma haematobium, Onchocerca volvulus*

4.4.2 Laboratory Diagnosis

Patients with dacryoadenitis should have imaging of the orbit with computed tomography and diagnostic B-scan ultrasonography. The adjacent bony fossa is not affected in these cases. Magnetic resonance imaging (MRI) may be ordered. In infectious dacryoadenitis, efforts should be made to identify the etiologic agents. Cultures of the discharge should be obtained. Complete blood count and differential and blood cultures may be taken. Laboratory confirmation may not be necessary when typical systemic or cutaneous findings suggest the diagnosis of mumps or herpes zoster ophthalmicus. Blood specimens for Epstein-Barr virus may be obtained in suspected cases of infectious mononucleosis dacryoadenitis. Care must be taken to rule out the possibility of other diseases such as benign mixed tumor or adenocarcinoma of the lacrimal gland. Chest x-ray or CT scan, interferon-gamma release assay (IGRA) and Purified Protein Derivative (PPD) skin testing should be done. Serologic tests for syphilis should be performed. The differential diagnosis of dacryoadenitis should include noninfectious inflammatory condition such as Sjögren's syndrome, benign lymphoepithelial lesions, sarcoidosis, amyloidosis, Graves's disease, lymphoma, and leukemia.

4.4.3 Treatment

Treatment of viral dacryoadenitis is symptomatic. In patients with herpes simplex or herpes zoster infections, the treatment of choice is oral valacyclovir 1 g twice daily for a period of 1 week. In patients with bacterial dacryoadenitis, the organism should be identified and cultured from the upper fornix or from draining abscess. Discharge should be taken and subjected to Gram stain and cultures. The sensitivity of the organism should guide the treatment. Empiric therapy may be started if *Neisseria gonorrhoeae* is suspected; Ceftriaxone 1 gm intramuscularly. daily for 5 days should be given together with doxycycline 100 mg orally twice a day. Alternative therapy includes azithromycin 500 mg orally daily for 2 weeks. *Staphylococcus aureus* infections may be treated with vancomycin, *Haemophilus influenzae* may be treated with Ampicillin with clavunate or cefuroxime, and streptococcal dacryoadenitis is treated with Augmentin or first-generation cephalosporins. Chronic dacryoadenitis caused by tuberculosis should be treated with antituberculous drugs including isoniazid, pyrazinamide, and rifampin (Chapter 2 Table 2.1).

Compliance with Ethical Requirements

Conflict of Interest The author declares that he has no conflict of interest.

Informed Consent No human studies were carried out by the authors for this article.

Animal Studies No animal studies were carried out by the authors for this article.

References

1. Tabbara KF, Hyndiuk RA, editors. Infections of the eye. Boston: Little, Brown and Company Publishers; 1996.
2. Tabbara KF, Okumoto M. Ocular ferning test: a qualitative test for mucus deficiency. Ophthalmology. 1982;89:712–4.
3. Tabbara KF, Okumoto M. Fungal growth in aphakic soft contact lenses. Letter to the editor. Am J Ophthalmol. 1981;92:591.
4. Tabbara KF. Aspergillus fumigatus colonization of punctal plugs. Am J Ophthalmol. 2007;143(1):180–1.
5. Tabbara KF, Bobb AA. Lacrimal system complications in trachoma. Ophthalmology. 1980;87:298–301.
6. Yuksel D, Hazirolan D, Sungur G, Duman S. Actinomyces canaliculitis and its surgical treatment. Int Ophthalmol. 2012;2(2):183–6.
7. Kamal S, Bodh SA, Goel R, Kumar S. Clinical significance of microbial growth on the surfaces of silicone tubes removed from dacryocystorhinostomy patients. Am J Ophthalmol. 2012;153(1):189–90.
8. Ban Y, Ideta S, Dogru M, Ogawa Y, Goto E, Shimazaki J. Surgical management of severe canaliculitis due to intracanalicular plug migration using fish-hook-type retractors: a report of two patients. Jpn J Ophthalmol. 2011;55(1):68–70.
9. Joganathan V, Mehta P, Murray A, Durrani OM. Complications of intracanalicular plugs: a case series. Orbit. 2010;29(5):271–3.
10. Varley CD, Gross ND, Marx DP, Winthrop KL. Tuberculosis of the nasolacrimal duct. Ophthal Plast Reconstr Surg. 2011;27(5):e129–31.
11. Isenberg SJ, Apt L, Del Signore M, Gichuhi S, Berman NG. A double application approach to ophthalmic neonatorum prophylaxis. Br J Ophthalmol. 2003;87:1449–52.
12. Moscovici BK, Romero IL, Vital Filho J, Bison SH. Epstein-Barr virus bilateral dacryoadenitis: case report. Arq Bras Oftalmol. 2009;72(6):826–8.
13. Barros MB, Costa DL, Schubach TM, do Valle AC, Lorenzi NP, Teixeira JL, Schubach Ade O. Endemic of zoonotic sporotrichosis: profile of cases in children. Pediatr Infect Dis J. 2008;27(3):246–50.
14. Faden HS. Dacryocystitis in children. Clin Pediatr (Phila). 2006;45(6):567–9.
15. de Palma P, Ravalli L, Modestino R, Grisanti F, Casillo F, Marzola A. Primary lacrimal sac B-cell immunoblastic lymphoma simulating an acute dacryocystitis. Orbit. 2003;22(3):171–5.
16. Marchese-Ragona R, Marioni G, Staffieri A, de Filippis C. Acute infectious mononucleosis presenting with dacryoadenitis and tonsillitis. Acta Ophthalmol Scand. 2002;80:345–6.
17. Mawn LA, Sanon A, Conlon MR, Nerad JA. Pseudomonas dacryoadenitis secondary to a lacrimal gland ductule stone. Ophthal Plast Reconstr Surg. 1997;13:135–8.
18. Bouza E, Merino P, Muñoz P, Sanchez-Carrillo C, Yáñez J, Cortés C. Ocular tuberculosis. A prospective study in a general hospital. Medicine (Baltimore). 1997;76:53–61.
19. Levin LA, Avery R, Shore JW, Woog JJ, Baker AS. The spectrum of orbital aspergillosis: a clinicopathological review. Surv Ophthalmol. 1996;41:142–54.

5 Infections of the Eyelids

Moncef Khairallah and Rim Kahloun

5.1 Introduction

Eyelids protect the anterior surface of the globe from local injury. Additionally, they aid in regulation of incident light reaching the eye and in tear film maintenance [1]. Infections of the eyelids occur in case of disequilibrium between local defenses and aggressive factors [2, 3]. They represent a heterogeneous group of disorders having a cutaneous and ocular expression and may need close collaboration between an ophthalmologist and a dermatologist for optimal management.

5.2 Bacterial Infections of the Eyelids

5.2.1 Hordeolum

Hordeolum is a common disorder of the eyelid due to an acute focal infection, usually staphylococcal in origin, which involves either the glands of Zeis (external hordeola or styes) or, less frequently, the meibomian glands (internal hordeola). It typically presents in the form of focal abscess manifesting as a painful, warm, swollen, red lump on the eyelid (Fig. 5.1). Bilateral involvement, as well as multiplicity of lesions, may occur. The main risk factors for developing hordeola include chronic blepharitis, meibomian gland dysfunction, ocular rosacea, and diabetes [4–6].

The differential diagnosis of hordeolum includes acute chalazion, basal cell carcinoma, sebaceous gland carcinoma, and squamous cell carcinoma of the eyelid.

Hordeola usually have a self-limited course with a spontaneous rupture and drainage in 1–2 weeks. An internal hordeolum may evolve into a chalazion.

Medical therapy for hordeola includes eyelid hygiene, warm compresses and massages of the lesions for 10 min four times per day, and topical antibiotic ointment in the inferior fornix if the lesion is draining or if there is an accompanying blepharoconjunctivitis [7, 8]. Systemic antibiotics may be indicated if the hordeola is complicated by preseptal cellulitis. Oral doxycycline may also be added if there is a history of multiple or recurrent lesions or if there is significant and chronic meibomitis [9].

5.2.2 Chalazion

Chalazia appear most commonly as chronic subcutaneous nodules within the eyelid. A chalazion results from the obstruction of the meibomian gland leading to blockage of the gland's duct at

M. Khairallah, MD (✉) • R. Kahloun, MD
Department of Ophthalmology, Fattouma Bourguiba University Hospital, Monastir, Tunisia

Faculty of Medicine, University of Monastir, Monastir, Tunisia
e-mail: moncef.khairallah@rns.tn

K. Tabbara et al. (eds.), *Ocular Infections*, Essentials in Ophthalmology,
DOI 10.1007/978-3-662-43981-4_5, © Springer-Verlag Berlin Heidelberg 2014

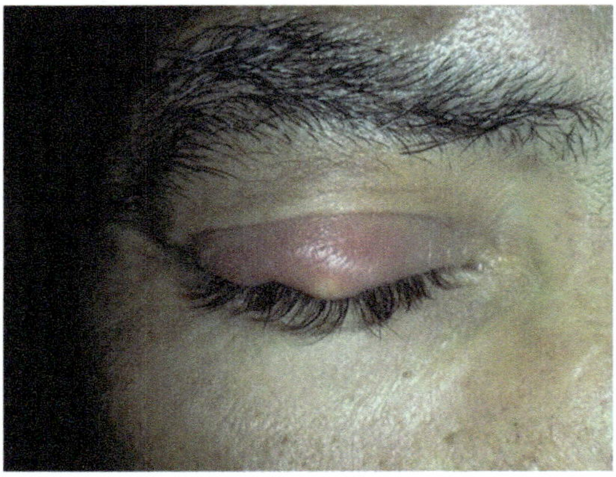

Fig. 5.1 Hordeolum on the upper eyelid

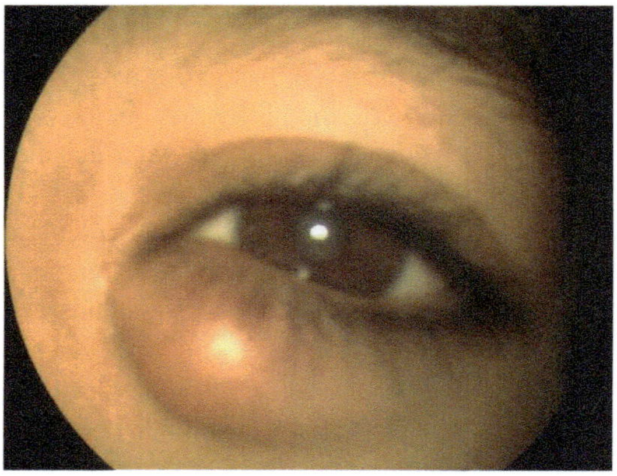

Fig. 5.2 Chalazion on the lower eyelid

the eyelid margin and then release of the contents of the gland into the surrounding eyelid soft tissue [10, 11]. A chalazion arises as a mild to moderately tender red swelling of the upper or lower eyelid (Fig. 5.2). At various locations and stages, multiple lesions may appear. Clinical onset of a chalazion occurs over days, with the redness and tenderness subsiding while the lump remains [10]. Patients usually present when the lump becomes symptomatic, either due to cosmetic reasons or if the chalazion is of a considerable size, because it is causing ptosis, astigmatism, and/ or vision loss [12].

Patients with underlying conditions such as rosacea, seborrheic dermatitis or blepharitis, and diabetes are more prone to multiple and recurrent chalazia.

If left untreated, chalazia may spontaneously resolve over many months. Management includes

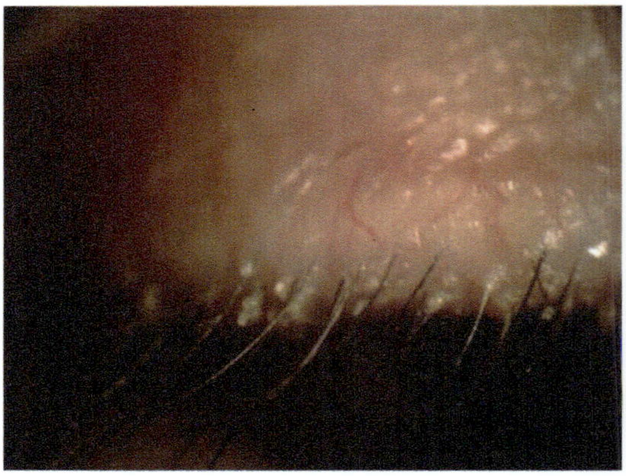

Fig. 5.3 Staphylococcal blepharitis with collarettes surrounding the eyelashes

warm compresses application with topical corticosteroids and antibiotic, if signs of infection are present. If the lesion persists in spite of medical therapy, it may be incised and drained [11]. Steroid injections can be applied either intralesionally or subcutaneously and are considered to be a simple and effective treatment with reported success and resolution in 50–95 % of cases [12–17].

5.2.3 Bacterial Blepharitis

Anterior bacterial blepharitis affecting the base of the eyelashes is often caused by staphylococcal infection (*Staphylococcus epidermidis*, *Staphylococcus aureus*). Other causative organisms include *Propionibacterium acnes*, *Corynebacteria*, and *Moraxella*. Blepharitis predominantly involves young to middle-aged women and is associated with keratoconjunctivitis sicca in up to 50 % of patients [18]. There is a wide variety of ocular symptoms including sore eyelids, eyes feeling irritated, itchy, burning, or gritty, red eyes, dry or watery eyes, increased frequency of blinking, foreign body sensation, photophobia, contact lens intolerance, and eyelids sticking together, particularly in the morning [18]. Signs include swollen eyelids, inflamed lid margins with redness, thickening, and collarettes surrounding the eyelashes (Fig. 5.3), scaling, crusting, irregularity, and/or ulceration of the lid margins, altered eyelash appearance, individual lash poliosis, and lashes broken, misdirected, or crusted with fibrinous or sebaceous matter, as well as secondary alterations to the conjunctiva and cornea. Hordeolum and multiple and recurrent chalazia may occur in the course of bacterial blepharitis [18]. Staphylococcal blepharitis may be also associated to seborrheic blepharitis.

The clinical diagnosis of staphylococcal blepharitis may be confirmed by culture, which usually reveals many *S. aureus* organisms on the lid margins.

A combination of lid hygiene with warm compresses, lid scrubs, and antibiotherapy is required. Erythromycin or bacitracin ointments and fusidic acid gel have been the most frequently used agents for blepharitis. Aminoglycosides such as gentamycin or tobramycin eyedrops or ointment are also useful but do not have the same broad coverage against gram-positive bacteria [18]. Topical vancomycin 50 mg/mL four times daily has been used to treat resistant *Staphylococcus* [18]. Fluoroquinolones such as ciprofloxacin ophthalmic solution 0.3 % and topical levofloxacin 0.5 % proved their efficacy in the management of bacterial blepharitis [18–20]. The fourth-generation fluoroquinolones are also used for the treatment of bacterial blepharitis [21]. Corticosteroid-antibiotic combinations are also available in either ointment or eyedrop form [22, 23]. Most experts recommend corticosteroids for short-term use only (less than 2 weeks) in an effort to "jump start" therapy for moderate-to-severe anterior blepharitis or blepharoconjunctivitis. One of the more recent additions to the management of blepharitis is topical azithromycin [24, 25]. Prevention is based on careful cleaning of the eyelids which is the most effective way to prevent bacterial blepharitis and its recurrence.

5.2.4 Erysipelas

Erysipelas is a bacterial skin infection most often caused by Group A *Streptococcus*. Patients typically develop symptoms including high fever, shaking, chills, fatigue, headaches, vomiting, and general illness within 48 h of the initial infection. Eyelid involvement appears as erythematous swollen, warm, hardened, and painful skin lesion with sharply demarcated raised edge that enlarges rapidly. More severe infections can result in vesicles, bullae, and petechiae, with possible skin necrosis [26, 27]. Lymph nodes may be swollen, and lymphedema may occur.

Penicillin administered orally or intramuscularly is sufficient for most cases of classic erysipelas and should be given for 10–20 days. A first-generation cephalosporin or macrolide, such as erythromycin or azithromycin, may be used if the patient has an allergy to penicillin [28].

5.2.5 Impetigo

Impetigo of the eyelid is caused by superinfection of skin disorder such as eczema, poison ivy, insect bites, and cuts or scrapes due to minor trauma by *Staphylococcus aureus* or *Streptococcus pyogenes*. The infection is more common in children younger than 6 years of age [29, 30]. Impetigo contagiosa of the eyelid is usually associated with infection of the face. Impetigo begins as tiny blisters, which eventually burst and leave small wet patches of red skin that may weep fluid. Gradually, a tan or yellowish-brown crust covers the affected area.

Cleansing of the affected area and local antibiotics ointments are generally effective. Systemic antibiotics are sometimes necessary.

5.2.6 Preseptal Cellulitis

The term preseptal cellulitis refers to an infectious process in the eyelids that is isolated to regions anterior to the orbital septum (Chap. 3).

5.3 Other Bacterial Infections of the Eyelids

5.3.1 Tuberculosis

The *Mycobacterium tuberculosis* can infect the eyelid as a primary infection or by spread of lupus vulgaris from the face. Lupus vulgaris is characterized by reddish-brown nodules that blanch to an "apple-jelly" color when pressure is applied and may appear on the skin of the eyelids. Tuberculosis can also manifest as a "cold abscess," a soft, fluctuant mass without acute inflammation, or simulate a chalazion [31–35].

Diagnosis is based on epidemiological data, Mantoux test, and QuantiFERON and proved by histopathologic examination of lesion-exeresis biopsy showing granulomatous inflammation with areas of caseation, Langhans giant cells, and acid-fast bacilli [36].

Tuberculosis of the eyelid must be treated with the systemic antituberculous drugs isoniazid, pyrazinamide, and rifampin. Ethambutol or streptomycin may be added as a third drug if isoniazid resistance is suspected [31, 34].

5.3.2 Leprosy

Leprosy is a chronic disease caused by the bacteria *Mycobacterium leprae* and *Mycobacterium lepromatosis*. Thinning or loss of the eyebrows or eyelashes associated with a multiple upper eyelid crease pattern and trichiasis is common in leprosy [37]. Lagophthalmos or anesthetic, infiltrated macules or nodules can also be seen [38].

A combination of systemic dapsone and rifampin is the therapy of choice. The lagophthalmos is treated by a tarsal-strip procedure or a tarsorrhaphy or by surgery [39, 40].

5.3.3 Syphilis

Syphilis is a sexually transmitted disease, caused by the spirochete bacterium *Treponema pallidum*. Eyelid involvement may occur by direct contact with an infected person. The chancre of primary acquired syphilis rarely occurs on the lid or lid margin. The skin of the eyelids can develop a macular or papular eruption in association with the generalized rash of secondary syphilis [41]. Pustules and ulcerative lesions can also occur, along with temporary syphilitic alopecia of the eyebrows and lashes. The skin eruption spontaneously fades as the secondary stage ends. In rare cases, benign tertiary syphilis involves the eyelid in the form of a gumma that begins as a deep swelling with minimal surrounding inflammation and eventually ulcerates to form exuberant granulation tissue. Congenital syphilis can involve the eyelid in the form of eruption, ulceration, or a gumma [42]. Temporary madarosis is also possible.

Penicillin G 12–24 million units per day for 6–21 days remains the treatment of choice in syphilis [42].

5.3.4 Anthrax

Anthrax is caused by *Bacillus anthracis*. Humans become infected as they come into contact with infected animals or animal products. Eyelid involvement present as a localized itchy erythematous papule of the eyelid that enlarges within 24–48 h, developing into an ulcer surrounded by vesicles that evolves into black, necrotic, central eschar characteristic of the disease [43, 44].

Treatment consists of ten million units of penicillin G given intravenously each day for a period of 7 days [43, 44]. With treatment, progressive healing of the skin occurs with or without complications that may include persistent cicatricial ectropion, lagophthalmos, palpebral symphysis, or restriction of upper eyelid movement.

5.4 Viral Infections of the Eyelids

5.4.1 Herpes Simplex Virus Blepharitis

Herpes simplex virus blepharitis is encountered primarily in children, although adults may also manifest this disorder. It usually presents in the form of small vesicles or pustules along the lid margin and/or periocular skin with associated regional lymphadenitis [45] (Fig. 5.4). Within the first week of infection, the vesicles may ulcerate or harden into crusts, although they will ultimately resolve without scarring [45–48].

The course of herpetic blepharitis is usually self-limiting within 2–3 weeks. The use of warm saline compresses with a topical drying agent is

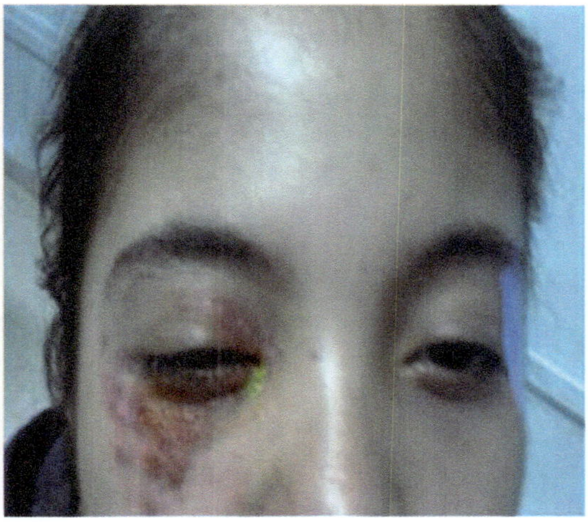

Fig. 5.4 Herpes simplex infection in a young patient involving the superior and inferior eyelids, with erythema-vesiculous lesions

usually sufficient to palliate the patient. If the lesions are extensive, the concomitant use of topical antibiotic ointment is considered prudent to prevent a secondary bacterial infection [45]. The use of antivirals is advocated by some practitioners for severe cases.

5.4.2 Herpes Zoster Ophthalmicus

Herpes zoster ophthalmicus (HZO) is characterized by reactivation of the varicella-zoster virus infection. Early in the course of disease, the eyelids may become hyperemic and edematous [49–51]. HZO presents as an acute, painful, vesicular eruption distributed along a single dermatome. The rash evolves from an erythematous lesion, with macules, papules, vesicles, pustules, and crusts developing subsequently (Fig. 5.5a).

The affected dermatome often heals within 2 weeks. As the inflammation resolves, there may be residual ptosis, lid scarring, deep scalp pitting, entropion, ectropion, loss of normal pigmentation, lid necrosis, loss of eyelid mobility (Fig. 5.5b), and lagophthalmos [52].

HZO is treated with acyclovir (800 mg five times daily for 7–10 days), valacyclovir (1 g three times daily for 7 days), or famciclovir (500 mg three times daily for 7 days). Palliative treatment of skin lesions with cool compresses and mechanical

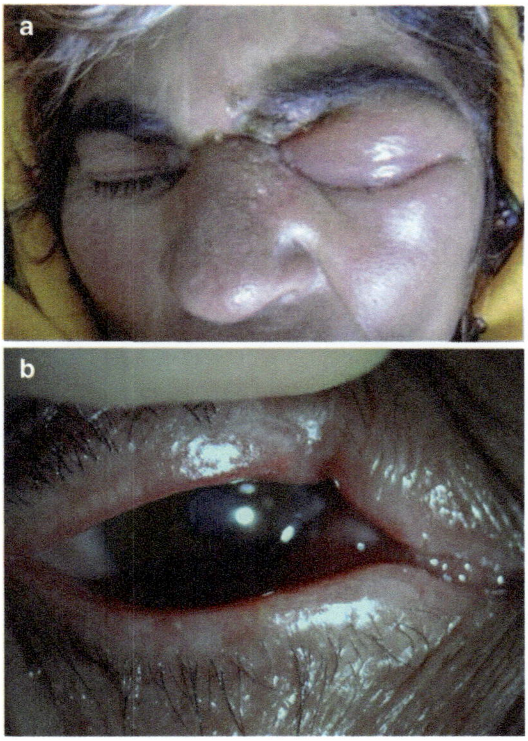

Fig. 5.5 (**a**) Acute herpes zoster ophthalmicus infection with eyelid edema and vesicles in a dermatomal pattern. (**b**) Cicatricial changes of the upper eyelid margin in a patient with history of herpes zoster ophthalmicus infection

cleansing is useful [51]. Oral antiviral medication, if started within 72 h of the onset of the acute HZO rash, significantly shortens the periods of acute pain, virus shedding, rash, acute and reduce the rate of late-onset anterior segment complications and severity of postherpetic neuralgia [53].

5.5 Other Viral Infections of the Eyelids

5.5.1 Molluscum Contagiosum

Molluscum contagiosum infections are characterized by elevated, round, waxy, pearly white, noninflammatory lesions with umbilicated centers [54, 55].

Removal or expression of the nodule, allowing permeation of blood into its substance, is curative.

5.5.2 Kaposi's Sarcoma

Kaposi's sarcoma is a tumor caused by human herpesvirus 8 that usually occurs in patients with AIDS. Kaposi's sarcoma of the eyelid appears as multiple purple to red nodules [54]. It can mimic a chalazion.

Therapeutic options include cryotherapy, surgical excision, radiation, and/or chemotherapy.

5.6 Fungal Infections of the Eyelids

5.6.1 Candidiasis

Candidal infections of the eyelid, usually associated with candidal infections elsewhere in the body, typically occur in immunocompromised patients. It may present as small ulcers, vesicles, or pustules at the bases of the eyelashes [56, 57]. Small granulomas are often found on the lid margin.

Candidiasis may be treated with fluconazole or itraconazole. Amphotericin B, voriconazole, or posaconazole are recommended in case of severe systemic-associated disease. Topical glucocorticoids and broad-spectrum antibiotics should be discontinued.

5.6.2 Eyelids Dermatophytosis

Dermatophytosis of the eyelids or tinea is an infection caused by a dermatophyte, which is most commonly of the *Trichophyton* genus. Tinea can affect the eyelid primarily or spread to the eyelid from other parts of the face. The early lesions begin as flattened, reddish papules that spread peripherally while the central area heals. The fully developed lesion has a ring-like appearance, with a reddish, scaly, sharply defined border and a central pinkish scaly area [58, 59]. Loss of the eyelashes is characteristic of these fungal infections, similar to the hair loss that occurs in kerions associated with tinea capitis [58].

Diagnosis is established by microscopic examination of edge scrapings with a drop of potassium hydroxide preparation and/or culture positive for fungal elements [58–60].

Treatment of eyelids dermatophytosis involves the use of topical imidazole preparations, including ketoconazole, bifonazole, miconazole, econazole, and clotrimazole. For cases that are widespread or recalcitrant to topical therapies, treatment with systemic antifungals including ketoconazole, itraconazole, or fluconazole can be considered [59, 61, 62].

5.6.3 Blastomycosis

Blastomycosis is caused by the dimorphic fungus *Blastomyces dermatitidis*. Blastomycosis of the eyelids is rare and occurs in approximately 25 % of patients with systemic blastomycosis. Eyelid involvement is characterized by granulomatous ulcers with thick crusts and an underlying purplish color [63–66]. Blastomycosis of the eyelid may be mistaken for a chalazion, basal cell, or squamous cell carcinoma [64].

Preferred therapy is itraconazole 200–400 mg/day for 6 months. Amphotericin B is used in children, patients who are pregnant or immunocompromised, patients with more severe blastomycosis or central nervous system blastomycosis, and patients who do not improve with oral azole therapy [64, 65, 67].

5.6.4 Cryptococcosis

Cryptococcosis, caused by *Cryptococcus neoformans*, arises in immunosuppressed patients and can affect the skin of the eyebrow, forehead, and eyelids. Eyelid manifestations include papules, nodules, infiltrative plaques, pustules, ulcers, or subcutaneous abscesses [68, 69].

In patients with localized lesions, treatment is based on fluconazole 400 mg per os once/day for 3–6 months. For more severe disease, amphotericin B 0.5–1.0 mg/kg IV once/day with flucytosine 25 mg/kg per os q 6 h is given for several weeks.

5.7 Parasitic Infections of the Eyelids

5.7.1 Onchocerciasis

Onchocerciasis, also named river blindness or Robles disease, is a parasitic disease caused by the microfilariae *Onchocerca volvulus*. Onchocerciasis is endemic in many areas of sub-Saharan Africa and in isolated foci in Central and South America [70, 71]. Eyelids onchocerciasis is characterized by eyelid edema in the early phase of the infection. Later, severe pruritic dermatitis and intense photophobia can occur, followed by the development of subcutaneous nodules that occasionally involve the eyelid, especially in patients from Central and South America. Diagnosis of onchocerciasis is done by identification of worms from skin or subcutaneous nodules obtained by biopsy.

Treatment consists of ivermectin medical therapy given in a single oral dose of 150 μg/kg [72].

5.7.2 Leishmaniasis

Mucocutaneous leishmaniasis is caused by *Leishmania braziliensis* and *Leishmania mexicana*. The microorganism is transmitted by the bite of infected phlebotomine sand flies. Eyelid involvement presents as highly polymorphous lesions, such as swelling lesions, papules, plaques, nodules, and sometimes ulcerative or covered by crusts and scaling, erosions, ulcers, and blepharoconjunctivitis [73–77]. Ocular complications include palpebral scar, trichiasis, eyelash loss, lagophthalmos, epicanthus, trichiasis, and ectropion. If eyelid lesions remain untreated, the contiguous spread from the skin of the eyelid will extend to involve the conjunctiva, sclera, and even cornea, causing interstitial keratitis. Leishmania infection may simulate other conditions such as cysts, chalazion, dacryocystitis, tuberculosis, syphilis, sarcoidosis, and tumors [78, 79]. Diagnosis is primarily based on epidemiological data, history, and clinical findings. It can be confirmed by a positive leishmanin skin test, identification of the parasite by histopathologic sections, culture in NNN (Novy, McNeal, and Nicolle) medium, or by detection of the parasite DNA [73].

Pentavalent antimonial compounds such as Glucantime or sodium stibogluconate are the therapy of choice. The recommended dose is 20 mg/kg/day for at least 3 weeks [80].

5.7.3 Demodicidosis

Demodicidosis of the eyelids is caused by *Demodex folliculorum,* found in the eyelash follicle or *Demodex brevis* that burrows deep in sebaceous and meibomian glands [81]. Demodex is spread by direct contact and probably by dust containing eggs. Infection of Demodex often occurs in the course of chronic blepharitis, considered to be involved in its pathogenesis [82–84].

Lashes with cylindrical dandruff are pathognomonic for ocular demodex infestation [85]. Demodex has also been associated with intermittent trichiasis and meibomian gland dysfunction.

Diagnosis is based on identification and count of eyelashes with cylindrical dandruff using the light microscope [85, 86]. Fluorescein 0.25 % drops can improve the visibility of the mites [86].

A wide range of antiseptic solutions such as salicylic acid, topical 1 % mercury oxide ointment, selenium sulfide, metronidazole, crotamiton, lindane, tea tree oil, and ivermectin (single dose of 200 μg/kg) with or without associated topical permethrin [87] were used to control and eradicate *D. folliculorum* and its cysts. Weekly lid scrub with 50 % tea tree oil and daily lid scrub with tea tree shampoo is effective in eradicating ocular Demodex [88–90].

5.7.4 Myiasis

External myiasis occurs when the eyelids and conjunctiva are infested by fly larvae. External myiasis is associated most frequently with larvae of the *Oestrus ovis*, *Dermatobia hominis*, *Hypoderma bovis*, and *Calliphoridae*. Myiasis of the eyelid had also been reported due to *Cuterebra* and *Dermatobia hominis*, *Cordylobia anthropophaga*, and *Cordylobia rhodaini* [91, 92].

Eyelid myiasis presents as furuncle-like lesions draining serosanguineous fluid and unresponsive to antibiotics [91–94]. It may also present with movable mass and a draining fistula that intermittently produces yellowish discharge [95]. Diagnosis and estimation of the number of parasites in the lesion can be made with Doppler ultrasound [96].

Treatment modalities include asphyxiation of the larvae with paraffin or petroleum jelly, or plasters or injecting a local anesthetic under the larva itself leading to its extrude through the skin [95, 97]. Adjuvant oral ivermectin (single oral dose of ivermectin 200 μg/kg) has also been used successfully [98]. Surgical removal of larva may be performed; the larva should be totally removed, as its rupture can lead to a severe inflammatory response [99].

5.7.5 Phthiriasis Pubis Blepharitis

Phthiriasis palpebrarum is a rare eyelid infestation caused by *Phthirus pubis* which is transferred by hand contact from the genital area to the eye [100, 101]. The organism produces itching and erythema of the lid margin [102]. Nits, which are transparent, oval, and cemented to the eyelashes, are characteristically found. The adult organism is gray and is often overlooked because of its transparency. Phthiriasis palpebrarum may be a rare cause of blepharoconjunctivitis with marked conjunctival inflammation, preauricular lymphadenopathy, and secondary infection at the site of lice bite [103].

Phthiriasis palpebrarum is often confused with seborrheic blepharitis or lid eczema [102].

Most commonly used management options for phthiriasis palpebrarum include mechanical removal, cryotherapy, argon laser photocoagulation, fluorescein eyedrops 20 %, physostigmine 0.25 %, lindane 1 %, petroleum gel, yellow mercuric oxide ointment 1 %, malathion drops 1 % or malathion shampoo 1 % or pilocarpine gel 4 %, and oral ivermectin [101, 104–106].

Compliance with Ethical Requirements

Conflict of Interest The authors declare that they have no conflict of interest.

Informed Consent No human studies were carried out by the authors for this article.

Animal Studies No animal studies were carried out by the authors for this article.

References

1. Most SP, Mobley SR, Larrabee Jr WF. Anatomy of the eyelids. Facial Plast Surg Clin North Am. 2005;13(4):487–92, v.
2. American Academy of Ophthalmology. Infectious diseases of the external eye: clinical aspects. In: External disease and cornea, vol. 8. San Francisco: LEO; 2006–2007.
3. American Academy of Ophthalmology. Eyelids. In: Ophthalmic pathology and intraocular tumors, vol. 4. San Francisco: LEO; 2007–2008.
4. Raskin EM, Speaker MG, Laibson PR. Blepharitis. Infect Dis Clin North Am. 1992;6(4):777–87.
5. Kiratli HK, Akar Y. Multiple recurrent hordeola associated with selective IgM deficiency. J AAPOS. 2001;5(1):60–1.
6. Lederman C, Miller M. Hordeola and chalazia. Pediatr Rev. 1999;20(8):283–4.
7. Panicharoen C, Hirunwiwatkul P. Current pattern treatment of hordeolum by ophthalmologists in Thailand. J Med Assoc Thai. 2011;94(6):721–4.
8. Lindsley K, Nichols JJ, Dickersin K. Interventions for acute internal hordeolum. Cochrane Database Syst Rev. 2010;(9):CD007742.
9. Ehrenhaus MP. Hordeolum. http://emedicine.medscape.com/article/1213080-treatment.
10. Papier A, Tuttle DJ, Mahar TJ. Differential diagnosis of the swollen red eyelid. Am Fam Physician. 2007;76(12):1815–24.
11. Gilchrist H, Lee G. Management of chalazia in general practice. Aust Fam Physician. 2009;38(5):311–4.
12. Ben Simon GJ, Huang L, Nakra T, Schwarcz RM, McCann JD, Goldberg RA. Intralesional triamcinolone acetonide injection for primary and recurrent chalazia: is it really effective? Ophthalmology. 2005;112(5):913–7.
13. Yağci A, Palamar M, Eğrilmez S, Sahbazov C, Ozbek SS. Anterior segment ischemia and retinochoroidal vascular occlusion after intralesional steroid injection. Ophthal Plast Reconstr Surg. 2008;24(1):55–7.
14. Hosal BM, Zilelioğlu G. Ocular complication of intralesional corticosteroid injection of a chalazion. Eur J Ophthalmol. 2003;13(9–10):798–9.

15. Thomas EL, Laborde RP. Retinal and choroidal vascular occlusion following intralesional corticosteroid injection of a chalazion. Ophthalmology. 1986;93(3):405–7.
16. Cohen BZ, Tripathi RC. Eyelid depigmentation after intralesional injection of a fluorinated corticosteroid for chalazion. Am J Ophthalmol. 1979;88(2):269–70.
17. Goawalla A, Lee V. A prospective randomized treatment study comparing three treatment options for chalazia: triamcinolone acetonide injections, incision and curettage and treatment with hot compresses. Clin Experiment Ophthalmol. 2007;35(8):706–12.
18. Jackson WB. Blepharitis: current strategies for diagnosis and management. Can J Ophthalmol. 2008; 43(2):170–9.
19. Adenis JP, Colin J, Verin P, Riss I, Saint-Blancat P. Ciprofloxacin ophthalmic solution in the treatment of conjunctivitis and blepharitis: a comparison with fusidic acid. Eur J Ophthalmol. 1996;6(4):368–74.
20. Yactayo-Miranda Y, Ta CN, He L, Kreutzer TC, Nentwich MM, Kampik A, Mino de Kaspar H. A prospective study determining the efficacy of topical 0.5 % levofloxacin on bacterial flora of patients with chronic blepharoconjunctivitis. Graefes Arch Clin Exp Ophthalmol. 2009;247(7):993–8.
21. Belfort Jr R, Gabriel L, Martins Bispo PJ, Muccioli C, Zacharias Serapicos PC, Clark L, Bell B, Bartell J, Stroman DW, Höfling-Lima AL. Safety and efficacy of moxifloxacin-dexamethasone eyedrops as treatment for bacterial ocular infection associated with bacterial blepharitis. Adv Ther. 2012;29(5):416–26.
22. Donshik P, Kulvin SM, Mckinley P, Skowron R. Treatment of chronic staphylococcal blepharoconjunctivitis with a new topical steroid anti-infective ophthalmic solution. Ann Ophthalmol. 1983;15(2):162–7.
23. Shulman DG, Sargent JB, Stewart RH, Mester U. Comparative evaluation of the short-term bactericidal potential of a steroid-antibiotic combination versus steroid in the treatment of chronic bacterial blepharitis and conjunctivitis. Eur J Ophthalmol. 1996;6(4):361–7.
24. Haque RM, Torkildsen GL, Brubaker K, Zink RC, Kowalski RP, Mah FS, Pflugfelder SC. Multicenter open-label study evaluating the efficacy of azithromycin ophthalmic solution 1 % on the signs and symptoms of subjects with blepharitis. Cornea. 2010;29(8):871–7.
25. John T, Shah AA. Use of azithromycin ophthalmic solution in the treatment of chronic mixed anterior blepharitis. Ann Ophthalmol (Skokie). 2008;40(2):68–74.
26. Chang FB. Painful rash on face. J Fam Pract. 2010;59(8):459–62.
27. Szołdra-Seiler A, Horbacz-Jary G. Head phlegmon as a complication of eyelids erysipelas – two cases in one family. Otolaryngol Pol. 2008;62(6):779–81.
28. Bonnetblanc JM, Bédane C. Erysipelas: recognition and management. Am J Clin Dermatol. 2003;4(3):157–63.
29. Cole C, Gazewood J. Diagnosis and treatment of impetigo. Am Fam Physician. 2007;75(6):859–64.
30. Durkin SR, Selva D, Huilgol SC, Guy S, Leibovitch I. Recurrent staphylococcal conjunctivitis associated with facial impetigo contagiosa. Am J Ophthalmol. 2006;141(1):189–90.
31. Thompson MJ, Albert DM. Ocular tuberculosis. Arch Ophthalmol. 2005;23:844–9.
32. Zorić LD, Zorić DL, Zorić DM. Bilateral tuberculous abscesses on the face (eyelids) of a child. Am J Ophthalmol. 1996;121(6):717–8.
33. Chowdhury MM, Varma S, Howell S, Holt PJ, Statham BN. Facial cutaneous tuberculosis: an unusual presentation. Clin Exp Dermatol. 2000;25(1):48–50.
34. Baha Ali T, Allali B, Essalime K, Lamari H, Zaghloul K. Primary palpebral tuberculosis (case report). Bull Soc Belge Ophtalmol. 2006;299:21–5.
35. Gannoune A, Naji A, Eladioui K, Benjelloun A. Primary palpebral tuberculosis. Rev Stomatol Chir Maxillofac. 2009;110(1):42–4.
36. Demirci H, Shields CL, Shields JA, Eagle Jr RC. Ocular tuberculosis masquerading as ocular tumors. Surv Ophthalmol. 2004;49(1):78–89.
37. Guimarães FC, Cruz AA. Eyelid changes in long-standing leprosy. Ophthal Plast Reconstr Surg. 1998;14(4):239–43.
38. Khandpur S, Robertson SJ, Rao PS. Ocular morbidity in leprosy patients with lagophthalmos. Indian J Lepr. 2009;81(1):1–4.
39. Das P, Kumar J, Karthikeyan G, Rao PS. Efficacy of temporalis muscle transfer for correction of lagophthalmos in leprosy. Lepr Rev. 2011;82(3):279–85.
40. Lavilla L, Castillo J, Domínguez AM, Rodríguez NA, Ascaso FJ, Cristóbal JA. Surgical treatment of bilateral paralytic lagophthalmos using scapha graft in a case of lepromatous leprosy. Lepr Rev. 2009; 80(4):448–52.
41. Jeyakumar W, Chithra A, Shanmugasundararaj A. Primary syphilis of the eyelid: case report. Genitourin Med. 1989;65(3):192–3.
42. Kiss S, Damico FM, Young LH. Ocular manifestations and treatment of syphilis. Semin Ophthalmol. 2005;20(3):161–7.
43. Celebi S, Aykan U, Alagöz G, Esmerligil S. Palbebral anthrax. Eur J Ophthalmol. 2001;11(2):171–4.
44. Amraoui A, Tabbara KF, Zaghloul K. Anthrax of the eyelids. Br J Ophthalmol. 1992;76(12):753–4.
45. Liu S, Pavan-Langston D, Colby KA. Pediatric herpes simplex of the anterior segment: characteristics, treatment, and outcomes. Ophthalmology. 2012;119(10):2003–8.
46. Gupta PC, Pavan-Langston D. Herpetic simplex eye disease in the pediatric population. Int Ophthalmol Clin. 2008;48(2):209–14.
47. Toma HS, Murina AT, Areaux Jr RG, Neumann DM, Bhattacharjee PS, Foster TP, Kaufman HE, Hill JM. Ocular HSV-1 latency, reactivation and recurrent disease. Semin Ophthalmol. 2008;23(4):249–73.

48. Du Toit N, Van der Merwe J. Herpetic ulcer of the eyelids in an immunocompromised patient. S Afr Med J. 2012;102(6):472–3.
49. Kaufman SC. Anterior segment complications of herpes zoster ophthalmicus. Ophthalmology. 2008; 115(2 Suppl):S24–32.
50. Weinberg JM. Herpes zoster: epidemiology, natural history, and common complications. J Am Acad Dermatol. 2007;57(6 Suppl):S130–5.
51. Shaikh S, Ta CN. Evaluation and management of herpes zoster ophthalmicus. Am Fam Physician. 2002;66(9):1723–30.
52. Liesegang TJ. Herpes zoster ophthalmicus natural history, risk factors, clinical presentation, and morbidity. Ophthalmology. 2008;115(2 Suppl):S3–12.
53. Pavan-Langston D. Herpes zoster antivirals and pain management. Ophthalmology. 2008;115(2 Suppl): S13–20.
54. Biswas J, Sudharshan S. Anterior segment manifestations of human immunodeficiency virus/acquired immune deficiency syndrome. Indian J Ophthalmol. 2008;56(5):363–75.
55. Jeng BH, Holland GN, Lowder CY, Deegan 3rd WF, Raizman MB, Meisler DM. Anterior segment and external ocular disorders associated with human immunodeficiency virus disease. Surv Ophthalmol. 2007;52(4):329–68.
56. Klotz SA, Penn CC, Negvesky GJ, Butrus SI. Fungal and parasitic infections of the eye. Clin Microbiol Rev. 2000;13(4):662–85.
57. Offret H, Quillard J. Palpebral mycosis. J Fr Ophtalmol. 1995;18(10):614–6.
58. Basak SA, Berk DR, Lueder GT, Bayliss SJ. Common features of periocular tinea. Arch Ophthalmol. 2011;129(3):306–9.
59. Bélair ML, Mathieu-Millaire F, Mabon M. Periocular dermatophytosis in an 11-year-old boy. Can J Ophthalmol. 2005;40(2):183–4.
60. Machado AP, Hirata SH, Ogawa MM, Tomimori-Yamashita J, Fischman O. Dermatophytosis on the eyelid caused by Microsporum gypseum. Mycoses. 2005;48(1):73–5.
61. Huang WW, Tharp MD. A case of tinea versicolor of the eyelids. Pediatr Dermatol. 2012. doi:10.1111/j.1525-1470.2012.01753.x.
62. Demirci H, Nelson CC. Dermatophyte infection of the eyelid in a neonate. J Pediatr Ophthalmol Strabismus. 2006;43(1):52–3.
63. Pemberton JD, Vidor I, Sivak-Callcott JA, Bailey NG, Sarwari AR. North American blastomycosis of the eyelid. Ophthal Plast Reconstr Surg. 2009;25(3): 230–2.
64. Rodriguez RC, Cornock E, White VA, Dolman PJ. Eyelid blastomycosis in British Columbia. Can J Ophthalmol. 2012;47(3):e1–2.
65. Altman JS, Tonelli DG, Bukhalo M. Red, scaly lesion on the upper eyelid. Am Fam Physician. 2007;76(10):1533–4.
66. Bartley GB. Blastomycosis of the eyelid. Ophthalmology. 1995;102(12):2020–3.
67. Bradsher RW, Chapman SW, Pappas PG. Blastomycosis. Infect Dis Clin North Am. 2003;17:21–40.
68. Souza MB, Melo CS, Silva CS, Santo RM, Matayoshi S. Palpebral cryptococcosis: case report. Arq Bras Oftalmol. 2006;69(2):265–7.
69. Coccia L, Calista D, Boschini A. Eyelid nodule: a sentinel lesion of disseminated cryptococcosis in a patient with acquired immunodeficiency syndrome. Arch Ophthalmol. 1999;117(2):271–2.
70. Ament CS, Young LH. Ocular manifestations of helminthic infections: onchocersiasis, cysticercosis, toxocariasis, and diffuse unilateral subacute neuroretinitis. Int Ophthalmol Clin. 2006;46(2):1–10.
71. Sabrosa NA, Zajdenweber M. Nematode infections of the eye: toxocariasis, onchocerciasis, diffuse unilateral subacute neuroretinitis, and cysticercosis. Ophthalmol Clin North Am. 2002;15(3):351–6.
72. Babalola OE. Ocular onchocerciasis: current management and future prospects. Clin Ophthalmol. 2011;5:1479–91.
73. Oliveira-Neto MP, Martins VJ, Mattos MS, Pirmez C, Brahin LR, Benchimol E. South American cutaneous leishmaniasis of the eyelids: report of five cases in Rio de Janeiro State, Brazil. Ophthalmology. 2000;107(1): 169–72.
74. Sadeghian G, Nilfroushzadeh MA, Moradi SH, Hanjani SH. Ocular leishmaniasis: a case report. Dermatol Online J. 2005;11(2):19.
75. Satici A, Gurler B, Aslan G, Ozturk I. Ocular involvement in cutaneous leishmaniasis four cases with blepharoconjunctivitis. Eur J Epidemiol. 2004;19(3):263–6.
76. Durdu M, Gökçe S, Bagirova M, Yalaz M, Allahverdiyev AM, Uzun S. Periocular involvement in cutaneous leishmaniasis. J Eur Acad Dermatol Venereol. 2007;21(2):214–8.
77. Jafari AK, Akhyani M, Valikhani M, Ghodsi ZS, Barikbin B, Toosi S. Bilateral cutaneous leishmaniasis of upper eyelids: a case report. Dermatol Online J. 2006;12(1):20.
78. Mencía-Gutiérrez E, Gutiérrez-Díaz E, Rodríguez-Peralto JL, Monsalve-Córdova J. Old World eyelid cutaneous leishmaniasis: a case report. Dermatol Online J. 2005;11(3):29.
79. Veraldi S, Bottini S, Currò N, Gianotti R. Leishmaniasis of the eyelid mimicking an infundibular cyst and review of the literature on ocular leishmaniasis. Int J Infect Dis. 2010;14 Suppl 3: e230–2.
80. Herwaldt BL, Berman JD. Recommendations for treating leishmaniasis with sodium stibogluconate (Pentostam) and review of pertinent clinical studies. Am J Trop Med Hyg. 1992;46:296–306.
81. English FP, Nutting WB. Demodicosis of ophthalmic concern. Am J Ophthalmol. 1981;91:362–72.
82. Rodríguez AE, Ferrer C, Alió JL. Chronic blepharitis and Demodex. Arch Soc Esp Oftalmol. 2005; 80(11):635–42.
83. Czepita D, Kuźna-Grygiel W, Czepita M, Grobelny A. Demodex folliculorum and Demodex brevis as a

cause of chronic marginal blepharitis. Ann Acad Med Stetin. 2007;53(1):63–7.
84. Czepita D, Kuźna-Grygiel W, Kosik-Bogacka D. Demodex as an etiological factor in chronic blepharitis. Klin Oczna. 2005;107(10–12):722–4.
85. Gao Y-Y, Di Pascuale MA, Li W, Liu D, Baradaran-Rafii A, Elizondo A, Kuo IC, Kawakita T, Raju VK, Tseng SCG. High prevalence of ocular demodex in lashes with cylindrical dandruffs. Invest Ophthalmol Vis Sci. 2005;46:3089–94.
86. Kheirkhah A, Blanco G, Casas V, Tseng SC. Fluorescein dye improves microscopic evaluation and counting of demodex in blepharitis with cylindrical dandruff. Cornea. 2007;26:697–700.
87. Holzchuh FG, Hida RY, Moscovici BK, Villa Albers MB, Santo RM, Kara-José N, Holzchuh R. Clinical treatment of ocular Demodex folliculorum by systemic ivermectin. Am J Ophthalmol. 2011;151(6):1030–1034.e1.
88. Gao YY, Xu DL, Huang J, Wang R, Tseng SC. Treatment of ocular itching associated with ocular demodicosis by 5 % tea tree oil ointment. Cornea. 2012;31(1):14–7.
89. Gao YY, Di Pascuale MA, Elizondo A, Tseng SC. Clinical treatment of ocular demodecosis by lid scrub with tea tree oil. Cornea. 2007;26(2):136–43.
90. Gao YY, Di Pascuale MA, Li W, Baradaran-Rafii A, Elizondo A, Kuo CL, Raju VK, Tseng SC. In vitro and in vivo killing of ocular Demodex by tea tree oil. Br J Ophthalmol. 2005;89(11):1468–73.
91. Lee EJK, Robinson F. Furuncular myiasis of the face caused by larva of the Tumbu fly (Corylobia anthropophaga). Eye. 2007;21:268–9.
92. Jun BK, Shin JC, Woog JJ. Palpebral myiasis. Korean J Ophthalmol. 1999;13(2):138–40.
93. Caça I, Satar A, Unlü K, Sakalar YB, Ari S. External ophthalmomyiasis infestation. Jpn J Ophthalmol. 2006;50(2):176–7.
94. Bal S, Amitava AK. Palpebral myiasis. J Pediatr Ophthalmol Strabismus. 2000;37(5):309–10.
95. Missotten GS, Kalpoe JS, Bollemeijer JG, Schalij-Delfos NE. Myiasis of the upper eyelid. J AAPOS. 2008;12(5):516–7.
96. Quintanilla-Cedillo MR, León-Urena H, Contreras-Ruiz J, Arenas R. The value of Doppler ultrasound in diagnosis in 25 cases of furunculoid myiasis. Int J Dermatol. 2005;44:34–7.
97. Swetter SM, Stewart MI, Dmoller BR. Cutaneous myiasis following travel to Belize. Int J Dermatol. 1996;35:118–20.
98. Wakamatsu TH, Pierre-Filho PTP. Ophthalmomyiasis externa caused by Dermatobia hominis: a successful treatment with oral ivermectin. Eye. 2006;20:1088–90.
99. Denion E, Dalens PH, Couppié P, Aznar C, Sainte-Marie D, Carme B, et al. External ophthalmomyiasis caused by Dermatobia hominis. A retrospective study of nine cases and a review of the literature. Acta Ophthalmol Scand. 2004;82:576–84.
100. Mansour AM. Photo essay: phthiriasis palpebrarum. Arch Ophthalmol. 2000;118(10):1458–9.
101. Couch JM, Green WR, Hirst LW, Cruz Z. Diagnosing and treating Phthirus pubis palpebrarum. Surv Ophthalmol. 1982;26(4):219–25.
102. Turgut B, Kurt J, Catak O, Demir T. Phthriasis palpebrarum mimicking lid eczema and blepharitis. J Ophthalmol. 2009;2009:803951.
103. Lin Y-C, Kao S-C, Kau H-C, Hsu W-M, Tsai C-C. Phthiriasis palpebrarum: an unusual blepharoconjunctivitis. Chin Med J (Engl). 2003;65(10):498–500.
104. Ashkenazi I, Desatnik HR, Abraham FA. Yellow mercuric oxide: a treatment of choice for Phthriasis palpebrarum. Br J Ophthalmol. 1991;75(6):356–8.
105. Yoon KC, Park HY, Seo MS, Park YG. Mechanical treatment of phthiriasis palpebrarum. Korean J Ophthalmol. 2003;17(1):71–3.
106. Burkhart CN, Burkhart CG. Oral ivermectin therapy for phthiriasis palpebrum. Arch Ophthalmol. 2000;118(1):134–5.

Infectious Conjunctivitis

6

Khalid F. Tabbara

6.1 Introduction

Many types of organisms including bacteria, viruses, fungi and parasites cause infectious conjunctivitis in man. Unlike the cornea, where most infections except viral infections require disruption of the integrity of the anatomic surface, the conjunctiva may be invaded by a variety of infectious agents without trauma. The majority of infections of the conjunctiva are self-limited while other types of infections require antibiotic therapy to prevent local or systemic complications.The conjunctiva has defense mechanisms and is protected from the environmental noxious agents. The integrity of the conjunctival epithelium, the toll-like receptors, the substantia propia with its lymphoid tissue, the continuous blinking and the constituents of tears help to protect the conjunctiva from invasion by organisms. The tears are important defense mechanisms, and contain antimicrobial constituents, betalysine, lysozyme, lactoferrin, immunoglobulins. In addition, the flushing action of tears can remove free organisms from the surface of the conjunctiva. Macrophages and lymphocytes reside in the substantia propia of the conjunctiva. Goblet cells produce mucin in the tear film and the mucus can serve as a barrier to bacterial adhesions to the epithelium of the conjunctiva and can trap organisms. Furthermore, the temperature of the conjunctiva is less than the body temperature and this discourages the growth of some organisms. Dry eye syndrome and mechanical trauma may cause disruption of the anatomic integrity of the epithelium rendering the conjunctiva more susceptible to infectious agents. The topical use and abuse of topical corticosteroids may predispose to ocular surface infections.

Toll-like receptors (TLRs) are found on the surface of the conjunctiva and serve as innate nonspecific defense against infections. Several TLRs play a key role in innate immunity in man. The TLRs resemble receptors that were first identified in the *Drosophila* and play an essential role in the immunity of the fly. TLRs recognize molecules derived from pathogens after breaching the epithelial surface of the conjunctiva. The most important TLR is TLR-4.

Lipopolysaccharides of Streptococci have the ability to abolish the function of the TLR-4. TLRs are activated by lipopolysaccharides of bacteria and by DNA of viruses. Other molecules that can inactivate TLRs include flagellin, lipopeptides, and lipoproteins. The TLRs have the ability to activate antigen-presenting cells,

K.F. Tabbara, MD, ABO, FRCOphth
Department of Ophthalmology, The Eye Center and The Eye Foundation for Research in Ophthalmology, Riyadh, Saudi Arabia

Department of Ophthalmology, College of Medicine, King Saud University, Riyadh, Saudi Arabia

The Wilmer Ophthalmological Institute of The Johns Hopkins University School of Medicine, Baltimore, MD, USA
e-mail: kftabbara@yahoo.com

K. Tabbara et al. (eds.), *Ocular Infections*, Essentials in Ophthalmology,
DOI 10.1007/978-3-662-43981-4_6, © Springer-Verlag Berlin Heidelberg 2014

such as Langerhans cells, T cells, and macrophages, and can bind to interleukin-1 (IL-1).

Infectious conjunctivitis is classified according to the causative agents and this include: bacteria, viruses, chlamydia, fungi and parasites [1–6].

6.2 Bacterial Conjunctivitis

6.2.1 Hyperacute *Neisseria* Conjunctivitis

Infectious conjunctivitis can be classified clinically into three forms: Hyperacute conjunctivitis, acute conjunctivitis, and chronic conjunctivitis. Hyperacute conjunctivitis is a rapidly progressive infection of the conjunctiva characterized by swelling of the eyelid, conjunctival hyperemia, and profuse purulent discharge with chemosis. The onset of symptoms is abrupt in one or both eyes. The most common cause of this type of conjunctivitis is *Neisseria gonorrhoeae* or *Neisseria meningitidis*. This form of conjunctivitis may be associated with preauricular lymph node. Membrane or pseudomembrane may be present. Peripheral corneal infiltrates, ulceration and thinning may lead to perforation in a few days.

Neisseria gonorrhoeae in adults is a sexually transmitted disease and may cause of ophthalmia neonatorum. On the other hand, *Neisseria meningitidis* may occur in children and adults. Both infections are serious and require rapid intervention with systemic treatment. In cases of *Neisseria meningitidis*, the ocular infection may lead to meningitis. Systemic infections occur in 10 % of the cases.

The differential diagnosis of hyperacture conjunctiviotis included viruses such as Herpes virus and Adenovirus.

6.2.2 Laboratory Investigations

In cases of purulent conjunctivitis, there is urgent need to obtain conjunctival swab and scrapings for cultures and stains. Conjunctival swabs are placed on blood agar and Thayer-Martin medium. The culture should be incubated in a 5–10 % carbon dioxide atmosphere. *Neisseria* is fastidious and dies quickly at room temperature. Fermentation test can be done to differentiate *Neisseria gonorrhoeae* from *Neisseria meningitidis. Neisseria gonorrhoeae* ferments glucose, while *Neisseria meningitidis* can ferment both glucose and maltose but not lactose. Antibiotic sensitivities should be determined. Conjunctival scrapings are stained with Gram and Giemsa stain. Typical intracytoplasmic Gram negative diplococcic may be seen in the polymorphonuclear cells.

6.2.3 Treatment

The treatment of *Neisseria* conjunctivitis should be considered an ophthalmic emergency. Patients should be admitted to the hospital and started on aggressive topical and systemic therapy. Topical treatment consists of irrigation of the eye with saline every 2 h during the day. Topical antibiotics in the form of azithromycin 0.15 % eyedrops (Azyter®, Laboratoires Théa, Clermont-Ferrand, Cedex, France) are instilled every 2 h or topical moxifloxacin 0.5 % eyedrops every 1 h. In adult form of *Neisseria gonorrhoeae* conjunctivitis, the patient and the sexual consent should be treated. The combination of therapy consists of doxycycline 100 mg orally twice daily may be given for 2 weeks and ceftriaxone 1 g intramuscularly or intravenously daily for 5 days. In neonates, cefotaxime 25 mg/kg every 12 h for 7 days should be given together with topical azithromycin eyedrops and erythromycin ointment with copious irrigation of the discharge. Adult patients with gonococcal conjunctivitis are at high risk of concomitant chlamydial genital infection and should therefore be treated with either doxycycline or azithromycin. *Neisseria meningitidis* infections may be prevented by vaccination.

6.3 Acute Bacterial Conjunctivitis

Acute bacterial conjunctivitis is common in children and adults. The most frequently encountered bacteria in acute bacterial conjunctivitis are *haemophilus influenzae*, *Alpha-hemolytic Streptococci*, *Staphylococcus aureus*, and *Streptococcus pneumoniae*. Other organisms such as *Proteus*, *Pseudomonas*, *Moraxella*, *Shigella*, *Klebsiella, and Listeria monocytogenes* have been isolated from cases with acute conjunctivitis.

6.3.1 Clinical Findings

The onset of acute bacterial conjunctivitis is sudden. Patients complain of irritation, foreign-body sensation, itching, soreness, and sticky lids in the morning. Morning discharge with transient blurring of vision may occur. The symptoms may be unilateral or bilateral. Membranes and pseudomembranes are uncommon in bacterial infections except in patients with Streptococcal or diphterial infections. The discharge is purulent or mucopurulent. Biomicroscopy reveals lid swelling with conjunctival hyperemia with discharge in the lower fornix and outer canthi. The cornea may be involved by peripheral corneal infiltrates or corneal ulcers. In general, acute bacterial conjunctivitis has a self-limited course, but treatment with topical antibiotics is essential to prevent complications specifically in patients with a compromised ocular surface such as patients with dry eye syndrome. Patients with *Listeria conjunctivitis* should be treated topically and systemically to prevent intraocular and systemic spread. Listerial keratoconjunctivitis may be complicated by endophthalmitis [7].

6.3.2 Laboratory Diagnosis

Conjunctival scrapings are obtained for stains and cultures. Standard laboratory procedures include obtaining two conjunctival scrapings placed onto clean slides. Conjunctival swabs are placed on blood agar, chocolate agar, and thioglycolate. The slides are stained with Gram and Giemsa stains. Gram stain may show polymorphonuclear cells and organisms, either Gram-negative or Gram-positive organisms. Giemsa stain may reveal the organisms as well as polymorphonuclear cells.

6.3.3 Gram Stain

Intracellular diplococci organisms may be seen in the stained slides of patients with *Neisseria* infections, and Gram-negative rods with epithelial parasitism may be seen in patients with *Haemophilus* spp. infection.

6.3.4 Treatment

Empiric topical treatment with antibiotics should be rendered to patients with acute conjunctivitis. A fourth-generation fluoroquinolone such as moxifloxacin 0.5 %, gatifloxacin 0.3 % eyedrops, or besifloxacin 0.6 % ophthalmic suspension may be given every 2 h on the first day followed by one drop every 6 h for a period of 1 week. Recent studies [1] have shown that besifloxacin 0.6 % is as effective as moxifloxacin ophthalmic solution 0.5 % in the treatment of bacterial conjunctivitis and can be given for 5 days. In cases of streptococcal infections, it is recommended to use topical azithromycin 0.15 % eyedrops (Azyter®, Laboratoires Théa, Clermont-Ferrand, Cedex, France) are instilled every 2 h for 1 day followed by twice daily for 5 days.

Children with acute conjunctivitis may sometimes develop otitis media. *Haemophilus influenzae* is the most common organism responsible for this syndrome and least commonly *Streptococcus pneumoniae*. In children, otitis media and conjunctivitis should be treated with systemic antibiotics. *Listeria monocytogenes* conjunctivitis should be treated with topical and systemic antibiotics [7].

6.4 Trachoma

Trachoma is a common cause of preventable blindness. The prevalence of active trachoma has decreased over the past two decades worldwide. The disease is caused by *Chlamydia trachomatis* serovars A, B, Ba, and C. *C. trachomatis* causes disease in humans only, and man is the only natural reservoir of this organism. In general, active trachoma is seen in communities with poor hygiene and inadequate sanitation. The transmission of trachoma is favored by the use of common fomites to wipe the face and the use of common bedding and person to person contact as well as the presence of flies which play a role in the eye to eye transmission. Trachoma causes chronic infection with inflammation leading to conjunctival cicatrization and corneal scarring. The subconjunctival cicatrization leads to entropion and trichiasis. The eyelashes disrupt the anatomic integrity of the corneal epithelium predisposing to corneal ulceration.

6.4.1 Clinical Findings

The principal diagnostic clinical criteria of trachoma include the presence of pannus, conjunctival follicles, conjunctival cicatrization, and limbal Herbert's pits. The clinical diagnosis of trachoma is made when two of the four criteria are present. The diagnosis of active trachoma is made when there is conjunctival edema and follicular reactions. The follicles may be pinhead and small and sometimes become large and necrotic. The corneal signs of trachoma include limbal follicles, Herbert's pits, and subepithelial keratitis with corneal vascularization. Fine epithelial punctate keratitis is seen, and occasionally a trachomatous peripheral corneal infiltration may form next to the superior pannus. This is referred to as trachomatous pustule. Several grading systems have been proposed. The grading of the intensity of trachoma helps in field surveys and was developed by the World Health Organization (WHO) Expert Committee on Trachoma [2]. The presence of limbal or conjunctival follicles suggests activity of the disease, but sometimes the follicles may be hidden by conjunctival edema.

6.4.2 Complications of Trachoma

Trachoma is a smoldering insidious inflammatory disease of the ocular surface that progresses over many years resulting in healing. Healing is associated with cicatrization of the conjunctiva which may eventuate in entropion with keratinization of the eyelid mucocutaneous junction and obstruction of the meibomian gland orifices. The entropion may lead to trichiasis, and eyelashes rub against the ocular surface. Conjunctival scarring may also cause shrinkage of the conjunctiva, symblepharon, and obliteration of the fornices. Scarring may lead to damage to the glands of Krause and Wölfring and sometimes cause obstruction of the lacrimal ductules leading to dry eye syndrome. Keratinization of the conjunctiva may occur with loss of the goblet cell population. Concretions may form due to subconjunctival epithelial entrapment. The lacrimal passages may be involved with submucosal lymphoid follicular reaction leading to necrosis, scarring, and obstruction of the nasolacrimal duct and canaliculi. Secondary bacterial infection is common in patients with trachoma. Obstruction of the nasal lacrimal duct may lead to subclinical chronic dacryocystitis commonly due to *Streptococcus pneumoniae* which may cause purulent conjunctivitis and keratitis in patients with trachoma. A number of conditions may be considered in the differential diagnosis of active trachoma including other causes of chronic follicular conjunctivitis such as viral conjunctivitis, the use of topical medications, molluscum contagiosum of the lid margin, *Moraxella* species, and oculoglandular disease caused by *Bartonella* species.

6.4.3 Treatment

The therapeutic regimen for active trachoma consists of a single-dose azithromycin 1,000 mg or azithromycin 500 mg orally daily for 3 days to be repeated in 1 week for adults. In cases of children, azithromycin suspension may be given 20 mg/kg/day for 3 days. Children may be treated with systemic therapy of erythromycin 40 mg/kg/day for 3 weeks. Alternative therapy consists of tetracycline 1 % ointment or erythromycin ointment 5 mg/g twice daily for 6–8 weeks.

In mass treatment campaigns, tetracycline 1 % ophthalmic ointment may be given twice daily for the first 5 days of each month for 6 months. Alternative therapy consists of doxycycline 100 mg orally twice daily for 3 weeks for adults. Oral tetracycline is not given in children.

Entropion and trichiasis should be treated surgically to prevent secondary infections of the ocular surface. Concretions may be removed with a needle under biomicroscopy, and obstruction of the nasolacrimal duct may be managed by dacryocystorhinostomy.

6.5 Inclusion Conjunctivitis

Inclusion conjunctivitis is a sexually transmitted disease caused by *C. trachomatis* serovars D, E, F, G, H, I, J, and K. The disease may be rarely caused by serovar B or C. Adult inclusion conjunctivitis is a common bilateral sexually transmitted disease.

Chlamydia agent may cause chronic infections and may lead to cervicitis in women and urethritis in men. The disease may be asymptomatic in women.

In humans, chlamydia has been recovered from approximately 50 % of patients with nongonococcal urethritis (NGU).

6.5.1 Clinical Findings

The disease is characterized by swelling and erythema of the eyelids with follicular reaction of the conjunctiva. There is hyperemia and chemosis. Superficial punctate keratitis may be observed, and corneal pannus formation occurs. In rare cases, phlyctenulosis may be seen.

6.5.2 Laboratory Diagnosis

Microscopic examination with Giemsa stain and scrapings of the conjunctiva may reveal a typical chlamydial inclusion bodies and cytology shows equal number of lymphocytes, polymorphonuclear cells and plasma cells. The agent can be cultured in tissue culture.

6.5.3 Treatment

The treatment of chlamydial inclusion conjunctivitis in adults consists of azithromycin 500 mg orally daily for 6 days. The sexual contact should also be treated. *Lymphogranuloma venereum* conjunctivitis is a rare chlamydial infection of the conjunctiva caused by *C. trachomatis* serovars L1, L2, L2a, and L3. This is a sexually transmitted disease.

6.6 Psittacosis

Psittacosis is a common infection in birds caused by Chlamydia psittaci. The disease may cause infections in human including conjunctivitis and pneumonia.

6.6.1 Clinical Findings

Patients with *C. psittaci* conjunctivitis develop hyperemia of the conjunctiva with follicular reaction and epithelial keratitis. Interstitial keratitis and uveitis may occur. No inclusion bodies are seen.

6.6.2 Treatment

The treatment of psittacosis requires six week course of oral doxycycline 100 mg orally twice daily. Pregnant woman may be given oral azithromycin.

6.7 Neonatal Conjunctivitis (Ophthalmia Neonatorum)

Ophthalmia neonatorum or conjunctivitis of the newborn is an acute conjunctivitis recognized in the first month of postnatal life. The disease is characterized by bilateral conjunctival hyperemia. Causes of neonatal conjunctivitis include *Neisseria gonorrhoeae*, *C. trachomatis*, herpes simplex type 2, bacteria, and silver nitrate.

6.7.1 Clinical Findings

Patients with neonatal conjunctivitis develop erythema of the lids, conjunctival hyperemia, and

Table 6.1 Treatment of conjunctivitis of the newborn

Chemical	
	Usually self-limiting; possibly irrigation with warm saline
Gonococcal	
	Hospitalization; isolation (at least 24 h after therapy is initiated)
	IV aqueous penicillin G 100,000 units/kg/day in four doses daily for 7 days
	Saline irrigation
	Topical antibiotics – not exceeded with IVR_x; effective against gonococcus
	Antibiotic sensitivities; if penicillin therapy fails, sensitivities used to dictate action[a]
Chlamydial	
	Oral erythromycin syrup, 30–50 mg/kg/day in four doses daily for 2 weeks (Optional: topical 1 % tetracycline *or* 10 % sulfonamide four to six times daily)
Herpetic	
	Topical trifluridine 1 % every 2 h for 7 days (not longer than 2 weeks) *or* acyclovir 10 mg/kg IV every 8 h for 10 days
Other bacteria	
	0.5 % erythromycin ointment *or* 1 % tetracycline ointment every 4 h for 7 days; smear is Gram-positive cocci
	0.3 % gentamicin *or* tobramycin 1 drop every 4 h for 7 days; smear is Gram-negative cocci

Adapted from Flach [3]

[a]Ceftriaxone 25–50 mg/kg IV *or* IM once daily for 7 days *or* gentamicin 5 mg/kg/day IM in two divided doses for 7 days

discharge. Neonates do not have subconjunctival lymphoid tissue, and therefore, conjunctival follicles are not seen in this age group. Edema of the palpebral and bulbar conjunctiva may be noted. In cases of purulent conjunctivitis, *Neisseria gonorrhoeae* should be ruled out, and this is an emergency because corneal perforation may occur within a few days if not treated early. Treatment of neonatal conjunctivitis [3] is shown in Table 6.1.

Conjunctival scrapings and cultures are essential in neonatal conjunctivitis. Corneal scrapings stained with Gram and Giemsa may show Gram-negative intracellular diplococci in polymorphonuclear cells in cases of *Neisseria gonorrhoeae*. In Chlamydial conjunctivitis, also known as inclusion blenorrhea, conjunctival scrapings show basophilic paranuclear cystoplasmic inclusion bodies. Lymphocytes, plasma cells, and macrophages with epithelial debris known as Leber's cells.

In herpetic conjunctivitis, multinucleated epithelial cells are seen with mononuclear cellular infiltration. In patients with other bacterial infections, Gram-positive or Gram-negative cocci or bacilli may be seen. Neonatal conjunctivitis due to chemical reaction may show neutrophils and occasional lymphocytes on Giemsa stain. Chemical conjunctivitis occurs to some degree in eyes treated prophylactically with 1 % silver nitrate. Silver nitrate 1 % eyedrops can bind to bacterial protein but at the same time adhere to conjunctival cellular protein and can cause irritation and inflammation.

6.8 Bartonella Conjunctivitis (Cat-Scratch Disease)

Bartonella conjunctivitis (cat-scratch disease) is a cause of Parinaud's oculoglandular conjunctivitis. The disease is usually unilateral, and the conjunctival granuloma occurs over the palpebral conjunctiva with preauricular lymph node. The most common cause is *Bartonella henselae*, but other infectious agents may cause Parinaud's oculoglandular conjunctivitis including *Pasteurella (Francisella) tularensis, Mycobacterium tuberculosis, Treponema pallidum, Yersinia* species, *Haemophilus ducreyi,* lymphogranuloma venereum, sporotrichosis, *Coccidioides immitis,* mumps, and Epstein-Barr virus (Table 6.2) [4]. *Bartonella* oculoglandular disease can lead to chronic conjunctivitis. The disease is caused by Gram-negative pleomorphic bacterium known as *Bartonella henselae*.

6.8.1 Clinical Findings

Patients with *Bartonella* oculoglandular disease have chronic conjunctivitis with localized granuloma which is unilateral associated with large preauricular lymph node. Conjunctival biopsy or scrapings may show Gram-negative bacteria in the lymph node. The bacilli could be detected with the

Table 6.2 Etiology of oculoglandular conjunctivitis

Cause	Organism	Disease
Bacteria	*Bartonella henselae*	Parinaud's oculoglandular conjunctivitis (cat-scratch disease)
	Francisella tularensis	Tularemia
	Mycobacterium tuberculosis	Tuberculosis
	Treponema pallidum	Syphilis
	Yersinia spp.[a]	Yersinia infection
	Haemophilus ducreyi[a]	Chancroid
	Listeria monocytogenes[a]	Listerellosis
Chlamydiae	Lymphogranuloma venereum agent	Lymphogranuloma venereum
	Inclusion conjunctivitis agent	Inclusion conjunctivitis
Fungi	*Sporotrichum schenckii*[a]	Sporotrichosis
	Coccidioides immitis	Coccidioidomycosis
	Actinomyces israelii[a]	Actinomycosis
	Blastomyces dermatitidis[a]	Blastomycosis
Virus	Mumps virus[a]	Mumps
	Epstein-Barr virus	Infectious mononucleosis

Adapted from Tabbara [4], p. 480
[a]Rare cases

Warthin-Starry silver impregnation stain in the tissue section of the lymph node. The organism is a Gram-negative pleomorphic bacterium. The bacterium is seen intracellularly and can be found in the biopsy specimen of conjunctival granuloma.

Bartonella oculoglandular disease is a form of subacute regional lymphadenitis which is usually preceded by history of a cat scratch or exposure to cats. The disease is characterized by a spectrum of signs ranging from mild self-limited adenopathy with a conjunctival nodule to severe systemic disease and hepatosplenomegaly. The disease may cause neuroretinitis and occurs more frequently in children than young adults.

Bartonellosis may be life-threatening in patients with HIV infection. The main symptoms in patients with *Bartonella* oculoglandular disease include unilateral hyperemia of the conjunctiva with discharge and photophobia. This may be associated with fever, malaise, anorexia, and headache. On examination, a large visible preauricular or submandibular lymph node may be noted. The lymph node is usually tender. Ptosis of the eyelid may occur due to swelling. The bulbar conjunctiva may show a localized granuloma with chemosis and hyperemia. These lesions may last from 2 weeks to 10 months and show progressive spontaneous healing. Treatment with antibiotics appears to shorten the course of the disease and prevents suppuration. Visual loss can occur in systemic disease due to neuroretinitis and retinal vasculitis.

6.8.2 Treatment

The treatment of *Bartonella* oculoglandular disease is systemic antibiotic in the form of doxycycline 100 mg orally twice daily for a period of 2–3 weeks. Children may be treated with rifamycin, trimethoprim sulfamethoxazole, or intramuscular gentamicin. Patients with hepatic involvement should be given intravenous gentamicin. Localized excision of the conjunctival granuloma may shorten the course of the disease. Symptomatic treatment of fever, chills, anorexia, malaise, and headaches may be rendered.

6.9 Borrelia Conjunctivitis

Borrelia conjunctivitis is a disease caused by the spirochete *Borrelia burgdorferi*. The disease is also known as Lyme disease. The disease has been recognized as the most common cause of tick-borne disease in the United States. The vector is the tick *Ixodes*, and the infection can lead to three clinical stages.

6.9.1 Clinical Findings

The first stage of Lyme disease occurs immediately after the patient is infected with the spirochete after a tick bite. The classic clinical manifestation of Lyme disease is an erythema chronicum migrans (ECM) of the skin at the site of the tick bite. This is a circumferential red rash that moves outward and eventually resolves spontaneously. During the second stage of the disease, patients may experience headaches with meningismus and neurologic symptoms. Patients may also develop cardiac arrhythmia and acute pericarditis. In stage three, the disease becomes chronic with neurologic ocular and joint symptoms. Facial palsy or other cranial nerves paresis may occur. The most common ocular manifestation of Lyme disease is conjunctivitis that occurs in stage 1 of the infection. The conjunctivitis appears as nonspecific acute conjunctivitis with redness, discharge, and discomfort. A chronic follicular conjunctivitis has been described in Lyme disease. Complete resolution of the conjunctivitis occurs.

6.9.2 Laboratory Diagnosis

Serologic tests for Lyme disease should be requested. Blood tests determine the presence of antibodies to *Borrelia burgdorferi*. The sensitivity of the assays is variable, and the negative test does not rule out the infection.

6.9.3 Treatment

The treatment of Lyme disease (stage 1) consists of doxycycline 100 mg orally twice daily, amoxicillin 500 mg orally three times daily, or cefuroxime 500 mg orally twice daily.

In patients who develop chronic Lyme disease, ceftriaxone is given intravenously every 24 h. In cases of arthritis, both doxycycline and amoxicillin should be combined.

6.10 Viral Conjunctivitis

Viral conjunctivitis is a common ocular condition caused by a variety of viruses. The most common cause of viral conjunctivitis is adenovirus. The disease has an abrupt onset and usually starts in one eye and later involves the other eye. Most cases of viral conjunctivitis have a self-limited course but may lead to corneal opacities and decrease in vision. There are different patterns of clinical presentation, and the disease manifestations may be variable and may have different sequelae in different patients. Most viruses that affect the conjunctiva lead to an acute unilateral follicular conjunctivitis with discharge followed by involvement of the second eye within 2 days to 1 week after the initial involvement. The disease is highly contagious, and several members of the same family may be involved.

6.10.1 Clinical Findings

Patients with viral conjunctivitis complain of foreign body sensation, tearing, irritation, and pain. Examination reveals swelling of the lids, with occasional ecchymosis, conjunctival hyperemia and chemosis, and subconjunctival hemorrhages. Small tender periauricular lymph node is noted. Hemorrhages may be seen in the conjunctiva. A true membrane or pseudomembrane may be seen over the conjunctiva, and the membrane may recur following removal. The cornea shows superficial epithelial keratitis in the first few days. The differential diagnosis of acute follicular viral conjunctivitis includes adenoviral keratoconjunctivitis, acute hemorrhagic conjunctivitis, primary herpes simplex virus conjunctivitis, Newcastle disease viral conjunctivitis, and rarely cytomegalovirus (CMV) or Epstein-Barr virus conjunctivitis. The follicles are usually seen in the lower fornix and lower palpebral conjunctiva. It takes several days for the follicles to appear. Follicles may get obscured by papillae, edema, and infiltration of the conjunctiva or by conjunctival membranes. The differential diagnosis of membranous or pseudomembranous conjunctivitis includes epidemic keratoconjunctivitis (EKC), pharyngoconjunctival fever, herpetic conjunctivitis, *Corynebacterium diphtheriae* conjunctivitis, ligneous conjunctivitis, Stevens-Johnson syndrome, ß (*beta*)-hemolytic streptococcal conjunctivitis, chlamydial conjunctivitis, chemical (alkali) burns, and topical drug-induced conjunctivitis.

The majority of cases of viral conjunctivitis are caused by adenovirus types 4, 7, 8, 19, 22, 37, and 53 [5]. Adenovirus keratoconjunctivitis is highly contagious and a significant health hazard because of the rapid spread of the disease. Economic loss occurs because of affliction of the young manpower in the population and usually affects people between the ages of 24 and 40 years. Seven to 10 days after the onset of the keratoconjunctivitis, focal epithelial keratitis develops leading to lesions at the level of Bowman's layer with subepithelial nummular infiltrates. These epithelial infiltrates consist of mononuclear cells mostly lymphocytes. The conjunctivitis lasts 2–3 weeks and is self-limited. Subepithelial infiltration may occur and may remain for many months, and some cases may persist up to 2 years. The number of subepithelial nummular opacities may vary in shape, size, location, and number. Diffuse subepithelial opacities may occur. Patients may have minimal subepithelial nummular opacity without affection of their visual acuity, and others may have numerous nummular opacities in the cornea that may be confluent and may coalesce causing decrease in visual acuity. Hyperopic shift may occur in some patients because of the superficial scarring of the cornea. Anterior self-limiting nongranulomatous uveitis occurs in severe adenoviral keratoconjunctivitis.

Membranous conjunctivitis may cause conjunctival scar and occasionally may lead to scarring of the lacrimal ductules leading to dry eye syndrome. The most commonly encountered adenoviruses include Ad4, Ad7, Ad8, Ad19, Ad22, Ad37, and Ad53 [6]. No specific antiviral therapy is available for adenovirus keratoconjunctivitis. The management is usually symptomatic with application of cold compresses and sunglasses. Topical nonsteroidal anti-inflammatory agents (NSAIDs) may help in relieving discomfort in the early stages of the disease. Topical diluted corticosteroids may also help in decreasing the signs and symptoms of viral conjunctivitis. Topical Povidone-iodine 0.4 % eyedrops and ganciclovir 0.15 % gel have been reported to be effective in the management of adenoviral keratoconjunctivitis [8–9].

Fluorometholone 0.05 % eyedrops or rimexolone 0.5 % eyedrops may be used four times daily in patients with severe subepithelial corneal infiltration. Topical cyclosporine 0.1 % eyedrops or tacrolimus 0.01 % eyedrops may be started 1 week after the onset of subepithelial opacities, and this can help in ameliorating the photophobia and irritation in patients with nummular subepithelial opacities due to adenoviral keratoconjunctivitis. Antibiotics are used in cases of secondary bacterial conjunctivitis.

Complications of adenoviral keratoconjunctivitis include dry eye syndrome, conjunctival scarring, punctal occlusion, hyperopic shiffs, nummular and diffuse corneal scarring.

Other causes of viral conjunctivitis include influenza virus conjunctivitis, acute hemorrhagic conjunctivitis secondary to adenovirus type 70, Epstein-Barr virus conjunctivitis, molluscum contagiosum of the skin of eyelids, and Human papilloma virus.

Compliance with Ethical Requirements

Conflict of Interest The author declares that he has no conflict of interest.

Informed Consent No human studies were carried out by the authors for this article.

Animal Studies No animal studies were carried out by the authors for this article.

References

1. McDonald MB, Protzko EE, Brunner LS, Morris TW, Haas W, Paterno MR, Comstock TL, Usner DW. Efficacy and safety of besifloxacin ophthalmic suspension 0.6% compared with moxifloxacin ophthalmic solution 0.5% for treating bacterial conjunctivitis. Ophthalmology. 2009;116(9):1615–23.
2. Dawson CR, Jones BR, Tarizzo ML. Guide to trachoma control. Geneva: World Health Organization; 1981. p. 12–20.
3. Flach AJ. Conjunctivitis of the newborn, chapter 30. In: Tabbara KF, Hyndiuk RA, editors. Infections of the eye. 2nd ed. Boston: Little Brown and Co; 1996. p. 471–8.

4. Tabbara KF. Parinaud's oculoglandular conjunctivitis (ocular cat-scratch disease), chapter 31. In: Tabbara KF, Hyndiuk RA, editors. Infections of the eye. 2nd ed. Boston: Little Brown and Co; 1996. p. 479–85.
5. Tabbara KF, Omar N, Hammouda E, Akanuma M, Ohguchi T, Ariga T, Tagawa Y, Kitaichi N, Ishida S, Aoki K, Ishiko H, Ohno S. Molecular epidemiology of adenoviral keratoconjunctivitis in Saudi Arabia. Mol Vis. 2010;16:2132–6.
6. Jin XH, Aoki K, Kitaichi N, Ariga T, Ishida S, Ohno S. Genome variability of human adenovirus type 8 causing epidemic keratoconjunctivitis during 1986–2003 in Japan. Mol Vis. 2011;17:3121–7.
7. Shoughy SS, Tabbara KF. Listeria monocytogenes endophthalmitis following keratoconjunctivitis. Clin Ophthalmol. 2014;24(8):301–4.
8. Clement C, Capriotti JA, Kumar M, Hobden JA, Foster TP, Bhattacharjee PS, Thompson HW, Mahmud R, Liang B, Hill JM. Clinical and antiviral efficacy of an ophthalmic formulation of dexamethasone povidone-iodine in a rabbit model of adenoviral keratoconjunctivitis. Invest Ophthalmol Vis Sci. 2011;52(1):339–44.
9. Tabbara KF, Al Balushi N. Topical ganciclovir in the treatment of acute herpetic keratitis. Clin Ophthalmol. 2010;4:905–12.

Infectious Keratitis

7

Khalid F. Tabbara and Charbel T. Bou Chacra

7.1 Introduction

Corneal infection or microbial keratitis is a common cause of ocular morbidity and visual loss. Microbial keratitis may be caused by viruses, bacteria, fungi, and parasites. The most common causative agent of corneal infection is viral, followed by bacteria, fungi, and parasites.

7.2 Pathogenesis of Corneal Infections

The viruses and parasites usually do not require breach of the corneal surface to establish an infection. On the other hand, bacteria and fungi require a break in the integrity of the epithelium barrier to gain entry and adhere to establish an infection. A few bacteria, however, such as *Neisseria, Corynebacterium, Haemophilus, and Listeria*, can invade the intact cornea and establish infections. The ocular surface is equipped with both specific and nonspecific defense mechanisms that prevent offending agents. Several systemic and local factors may predispose to corneal infections.

The main barrier to microorganisms that invade the cornea is the epithelial surface. The epithelium of the cornea serves as a physical and functional barrier to infections preventing entry of microbes and interfering with their growth through productions of microbial and antimicrobial agents. If the epithelium is breached and an organism gained access to the underlying tissue, the organism would encounter defense mechanisms of innate immunity which are designed to react rapidly against microbes. The ocular surface tear film contains substances that are effective in killing the organisms including lysozyme, lactoferrin, secretory immunoglobulin IgA, and other defense mechanisms. Neutrophils and macrophages ingest microbes and destroy them by producing substances that are microbiocidal. In addition, macrophages produce cytokines that recruit, activate, and upregulate immunocytes. On the other hand, natural killer cells kill virus-infected cells and produce cytokines including interferon gamma. Many forms of proteins are involved in the host defense including proteins of the complement system, the complement agent by microbes or by antigen antibody complexes. The complement system is aimed at

K.F. Tabbara, MD, ABO, FRCOphth (✉)
Department of Ophthalmology, The Eye Center and The Eye Foundation for Research in Ophthalmology, Riyadh, Saudi Arabia

Department of Ophthalmology, College of Medicine, King Saud University, Riyadh, Saudi Arabia

The Wilmer Ophthalmological Institute of The Johns Hopkins University School of Medicine, Baltimore, MD, USA
e-mail: kftabbara@yahoo.com

C.T. Bou Chacra, MD, FRCS (Glasg)
Department of Ophthalmology, The Eye Center and The Eye Foundation for Research in Ophthalmology, Riyadh, Saudi Arabia

K. Tabbara et al. (eds.), *Ocular Infections*, Essentials in Ophthalmology,
DOI 10.1007/978-3-662-43981-4_7, © Springer-Verlag Berlin Heidelberg 2014

killing microbes and lead to opsonization for the phagocytosis by macrophages and neutrophils. In addition to combating infections, innate immune responses stimulate subsequent adaptive immunity providing symptoms that are essential for initiating responses of antigen-specific T and B lymphocytes. Innate immunity works in concert with adaptive immune responses leading to the control of infection.

Antibodies bind to extracellular microbes blocking their ability to infect the host cells. The phagocytes ingest organisms and kill them, while helper T lymphocytes enhance the microbial killing of the phagocytes. Cytotoxic T lymphocytes, on the other hand, destroy cells that have been infected by microbes that are inaccessible to antibodies. The main goal of the adaptive response is to activate the defense mechanisms against microorganisms that invade the cornea.

Microorganisms that invade the epithelial cells of the cornea may be captured and processed by macrophages and dendritic cells that are residents in the epithelial surface and migrate from the limbus. Protein antigens of these microorganisms are processed by the antigen-presenting cells to generate peptides that are discreet on the surface of the antigen-presenting cells and then bind to the major histocompatibility complex molecules. Naive T cells recognize MHC complexes, and the T lymphocytes start to respond. Protein antigens are recognized by T lymphocytes, while polysaccharides and other nonprotein antigens are captured in the lymphoid organs.

The epithelial surface represents a barrier to infections and innate immunity provides the first line of defense against the offending organisms. There are multiple strategies of innate recognition of infection. The most common of which is recognition of molecules, highly characteristic of large groups of microbes or viruses. In the corneal epithelium, there are innate immune receptors known as Toll-like receptors (TLRs). Toll-like receptors recognize bacterial cell-wall components or cell membrane receptors. Their main function is to induce production of inflammatory cytokines such as tumor necrosis factor-alpha (TNF-α) and interleukin (IL-1) 1, whereas the intracellular TLRs cause production of type 1 interferon. Both TNF and IL-1 are the main inflammation-inducing cytokines. This helps in the fighting against infections but at the same time may lead to damage of the tissue leading to corneal scarring and, therefore, decrease in vision.

Toll-like receptors recognize pathogens on the epithelial surfaces. TLRs recognize the variety of molecules including bacterial cell-wall components and pathogen-derived nucleic acids. Nucleotide-binding oligomerization domain-containing protein 1 (NOD1) and nucleotide-binding oligomerization domain-containing protein 2 (NOD2) recognize proteoglycan substructures and promote innate immune responses as well. NOD1 and NOD2 are innate immune components found in the cytoplasm of cells. They recognize small fragments of bacterial cell-wall peptidoglycans which are transported across the host cell. NOD1 and NOD2 are synergistic with TLR signaling and bind to certain ligand to induce inflammatory cytokines.

Table 7.1 shows the factors that may predispose to ocular infections [1].

7.3 Bacterial Keratitis

Bacterial keratitis is a devastating infection of the cornea that may lead to rapid insult and loss of vision. Early diagnosis and prompt treatment are essential in minimizing the damage and improving the visual outcome. There are numerous bacteria that may cause bacterial keratitis. The most frequent causative organisms of bacterial keratitis include *Staphylococcus aureus*, *Staphylococcus epidermidis*, *Streptococcus pneumoniae*, *and Pseudomonas aeruginosa*. Other organisms that may cause bacterial keratitis include *Moraxella*, *Klebsiella*, *Proteus*, *Enterobacter*, *Serratia*, *Citrobacter*, *and Neisseria* species. In rare cases of bacterial keratitis, multiple organisms may be isolated.

This section covers the clinical findings of bacterial keratitis, diagnostic workup, and management.

Patients with bacterial keratitis usually present with history of pain, redness, photophobia,

Table 7.1 Predisposing factors for ocular infections

Exogenous factors	Endogenous local conditions	Systemic factors
Contact lens wear	Lid disorders	Alcoholism
Topical corticosteroids	1. Lagophthalmos	Allergies
Topical antibiotics	2. Entropion	Blood dyscrasias
Trauma	3. Ectropion	Collagen-vascular disease
Glaucoma medication	4. Blepharitis	Coma
	Lacrimal disorders	Dementia
	1. Keratitis sicca	Diabetes mellitus
	2. Dacryocystitis	Immune disorders
	Conjunctival disorders	Prematurity
	1. Vernal catarrh	Systemic steroids
	2. Trachoma	Nutritional deficiency
	3. Ocular pemphigoid	Psychosis
	4. Stevens-Johnson syndrome	
	5. Xerophthalmia	
	Corneal disorders	
	1. Neurotrophic keratitis	
	2. Penetrating keratoplasty	
	3. Bullous keratopathy	
	4. Herpetic eye disease	

tearing, irritation, foreign-body sensation, purulent discharge, and blepharospasm. Symptoms of lid swelling may be present.

7.3.1 Clinical Findings

Patients with bacterial keratitis present with hyperemia of the conjunctiva, ciliary injection, and purulent discharge. Biomicroscopy of the cornea reveals an epithelial defect with creamy-white infiltration surrounded by ground-glass appearance. The ulcer may be small or large. The cornea may show folds in Descemet's membrane with edema and keratic precipitates found on the endothelium. The anterior chamber demonstrates varying degrees of cells and flare. Fibrin or hypopyon may be present. It is important to examine the stroma carefully to assess the amount of necrosis that may lead to thinning of the cornea. This is true in patients with *Pseudomonas* infection where thinning of the stroma may be marked and sometimes a descemetocele may form which carries a poor prognosis. The descemetocele may lead to corneal perforation and iris adhesion to the cornea. Central corneal ulcers are usually infectious in nature, while noninfectious infiltrates may appear as single or multiple peripheral corneal infiltration ulcer secondary to immune-mediated reactions. Marginal ulcers that extent to the center may be infectious in nature. *Staphylococcus* corneal ulcers are usually round, well circumscribed with an epithelial defect and corneal infiltration. In some patients with *Staphylococcus* ulcer, multiple deep stromal infiltrates may be seen together with small infiltrates adjacent to the corneal ulcer. The surrounding cornea may show minimal edema. *Streptococcus pneumoniae* may appear as serpiginous ulceration that moves across the cornea with infiltration. On the other hand, *Pseudomonas aeruginosa* causes an aggressive and fulminant corneal ulcer which is rapidly progressing and may lead to corneal perforation if not treated early. The corneal ulcer is usually extensive with necrosis and yellow-green purulent discharge adherent to the surface. The corneal surrounding of the ulcer shows edema with ground-glass appearance and loss of its transparency. A hypopyon is usually present. Certain bacterial ulcers are indolent and insidious in nature such as *Moraxella*, *Nocardia*, and nontuberculous *Mycobacteria*. The corneal ulcers show a localized epithelial defect with infiltration. The ulcer tends to be round or oval, and the cornea surrounding the ulcer appears to be relatively clear unlike cases with *Pseudomonas* corneal ulcer. In cases of traumatic penetrating corneal laceration, the patient may be infected with *Bacillus* species or *Clostridium* species which may produce gas in the anterior chamber or corneal stroma. On the other hand, *Serratia marcescens* corneal ulcer may produce red pigment that appears in the stroma.

7.3.2 Diagnostic Laboratory Investigation

Simple corneal ulcers should always be scraped for cytological evaluation with Gram and Giemsa stains and for cultures. The corneal scrapings should be performed at the area of corneal infiltration obtaining adequate specimens. Part of the scraping specimen is placed on two slides for Gram and Giemsa staining, and another specimen should be placed onto culture plates, blood agar, and chocolate agar. Other media may be used, as indicated, such as Löwestein-Jensen medium, cooked meat, or brain-heart infusion medium. Corneal cultures are obtained in the office utilizing topical anesthetic such as proparacaine 0.5 %, tetracaine 0.1 %, or benoxinate 0.4 %. The corneal scrapings are obtained with the slit-lamp magnification using either Kimura spatula or a 25 g needle. The scrapings should be done aggressively in the bed of the ulcer as well as the leading edge of the infiltrate. Mucopurulent discharge should be avoided. A wire lid speculum may be used to prevent blinking during the procedure. Thioglycolate medium is use for anaerobic cultures. If fungi are suspected, Sabouraud's dextrose agar should be used. An additional slide may be prepared for periodic acid-Schiff (PAS) or Grocott-Gomori methenamine-silver nitrate stain. The corneal specimen should be cultured even in patients who are on antibiotics. Media with antibiotic removal device may be used. Molecular diagnostic techniques are available such as polymerase chain reaction (PCR). Molecular diagnostic tests may not be readily available in every institution but may prove to be helpful.

7.3.3 Management

Clinical severity of corneal ulcers is divided into three grades: mild, moderate, and severe. Mild corneal ulcers are those that are less than 2 mm in size, and the depth of the ulcer is less than 20 % or 100 μm of the corneal thickness. The infiltrates may be superficial next to the base of the ulcer. In cases with moderate corneal ulcers, the size of the ulcer is 2–5 mm, the depth of the ulcer is 20–50 % (100–275 μm) of the cornea, and the infiltrate is dense extending to the midstroma. In severe corneal ulcers, the ulcer size is more than 5 mm in size, the depth of the ulcer is more than 50 % (>275 μm) of corneal thickness, and the infiltration is dense reaching the deep layers of the corneal stroma. The sclera may be involved in patients with severe peripheral bacterial keratitis. After obtaining the corneal scrapings for culture and cytology, the patient should be started on combination of topical antibiotics to cover the most commonly encountered organisms while the patient is still in the office. The mainstay of treatment includes frequent aggressive administration of topical antibiotics. Certain antibiotics may have to be compounded and made available for the patient. Mild and moderate bacterial keratitis may be treated on an out-patient basis whereas patients with severe bacterial keratitis may have to be admitted to the hospital for the intensive in-patient management.

The patient should be treated with topical antibiotics every hour in addition to the pulse therapy which should be given three times a day and consists of one drop every minute for 5 min.

In moderate and severe corneal ulcers, treatment should be aggressive, and antibiotic eye drops should be administered every 15 min around the clock with an initial pulse therapy. It is of great importance to monitor the corneal thinning and stromal necrosis in cases of imminent perforations, shallowing of the anterior chamber, or sudden appearance of the hypopyon.

In patients with small perforations, tissue adhesive may be applied. In patients where there is rapid reepithelialization, it is recommended to re-scrape the cornea in order to increase the corneal penetration of the antimicrobial agents where the infiltration is persistent. Antibiotic therapy is modified when the culture is available. When the infiltration subsides and the epithelial defect heals, frequency of the antibiotics may be tapered. The size of the infiltration and the ulcer should be measured by slit beam. Optical coherence tomography (OCT) and external photography are helpful. The size of the infiltration and the epithelial defect are recorded and followed up closely. The size of the epithelial defect is usually smaller than the infiltration. Cycloplegic agents such as cyclopentolate 0.1 % eye drops may be given twice daily to minimize pain and blepharospasm. Oral analgesics may be required in patients with severe ocular pain. It is always recommended not to patch the infected eye, but a plastic clear shield may be applied.

Patients may be started on empirical therapy consisting of tobramycin 14 mg/ml and vancomycin 50 mg/ml eye drops. These can be given 5 min apart initially in the first hour followed by every hour. A pulse topical therapy may be given every 1 min for 5 times 3 times daily. Commercially available fluoroquinolones such as gatifloxacin, moxifloxacin, and besifloxacin may be used as initial empiric therapy in mild cases. Ciprofloxacin is approved for use in bacterial keratitis and has demonstrated clinical efficacy and safety in a large clinical trial [2]. Ciprofloxacin is potent against Gram-negative organisms such as *Pseudomonas* but has limited efficacy against staphylococci and streptococci.

The treatment for bacterial keratitis is the topical administration of commercially available antibiotics or fortified compounded antibiotics. Increasing the concentration of antibiotic solutions creates a larger diffusion grading across the cornea, and this serves to increase the corneal penetration of the antibiotic. Subconjunctival or subtenon injection of antibiotics is occasionally used in patients with moderate to severe corneal ulcers, ulcers with imminent perforation, patients with scleral extension of the corneal ulcers, and patients with associated endophthalmitis. Subconjunctival injection may also be indicated in patients who are not compliant. Repeated injections must be administered to maintain appropriate drug loads.

Intravenous administration of antibiotics is rarely indicated in patients with bacterial keratitis. *Neisseria* species and *Haemophilus* species are treated with systemic as well as topical antibiotics because of the possibility of systemic infection, particularly, in the pediatric age group.

The severe inflammation associated with bacterial keratitis may lead to damage to the corneal tissue, and this inflammatory reaction should be taken into consideration. Topical corticosteroids are contraindicated in the initial therapy of bacterial keratitis but once the infection is under control and the epithelium has healed, corticosteroids may be used with care. Clinical trials have shown that topical corticosteroids given 2 days after initiation of topical antibiotic therapy did not worsen the course of the disease. Topical corticosteroids, however, may inhibit the immune mechanisms of the ocular surface leading to persistence of the infection. The risks and benefits of topical corticosteroids should be weighed carefully.

7.4 Viral Keratitis

There are many viruses that lead to keratitis in man. Both DNA and RNA viruses may cause keratitis. The severity of keratitis varies from mild superficial punctate epithelial keratitis with or without conjunctivitis to severe form of stromal keratitis leading to scarring and loss of vision. Viruses that cause keratitis include herpes virus and varicella-zoster virus, adenovirus, human immunodeficiency virus, smallpox, vaccinia, *Molluscum contagiosum,* measles, mumps virus, mucacin disease virus, enterovirus, rubella virus, flaviviridae and myxoviridae group of viruses (Table 7.2).

Table 7.2 Non-herpetic viral keratitis

Virus	Ocular manifestations	
DNA viruses		
Adenovirus	Follicular conjunctivitis, epithelial keratitis, subepithelial nummular opacities	
Small pox (variola virus)	Corneal ulcers, corneal perforation	Skin vesicles, scars fever, death
Vaccinia virus	Corneal scars, keratitis, conjunctivitis blepharitis, superficial punctate keratitis (SPK)	Vesicles
Molluscum contagiosum	Lid umbilicated lesion, follicular conjunctivitis	
Papilloma virus	Limbal keratitis, conjunctival papilloma	Warts of lid margin
RNA viruses		
Measles virus	SPK, conjunctivitis secondary to bacterial infections	Koplik's spots
Mumps virus	SPK, acute conjunctivitis	Dacryoadenitis
New castle disease virus	SPK, follicular conjunctivitis	Parotiditis
Enterovirus 70 virus	Subconjunctival hemorrhage	
Coxsackie virus	Follicular conjunctivitis, subconjunctival hemorrhage	
Rubella virus	Congenital cataract, retinopathy, microphthalmia, iris atrophy Acquired follicular conjunctivitis, SPK	
Flaviviridae		
West Nile virus	Multifocal choroiditis, retinal vasculitis	
Dengue virus	Chorioretinitis, vasculitis	
Chikungunya virus		
Bunyaviridae	Subconjunctival hemorrhage	
Rift Valley fever	Retinitis, retinal vasculitis, optic neuritis, optic atrophy retinal hemorrhages	

7.5 Herpes Keratitis

Herpes simplex virus (HSV) and herpes zoster virus (HZV) are the most serious infections of the cornea that may lead to devastating complications and loss of vision. HSV is the most common infectious cause of unilateral visual loss from corneal disease [3]. Herpetic infections are common and afflict between 50 and 95 % of the population. HSV type 1 is transmitted by direct contact with infected secretions. Humans are the only known natural reservoir. The disease can be primary infection in an immunized individual or secondary disease due to recurrence of HSV which has been dormant in the trigeminal ganglion. Nearly 95 % of individuals older than 60 years of age harbor HSV in their trigeminal ganglia at autopsy. The majority of cases of herpetic infections are subclinical, and HSV has been isolated from tears and saliva of patients with no active disease [4]. Following a primary infection, the virus stays dormant in the trigeminal ganglion in cases of ocular surface infection. The ocular involvement is most commonly associated with type 1 HSV which causes disease in the distribution of the trigeminal ganglion: *Herpes keratitis*, *Herpes labialis*, *and Herpes gingivostomatitis*. HSV type 2, on the other hand, is associated with disease and in the distribution of the sacral ganglion leading *to Herpes vulvovaginitis* and *Herpes progenitalis*. Reports of HSV type 2 ocular disease have been shown in adults and suggest an oculogenital transmission of the virus. In neonates, HSV-2 is responsible for the 80 % of the herpetic infections. If the herpes virus is found in the birth canal, the risk of infection to a newborn is 40 %, and therefore, a cesarean section is preferable for delivery in such cases [5].

The most common manifestation of ocular herpes is herpetic keratitis. The newborn becomes susceptible to an infection with HSV at 6 months at the time of decline in maternal antibodies to the herpes virus. The initial episode of herpetic infection is referred to as primary infection and can occur between the ages of 1 and 5 years but is subclinical in the majority of cases. The primary infection may affect the eyelids, conjunctiva, and cornea presenting as lid swelling and edema with initial erythematous papular lesions progressing rapidly into vesicular eruptions and ulcerative stage 1. The conjunctiva may show follicular conjunctivitis, and the cornea reveals epithelial keratitis. The primary infection gives more severe symptoms than recurrent disease. The virus may be cultured from the conjunctiva. In patients who are immunologically compromised, a severe generalized infection may occur. Patients who are immunocompromised such as newborns, malnourished children, pregnant women in their last trimester, patients with atopic dermatitis, tuberculosis-acquired immunodeficiency syndrome, Wiskott-Aldrich syndrome, ataxia-telangiectasia, leukemia or lymphoma, severe burns, and patients on systemic immunosuppressive agents are susceptible to severe herpetic infection. The site of the primary infection determines the pathway of viral spread and site of viral latency. The most common site for the establishment of the latent infection is the trigeminal ganglion. Latency of HSV in the corneal nerves has been suggested [6].

7.6 Epithelial Disease

Following the primary infection, HSV stays latent in the trigeminal and sacral ganglia. Certain triggers have been shown to reactivate the herpetic infection. These triggers include fever, sunlight, cold wind, surgery, infection, menstruation, stress, cutting the root of the ganglion, trauma, and immunosuppression. Recurrent ocular disease may lead to herpetic dermatitis of the lids which tend to recur in the same geographic location where vesicle ulcerates leaving an erythematous base. Recurrent conjunctivitis leads to hyperemia and sometimes chemosis of the conjunctiva. The most common form of recurrence of the ocular disease is the cornea. Recurrent herpetic keratitis may lead to epithelial dendrites, geographic ulceration, and stromal invasion of the cornea by herpes virus [7]. Recurrent herpetic stromal disease may lead to infiltration and edema of the corneal stroma leading to stromal necrosis and melting. In severe cases, stromal keratitis may be associated with uveitis. Trauma to the trigeminal nerve of the cornea may induce viral recurrences in the peripheral tissue. HSV reactivation occurs in 90 % of patients after trigeminal root section, but not after trauma to previously denervated tissue. Herpetic disease may lead to dendrite formation in the cornea and geographic epithelial ulceration which if treated early may lead to minimal superficial corneal haze. Scrapings of the dendrites may show intra- and intercellular edema of the corneal epithelium with necrosis in the area of ulceration. Multinucleated epithelial cells and intranuclear eosinophilic inclusions may be seen. Virus may be isolated on culture from the smears, and PCR is usually positive. In the postinfectious period, epithelial defect may become indolent and the ulceration showing poor tendency towards healing. Viral replication does not occur in such lesions. Abnormal tear film function and decreased corneal sensation as well as antiviral toxicity may contribute to the development persistent postinfectious epithelial defect. Disciform keratitis may occur in some patients with recurrent herpetic keratitis. This is immune reaction to viral antigen.

Histologically, one may find lymphocytes and plasma cells within the stromal edema but usually no live virus. In some cases, herpes simplex viral particles may be seen in the corneal endothelium in cases of endotheliitis. Patients typically have well-circumscribed stromal edema with minimal infiltration and keratic precipitates.

Corneal immune rings and interstitial keratitis are also seen in herpetic keratitis. Uveitis and trabeculitis may occur, and some patients with keratouveitis may have an increase in the intraocular pressure which can be acute or chronic (Table 7.3).

Table 7.3 Causes of dendritic corneal lesions [8]

Herpes simplex virus
Varicella-zoster virus
Healing of epithelial defect
Richner-Hanhart syndrome (tyrosinemia type II)
Autoimmune polyendocrine syndrome type 1 (APS-1)
Keratosis follicularis
Thygeson's superficial punctate keratitis
Soft contact lens wear

Table 7.4 Differentiation between herpetic peripheral infiltration and staphylococcal peripheral infiltration

	Herpetic peripheral infiltrate	Staphylococcal peripheral infiltrate
Pain and photophobia	–	+
Early epithelial defect	+	–
Lucid interval	–	+
Decreased corneal sensation	+	–
Blepharitis	–	+
Cytology	Multinucleated cells	Polymorphonuclear cells

Patients with herpetic keratitis may present with unusual clinical presentation of peripheral corneal infiltration or a marginal ulcer. In these patients, differentiation from *Staphylococcus* marginal ulcer has to be made. Table 7.4 shows the differentiation between herpetic peripheral infiltration and staphylococcal peripheral infiltration [8].

The aftermath of interstitial herpetic keratitis is corneal scarring and vascularization with loss of vision. In patients who have been given topical steroids, secondary infection may occur or corneal descemetocele or perforation may ensue.

7.6.1 Laboratory Diagnosis

Corneal scrapings in corneal herpetic epithelial disease may be subjected to cytologic examination, PCR, culture, and electron microscopy. Giemsa-stained corneal scrapings may show multinucleated epithelial cells. Giemsa stain obscures nuclear details, and therefore, intranuclear inclusions typical of HSV infection cannot be seen. Specimens fixed with 95 % ethanol and stained with Papanicolaou (PA) method may demonstrate intranuclear inclusion bodies. Fluorescent antibody staining of the corneal scrapings can be done and may demonstrate the presence of herpetic antigens. Cultures taken from epithelial disease are usually positive, while cultures from geographic stromal or disciform lesions are much less likely to be positive. This denotes that the number of virus particles is low in such lesions. Cultures for bacteria and fungi should be obtained from patients with stromal infiltration where secondary infection is suspected.

7.6.2 Management of Epithelial Keratitis

The treatment epithelial dendrites or geographic corneal ulcers consists of applying topical anesthesia in the form of tetracaine 1 % or benoxinate 0.4 % and sweeping the epithelium with a sterile cotton applicator followed by topical application of acyclovir 3 % ophthalmic ointment 5 times daily or ganciclovir 0.15 % gel 5 times daily [9]. Antiviral therapy should be continued for a period of 7–10 days after. Antiviral agents such as idoxuridine, adenine arabinoside, and trifluridine are all toxic to the corneal epithelium and should be avoided [10]. An alternate therapy is trifluridine 1 % solution administered every 2 h. This dosage is used in the initial treatment period for 2–4 days and later decreased to 5 times daily. If there is lack of response or increase in the size of the ulcer, the therapy should be discontinued. Topical trifluridine may cause toxicity to the corneal epithelium.

7.7 Stromal Keratitis

In herpetic stromal keratitis, there is evidence of inflammatory response which requires the use of topical corticosteroids under antiviral coverage. Topical steroids can decrease the inflammation and minimize the damage to the stromal lamellae. At the same time, topical steroids may compromise the local immune response and may lead to viral replication. It is recognized from the study that delaying topical steroids did not have an adverse reaction on the corneal inflammation. It is, therefore, reasonable to start with antiviral agents initially and later add topical corticosteroids in the form of prednisolone acetate 1 % eye drops 4 times daily to be tapered over a period of 4–6 weeks [11, 12].

Patients with corneal thinning and perforation can complicate the stromal disease, and topical steroids may aggravate the corneal melting. It is, therefore, recommended to minimize the use of corticosteroids. One may shift from prednisolone acetate 1 % eye drops to fluorometholone 0.1 % eye drops to be used 3 or 4 times daily.

Soft contact lenses may promote epithelial healing and stop melting. If perforation occurs, cyanoacrylate glue may be used to seal small defect and reform the anterior chamber. Severe corneal scarring or corneal perforation may require tectonic graft or penetrating keratoplasty (PKP).

7.8 Disciform Keratitis

Disciform keratitis is an immune-mediated reaction to viral antigens [13]. The corneal epithelium is intact with central round corneal stromal infiltration and edema. Keratic precipitates may be present. Treatment of disciform keratitis includes topical prednisolone acetate 1 % eye drops 8 times daily for 3 days and later to be tapered to 4 times daily after 2–3 days. Steroids are given with appropriate topical or systemic antiviral therapy [13]. Topical therapy may consist of acyclovir 3 % ophthalmic ointment or ganciclovir 0.15 % gel. The corticosteroids and antiviral agents may later be tapered and adjusted according to the response of the corneal lesion. Disciform keratitis responds promptly to topical corticosteroids.

7.9 Penetrating Keratoplasty (PKP) in Herpetic Keratitis

Herpetic keratitis leads to upregulation of many cytokines and inflammatory response leading to upregulation of Class II antigens on the keratocytes and endothelial cell increasing the rate of graft rejection in patients undergoing PKP. The rate of rejection of the corneal graft in a patient with herpetic keratitis is high. Herpes virus in the trigeminal ganglion allows periodic shedding of the virus onto the cornea that may lead to recurrences of the herpetic disease in the corneal graft. Recurrence of herpetic keratitis in the corneal graft will increase the chances of corneal graft rejection because of the upregulation of many forms of cytokines and the expression of the HLA Class II antigen on the surface of the endothelial cells. It is estimated that 40–50 % of the corneal transplant cases may end up in corneal graft rejection. We have previously found out that preoperative oral valacyclovir at a dosage level of 500 mg orally twice daily for 2 days before the procedure and continued for up to 1 month after the procedure with topical ganciclovir 0.15 % gel given 4 times daily is safe and effective in the prevention of recurrences of herpetic disease *in* the corneal graft [14]. We had several cases that were kept on topical ganciclovir 0.15 % gel up to 2 years after the corneal transplantation with no evidence of recurrence or graft rejection [15]. Oral valacyclovir and topical ganciclovir 0.15 % are effective therapy for acute herpes simplex keratitis. Antiviral oral therapy and long-term prophylaxis is indicated in patients with keratitis and uveitis.

Herpetic keratitis is a recurrent disease, and prevention is essential in ameliorating the damage that occurs following recurrences of herpetic keratitis. Prophylactic therapy in herpetic keratitis consists of using valacyclovir 500 mg orally twice daily or topical ganciclovir 0.15 % gel twice daily. Sozen and associates [16] compared the efficacy of oral valacyclovir and topical acyclovir in the treatment of herpes simplex keratitis in a randomized prospective clinical trial. They found that systemic antiviral therapy is more effective in herpes simplex keratitis than topical acyclovir ointment.

7.10 Herpes Zoster Keratitis

Varicella-zoster virus is the cause of chicken pox and herpes zoster "shingles." The virus (*Herpesvirus varicellae*) is a distinct virus related to *Herpes* virus family. Other members of the

Herpes group include Herpes simplex, Cytomegalovirus (CMV), and Epstein-Barr virus (EBV). They are all morphologically similar and have icosahedral symmetry surrounding a spherical core of DNA. The initial infection of varicella-zoster virus leads to systemic varicella or chicken pox. Patient has a spontaneous recovery and sometimes the disease is asymptomatic. The virus remains latent in the body indefinitely and may reactivate later in life. Varicella occurs usually in childhood and is characterized disseminated cutaneous vesicular eruption that occurs after the onset of fever and flu-like illness.

7.11 Varicella Keratitis

Varicella-zoster virus may rarely cause keratitis in the primary form of the disease. It is characterized by conjunctivitis with watery discharge. A phlyctenule-like lesion may be seen at the limbus with punctate keratitis. Varicella may also cause dendritic keratitis [17]. The dendrites are fine linear and slightly elevated and nonulcerative. Disciform keratouveitis may occur occasionally [18].

7.11.1 Herpes Zoster Ophthalmicus

It is estimated that 20 % of unvaccinated adults develop disease at one time or another. Herpes zoster ophthalmicus (HZO) is much less common than varicella. It is postulated that with age there is decrease in the immunity to the varicella-zoster virus and this may lead to reactivation of the latent virus [19]. Other triggers to reactivation of latent varicella zoster are trauma, stress, systemic disease, surgery, immunosuppression, or disease such as leukemia and lymphoma.

Herpes zoster begins with a localized pain, tingling sensation, dysesthesia in the affected dermatome associated with fever and malaise. A cutaneous eruption occurs 3–4 days after with edematous and maculopapular eruption which becomes vesicular followed by ulceration and scarring [20]. The ophthalmic branch of the trigeminal nerve is involved and lead to swelling of the lids, conjunctival hyperemia. Involvement of the tip of the nose also known as, Hutchinson's sign, is evidence of nasociliary nerve distribution, and the ocular structures may be involved in 85 % of the cases. The cutaneous eruptions in Hutchinson's sign are *on* the tip of the nose [21]. The side of the midportion of the nose may also be involved. It should be kept in mind that herpes simplex dermatitis may have a dermatomal distribution and should be in the differential diagnosis of HZO. Recurrences of HZO is extremely rare but has been reported. The possible ocular manifestations of HZO are numerous. Herpes zoster can cause blepharitis, canaliculitis, episcleritis, conjunctivitis, keratitis, iridocyclitis, uveitis, retinal vasculitis, retinal necrosis, choroiditis, papillitis, and optic neuritis.

Herpes zoster keratitis may have variable ocular manifestations. The corneal epithelium shows punctate keratitis and fine with no terminal bulbs dendritic epithelial lesions and sometimes progress to geographic or neurotrophic corneal ulcerations. The corneal stroma may be involved showing disciform keratitis or nummular opacities. The nummular opacities are more frequently seen at the periphery. The lesions may cause corneal necrosis and melting, and corneal perforation may occur [22]. Lid corneal scarring and vascularization with lipid deposition in the cornea are seen. Zoster dendrites do not have terminal bulbs and are usually small, linear, and less ulcerative than herpetic keratitis caused by herpes simplex. The dendrites are softer and less branching than the herpes simplex dendrites. They tend to be small and in starfish configuration. Corneal sensation is diminished. Herpes zoster may cause disciform keratitis and sometimes keratouveitis [23]. The anterior uveitis may be associated with sector iris atrophy.

7.11.2 Laboratory Investigations

Corneal scrapings of the epithelial dendrites do not show viral particles. Multinucleated epithelial cells may be seen on Giemsa-stained corneal scrapings. Several predisposing diseases including leukemia and lymphoma and Hodgkin's disease as well as other neoplastic diseases, tuberculosis, syphilis, immunodeficiency syndrome, and systemic immunosuppression have been associated with HZO. Most patients with ophthalmic zoster are otherwise healthy.

Systemic evaluation should be done in patients who are young or in patients who have history suggestive of existing systemic diseases.

7.11.3 Management

Topical management of herpes zoster keratitis consists of ganciclovir 0.15 % gel given initially 8 times daily for 1 week and later decreased to 5 times daily for another 2 weeks. Skin lesions may be treated with topical 5 % acyclovir skin ointment to be applied 5 times daily [24]. In patients with zoster keratitis, there is element of inflammatory reaction. Systemic steroids are indicated for vision-threatening lesions such as retinitis or optic neuritis. Dosage for oral prednisone for adults is 40–60 mg daily followed by quick tapering to lower levels adjusted according to the clinical response. The treatment with systemic steroids should also be combined with valacyclovir 1,000 mg 3 times daily for 1 week tapered to 1 g orally twice daily after 1 week.

Systemic antivirals are initiated for anterior and posterior uveitis especially in vision-threatening conditions like retinitis, optic neuritis [25], and glaucoma. Since authors advised to treat retinal neurosis in herpes zoster with intravitreal injection of ganciclovir and dexamethasone.

Nonhealing postzoster epithelial defects are secondary to neurotrophic ulceration and should be treated with artificial tears and lubricating ointments, patching, and soft contact lenses. Topical preservatives such as benzalkonium chloride should be avoided [26]. Tarsorrhaphy or conjunctival flap may be indicated in cases with exposure keratitis. Amniotic membrane transplantation [27], topical autologous serum, and topical Cocicol eye drops may help in the healing of a persistent epithelial defect. Topical corticosteroids should be given in chronic stromal inflammation and anterior uveitis [26]. Autologous serum, topical exogenous nerve growth factor can also be used.

Corneal perforation of the cornea is treated with cyanoacrylate adhesive and soft contact lens. Keratoplasty may be considered at a later stage following complete healing and decrease in the inflammatory reaction.

Postzoster neuralgia [28] is a condition that may cause severe pain, tingling sensation, numbness, and paresthesias. The condition may be treated with oral analgesics or neuroleptics such as chlorpromazine, amitriptyline, gabapentin, or Lyrica. Because depression coexists with postzoster neuralgia, antidepressive therapy may enable the patients to tolerate the pain. Topical capsaicin 0.025 % dermatologic cream (Zostrix) or 8 % patch is reported to alleviate postzoster neuralgia in some cases. Capsaicin is applied 4 times daily to the skin of the affected dermatome. Lidocaine 5 % patch is more efficient than capsaicin topically [29].

7.12 Varicella-Zoster Vaccine (Zostavax)

Varicella-zoster vaccination is recommended for individuals over the age of 50 years. Vaccination helps in the prevention of herpes zoster ophthalmicus and postherpetic neuralgia.

Zostavax is a life-attenuated varicella-zoster virus that has been demonstrated to decrease the incidence of herpes zoster infection by 51 % over a period of 3 years. A total of 38,546 patients who were 60 years of age or older were enrolled prospectively in the study. The group clearly demonstrated that in the short term the vaccine can dramatically reduce the burden of HZV infections. The effects of this vaccine on children remain to be elucidated. It has postulated that decreasing the incidence of primary infection among children would effectively reduce the burden of herpes zoster. Vaccine may also be of help in patients with latent infection and may decrease the incidence of HZO [30].

7.13 Epstein-Barr Virus Keratitis

Epstein-Barr (EB) virus keratitis is another member of the *Herpesviridae* group. It is the most common cause of infectious mononucleosis syndrome characterized by lymphadenopathy, fever, pharyngitis, headache, hepatitis, skin rash, and sometimes arthritis and hepatomegaly and splenomegaly.

7.13.1 Clinical Findings

EB virus may cause nummular keratitis or well-circumscribed disciform lesions in the cornea. The lesions appear late in the course of the infectious mononucleosis syndrome. The disease may be associated with mild nonspecific conjunctivitis. EB virus also can cause dryness, oculoglandular syndrome, uveitis, and choroiditis. Occasionally, patients may develop optic (disk) nerve head edema (papillitis) and paresis of the oculomotor nerves [31].

7.13.2 Laboratory Investigations

Laboratory investigations include blood smears to determine the presence of atypical lymphocytes in the blood smears and positive neutrophil antibody response. PCR can be positive for an EB virus in case of uveitis, and EB virus and specific antibodies and core and capsid antigens may be detected [32].

7.13.3 Management

EB virus keratitis lesions may be treated with topical corticosteroids in the form of fluorometholone 0.1 % eye drops 4 times daily. The lesions may show spontaneous recovery and decrease in the redness and photophobia. No systemic therapy is indicated.

7.14 Cytomegalovirus Keratitis

Recent studies have shown that cytomegalovirus (CMV) can cause keratitis and anterior uveitis in immunocompetent hosts. The disease is usually unilateral and characterized by history of redness, photophobia, and decrease in vision. Patients develop increased intraocular pressure and endotheliitis with evidence of corneal edema and large keratic precipitates in a triangular fashion. No epithelial disease is noted in the cornea. Anterior corneal edema is observed. The anterior chamber shows cells and flare with evidence of iritis and cyclitis [33].

7.14.1 Laboratory Diagnosis

Aqueous specimens obtained from such patients may show CMV nucleotides by PCR [33].

7.14.2 Management

Patients with CMV (anterior) keratitis and uveitis may be treated with topical ganciclovir 0.15 % gel applied 8 times daily. The treatment is continued for 1 week and later decreased to 5 times daily or with systemic and intraocular ganciclovir [34]. Systemic valganciclovir and intravitreal ganciclovir has been used in some patients with CMV (retinitis) uveitis and keratitis [35].

Topical steroids in the form of prednisolone acetate 1 % eye drops 4 times daily may help the inflammatory reactions in the anterior chamber and decrease the corneal edema.

The intraocular pressure should be treated with beta-blockers, carbonic anhydrase inhibitors, and prostaglandin analogues. Oral therapy with valganciclovir (Valcyte) can be given at a dosage level of 450 mg tablets orally twice daily for 2 weeks. In severe cases like necrotizing retinitis, ganciclovir 0.5 mg/kg can be given intravenously every 12 h. Intravitreal ganciclovir can be given at a dosage level of 2 mg one injection twice a week for 2 weeks. Foscarnet can also be given. Formiversin was approved by the Food and Drug Administration (FDA) in 1998 for intravitreal injection. Ganciclovir intraocular implant was also used to treat CMV retinitis [36].

7.15 Fungal Keratitis

Fungal infection of the cornea, fungal keratitis or keratomycosis, is a serious ocular condition. It may eventuate in serious complications. Early diagnosis and prompt treatment are mandatory for arresting the disease process and inducing rehabilitation of the ocular surface. Fungal keratitis occurs in eyes with preexisting ocular surface disease. Fungal keratitis is difficult to diagnose and may present with a clinical picture similar to some bacterial infections or herpetic corneal disease. In such patients, a high index of suspicion is required, and laboratory identification of the fungal corneal pathogen is essential. Incomplete and inadequate therapy and inaccurate or delay in diagnosis may lead to poor outcome and visual loss. It is, therefore, conceded that successful management of fungal keratitis requires early diagnosis, prompt treatment, and close follow-up.

The use and abuse of corticosteroids may promote fungal replication and corneal invasion and lead to poor outcome. Fungal keratitis may be caused by filamentous fungi or by yeast. The disease is common in tropical climate and warm weather [37]. The disease is associated with outdoor activities and occupations. The most frequently encountered causes of fungal keratitis include *Fusarium* species, *Aspergillus* species, and *Candida* [37, 38]. Other causes of fungal keratitis include *Acremonium*, *Alternaria*, *Fusarium*, *Cephalosporium*, *Curvularia*, *Penicillium*, *Sporothrix*, *Mucor*, *Rhizopus*, and other fungi that are rarely seen. Predisposing factors to fungal keratitis include a compromised ocular surface, atopic disease, long-term use of topical corticosteroids, exposure keratopathy, keratoconjunctivitis sicca, neurotrophic keratitis, immunosuppression, agricultural occupation, vernal keratoconjunctivitis, trauma, older patients, herpetic keratitis, and soft contact lens use [38]. *Fusarium* is the most common genus of filamentous fungi responsible for fungal keratitis in the southern part of the United States, while *Aspergillus* species are more common in India [39] and Saudi Arabia [37].

7.15.1 Clinical Findings

Fungal keratitis is commonly found in patients who sustained superficial corneal trauma. The incubation period of the fungus may take 2–21 days depending on the type of organisms and the size of the inoculum as well as the immune status of the host. It should be kept in mind that there are no pathognomonic features of fungal keratitis. Certain findings, however, may suggest the presence of fungal keratitis. Fungal keratitis is an insidious slowly progressive ulceration of the cornea associated with corneal infiltration. The corneal infiltration consists of intrastromal abscess or discrete elevated plaque on the corneal epithelium. The fungal infiltration is characterized by feathery edges [40]. The ulcer base is usually dry, gray, or white texture. There is thickening and elevation of the borders with hypertrophic corneal epithelium. Stromal infiltration may radiate from the ulcer edge leading to small round satellite lesions [40]. A ring infiltration may be adjacent to the ulcer representing an immune response. The ulcer borders are irregular and elevated with fine branching infiltration. Folds in Descemet membrane may be seen, and stromal inflammation is observed. In some patients, an endothelial plaque composed of fibrin may be visualized over the endothelium. The plaque may be present in the absence of a hypopyon. The hypopyon is frequently observed in the anterior chamber and may contain fungal elements in contrast to bacterial keratitis which is usually sterile. The presence of keratoconjunctivitis sicca, neurotrophic keratitis, or herpetic keratitis should be ruled out in the absence of trauma. The fungal keratitis is usually an indolent form of keratitis that may last for days or weeks.

7.15.2 Laboratory Diagnosis

The clinical diagnosis of fungal keratitis should be confirmed by laboratory investigation. Following instillation of topical unpreserved anesthetic such as benoxinate 0.4 % or proparacaine hydrochloride 0.5 %, corneal scrapings are obtained for cytologic evaluation and cultures. Corneal scrapings are placed on precleaned glass slides, and one slide is immediately fixed in absolute methanol for 5 min. Corneal biopsy specimens are usually fixed in 10 % formalin solution for light microscopy and glutaraldehyde for electron microscopy. One slide is kept as reserve, while the other slides are stained with Gram stain, Giemsa stain, Grocott-Gomori methenamine-silver stain, and periodic acid-Schiff (PAS) stain. An anterior chamber paracentesis may be obtained in patients with suspected fungal endophthalmitis. Corneal scrapings are inoculated on blood agar, chocolate agar, thioglycolate broth, and Sabouraud's agar. A modification of Sabouraud (Emmond's medium) consisting of pH7.0 without cycloheximide may be used. Blood agar can support the growth of many fungi. Sabouraud's agar contains 50 μg of gentamicin to inhibit bacterial contamination. Sabouraud's agar plates are maintained at room temperature (25 °C). Liquid-infusion medium may be used as an adjunct to solid fungal media. The Grocott-Gomori methenamine-silver stain is a stain to identify fungi. PAS stain is useful for identifying fungal elements in tissue and cytological preparation. The carbohydrates in the fungal cell wall react with PAS and stain magenta. With this stain, the fungi appear pink with dark blue against the yellow background. Both Giemsa and Gram stains may also selectively stain fungi. The proteinaceous debris, however, may reduce the contrast between fungi and the background. Most fungi appear to be Gram positive. The use of potassium hydroxide 10 or 20 % is unreliable because of the presence of very few hyphae in the slides. Calcofluor white is another method of staining fungi. It makes the living and dead fungi visible under fluorescent microscope.

Fungal cultures should be checked daily. Growth may appear within 2–3 days. Delayed growth is unusual, and negative cultures do not rule out fungal keratitis. Keratectomy specimens or corneal biopsies may be obtained for histopathologic evaluations and staining with hematoxylin and eosin (H & E), Grocott-Gomori methenamine-silver stain and PAS stain. Confocal microscopy seems to be accurate and reliable diagnostic modality in the etiologic diagnosis of fungal keratitis [41].

7.15.3 Management

Fungal keratitis should be treated with topical agents that can penetrate the corneal tissue and reach the fungi in the stroma. Superficial yeast infection in the cornea such as *Candida* species may be treated with nystatin which is a polyene antifungal agent. It is found in a dermatologic preparation (Mycostatin ointment) containing 100,000 units per gram which is well tolerated when applied topically every 4–6 h. Nystatin, however, is a large molecular weight and, therefore, penetrates the cornea poorly.

Natamycin is a macrolide antibiotic produced by *Streptomyces natalensis* and is currently the only topical ophthalmic antifungal agent available commercially. Natamycin is a broad spectrum antifungal agent and has been used effectively in the treatment of fungal keratitis caused by *Fusarium*, *Cephalosporium*, *Aspergillus*, and *Candida* species [42]. Natamycin is poorly soluble in water but does form a stable microsuspension and adheres to the cornea at the site of epithelial defects. Natamycin demonstrates poor penetration and is less effective in the treatment of fungal keratitis with deep stromal infiltrates [43]. Natamycin 5 % ophthalmic suspension should be applied topically every hour. Intensive topical antifungal therapy is continued until clinical improvement is noted. Signs of improvement and resolution of the infection are demonstrated by rounding up the ulcer margin, decrease in the infiltrate, disappearance of the satellite lesions, healing of the epithelial defect, decrease in the corneal edema, and absorption of the hypopyon. Pain is decreased and the ocular inflammation subsides. Amphotericin B can be compounded as topical drops at the concentration level of 0.15 % eye drops. Amphotericin B is prepared in sterile water. Initial therapy may include topical administration every hour, and the medication may be gradually tapered after a favorable clinical response [44]. Amphotericin B is toxic to the tissues and can cause irritation and, therefore, should not be given subconjunctivally. Subconjunctival injection may lead to necrosis of the conjunctiva. Fluconazole (2 mg/ml) is available for injection and is well tolerated eye drops [45]. The intravenous injection can be prepared as topical and can be given subconjunctivally at the same concentration.

Fluconazole is effective in the treatment of *Candida* keratitis. Fluconazole may also be given orally 200 mg as loading dose than 150 mg/daily and 2 % subconjunctivally [46].

Voriconazole is effective against *Fusarium* [47], *Aspergillus*, and *Candida*. The drug can be prepared as 1 % eye drops and may be given every hour as initial loading dose and later shifted to every 2 h [48]. The drug is well tolerated. Voriconazole can be given subconjunctivally and also intravenously. Voriconazole 25 μgm in 0.1 ml can be given as an intrastromal injection at the site of the corneal infiltrates using a 30 g needle [49]. This can be done under topical anesthesia. Intrastromal injection has to be given every three days. Voriconazole 1 % eye drops can be prepared from the intravenous preparation (V Fend Pfizer, Inc.). Other imidazoles are miconazole which is available for injection 10 mg/ml and may be given topically and subconjunctivally 10 mg in 1 ml. Other imidazoles include ketoconazole and itraconazole. Ketoconazole can be given 200 mg orally per day but may cause hepatotoxicity, and liver function tests should be obtained. Miconazole may demonstrate good ocular penetration following topical, subconjunctival, or intravenous administration with no ocular or systemic toxicity. Miconazole may be helpful for deep fungal keratitis especially *Aspergillus*. Topical miconazole should be given 10 mg/ml eye drops every hour and subconjunctivally 10 mg in 1 ml.

In general, imidazole compound should not be combined with polyenes like amphotericin B because of their drug interaction. The imidazoles decrease the ergosterol synthesis which is the target of amphotericin B.

Corneal scrapings during treatment can help in debridement and also allow the antifungal agent to penetrate the corneal stroma. Corneal scraping can remove the dead cells and the necrotic tissue. Superficial keratectomy may be performed for small ulcers especially when they are covering the visual axis.

Conjunctival flap or amniotic membranes may be required in indolent fungal corneal ulcers not responsive to medical therapy. The conjunctiva flap should be thin and avascular and sutured with minimal tension to prevent retraction. Penetrating keratoplasty (PKP) may be performed at a later date following resolution of the infection and the ocular inflammation. Therapeutic PKP may be indicated in deep keratomycosis with impending corneal perforation [50]. Although PKP may be successful in eliminating residual infection and restoring the anatomic integrity of the globe, prognosis for visual recovery is poor [50]. Good visual outcome may be achieved with PKP in central corneal ulcers without hypopyon or significant anterior chamber reaction. Postoperative complications following PKP include peripheral anterior posterior synechiae, pupillary membranes, macular edema, retinal detachment, secondary glaucoma, cataract formation, as well as corneal graft rejection [50]. If there is no impending perforation, PKP may be performed several months after the conjunctival flap has healed and after dissecting away the flap from the cornea. Therapeutic keratoplasty is most successful when surgery is performed early enough to remove all the corneal pathology. Corneal cross-linking has been shown to be safe and effective in small early superficial fungal keratitis in experimental animals [51]. Finally, excimer laser lamellar keratectomy has been performed in experimental *Candida* keratitis and achieved sterilization on culture and histopathologically in all corneal tissues. These therapeutic modality should, however, be carried out early in superficial fungal keratitis.

7.16 Parasitic Keratitis

The most frequently encountered causes of parasitic keratitis include *Acanthamoeba, Leishmania, Microsporidia, and Onchocerca.*

7.16.1 Acanthamoeba Keratitis

Acanthamoeba species may cause an indolent form of parasitic keratitis. The organism has been identified as an important cause of ocular morbidity and has been increasing in prevalence over the past two decades [52]. *Acanthamoeba* is a free-living protozoa which is ubiquitous in nature and is found in soil, drinking water, stagnated water, swimming pools, and hot tubs. The most common species of *Acanthamoeba* that have been reported to cause

Acanthamoeba keratitis include *Acanthamoeba polyphaga*, *Acanthamoeba castellanii*, and *Acanthamoeba hatchetti.* It has also been isolated from animal feces. *Acanthamoeba* exists in two forms – the trophozoites form which is active motile and the dormant original double-walled structure which allows the amoeba to survive in hostile environment. The encysted form is triggered by food deprivation and desiccation. Several predisposing factors may lead to *Acanthamoeba* keratitis including poor hygiene with soft contact lens wearing, trauma, exposure to stagnated water, and immunocompromised patients. The majority of cases of *Acanthamoeba* keratitis have been reported in contact lens wearer [53, 54].

7.16.2 Clinical Findings

Patients with *Acanthamoeba* keratitis give history of pain, discomfort, irritation, tearing, and blurring of vision. In some patients, pain may be severe and much worse than what is expected in the clinical findings.

Biomicroscopy shows an indolent keratitis and may have variable clinical manifestations. Patients with *Acanthamoeba* keratitis may be mistaken for herpetic keratitis. Dendrite-like lesions may be seen or localized circumscribed geographic ulcer. In addition, patients may have infiltration of the cornea with peripheral ring infiltrates and severe inflammation with stromal keratitis which may lead to corneal stromal melting and descemetocele formation and perforation [55]. One characteristic finding in *Acanthamoeba* keratitis is the finding of perineuritis of the corneal nerves referred to as radial keratoneuritis. Satellite subepithelial infiltrates may be seen similar to those seen in patients with viral keratitis. The corneal epithelium may be irregular and elevated in the edges with recurrent erosions. The corneal infection may be associated with concurrent bacterial infections.

7.16.3 Laboratory Diagnosis

Corneal scrapings may be obtained and placed in liquid medium which can be centrifuged and examined by microscopy without staining. Occasionally, trophozoites are seen on the slide prepared from the sediment after centrifugation of corneal scrapings placed in Page's solution. *Acanthamoeba* can survive on cultured corneal epithelium and stromal keratocytes and can maintain its growth by nutritional support. In mixed infections, *Acanthamoeba* can thrive on bacteria, and it has been suggested that initial infections from contaminated soil or water may induced a mixed infection of *Acanthamoeba* and bacterial infection leading to the initial support of *Acanthamoeba* [56]. Corneal scrapings may be stained with Giemsa stain, Gram stain, and Wright stain. For patients with deep stromal involvement, corneal biopsy is necessary to make the diagnosis of *Acanthamoeba* keratitis. Hematoxylin-Eosin-stained sections of corneal biopsy specimens may show *Acanthamoeba* organisms both in trophozoites and the cysts. Trichrome stain, periodic acid-Schiff reagent, and Gomori methenamine-silver stain may also show the organism. Indirect fluorescent antibody staining techniques may be utilized to show the *Acanthamoeba* in the tissues [57]. Calcofluor white, a chemofluorescent stain is absorbed by the cellulose components of the cyst wall of *Acanthamoeba* and can highlight the organism in tissues [58]. *Acanthamoeba* may be cultured on blood agar, chocolate Agar, Sabouraud's agar, and Löwestein-Jensen agar at 25C or 37C. On the other hand, optimal recovery of the organism can be achieved by the inoculation of the corneal scrapings specimens on non-nutrient agar coated with a bacterial overlay of *Escherichia coli* (*E. coli*) which provides nutrition for the *Acanthamoeba*. The culture is positive when wavy cracks are seen on the surface of the agar plate indicating motile trophozoites that are engulfing the bacteria. *Acanthamoeba* may be stored in Page's solution if culture material is not available. Electron microscopy can show the trophozoites and the cyst of *Acanthamoeba.*

Confocal microscopy has also been helpful in the diagnosis of in vivo *Acanthamoeba* and in the diagnosis of corneal stromal cysts and trophozoites in vivo [59].

7.16.4 Management

Corneal debridement and removal of necrotic tissue can help in the healing of the ulcers, and the material can be used for diagnosis of *Acanthamoeba* keratitis. The debridement of *Acanthamoeba* keratitis should be with combination therapy of topical neomycin ointment, propamidine isethionate and one of the imidazoles (such as miconozole, fluconazole, ketoconazole or intraconazole); and polyhexamethylenebiguanide (PHMB) [60] or chlorhexidine 0.02% eyedrops. Bang and associates [61] have reported successful treatment of three eyes with resistant *Acanthamoeba* keratitis with 1 % voriconazole. Voriconazole can be given 25 μgm/0.1 ml intrastromally with a 30 g needle. Voriconazole has to be compounded for topical use at a dosage level of 1 or 2 % eye drops.

In patients with severe *Acanthamoeba* keratitis, corneal scarring may occur, and patients may require PKP at a later stage when the eye has no evidence of inflammation.

7.17 Microsporidia Keratitis

Microsporidium is a unicellular parasite that may cause disease in man. *Microsporidia* are primitive eukaryotes that lack mitochondria, initially recognized as protozoa and now regarded as fungi. Several intestinal organisms have shown to cause keratitis and keratoconjunctivitis. Immunocompetent and immunodeficient individuals may acquire the disease. *Microsporidia* are small, oval, obligate intracellular organisms widely distributed among both vertebrates and invertebrates [62]. They were believed to be protists under *Archezoa*, but now they are classified as fungi. They are opportunistic organisms. The ocular manifestations of microsporidiosis include superficial diffuse punctate keratitis, conjunctivitis, and stromal keratitis. Immunocompromised individuals may develop keratoconjunctivitis [63, 64]. The most commonly encountered genus is *Encephalitozoon encephalae dejune* while stromal keratitis is caused by *Nosema and Microsporidia.* The disease starts in the corneal epithelium with diffuse epithelial keratitis and later may progress to cause stromal keratitis. In *Nosema* keratitis, the deep stromal layers of the cornea may be involved and patients may show evidence of folds in Descemet membrane [65]. Extensive inflammatory reactions are noted in the cornea and patients may have marked decrease in vision.

7.17.1 Laboratory Diagnosis

Corneal scrapings are obtained from patients with keratitis, while patients with keratoconjunctivitis conjunctival scrapings may be obtained. Corneal scrapings are placed onto clean slides and stained with Giemsa and Gram stains and Acid-Fast stain [66]. Scrapings are also cultured to rule out bacterial or fungal infections. *Microsporidia* cannot be cultured but can be seen by special stains including 1 % acid-fast stain, modified trichrome stain, Gram stain, and Gomori methenamine-silver stain. The organism appears as small, oval bodies that are Gram negative. The corneal scrapings may be fixed with 2 % glutaraldehyde for electron microscopy and blood test for HIV 1 and 2 should be performed. PCR and indirect immunofluorescent antibody (IFA) staining method can also be used.

7.17.2 Management

Patients with *Microsporidia* keratitis should be given albendazole 400 mg orally twice daily for a period 4–6 weeks, and liver function test should be monitored. Patients may be treated with topical fumagillin 0.113 mg/ml eye drops initially every 2 h for a period of 2 weeks and later decreased in frequency to 4 times daily for a period of 6 weeks [67]. In addition, compounded fluconazole or voriconazole eye drops may be given [68].

7.18 Leishmaniasis

Leishmania species may cause systemic or cutaneous disease in man. *Leishmania donovani* causes visceral leishmaniasis kala-azar and patients with fever and hepatosplenomegaly [69], while *Leishmania tropica* causes localized papule (oriental sore) that becomes ulcerative over a few weeks or months at the site of inoculation by the insect vector, sand fly, *Phlebotomus* genus. Spontaneous healing ensues following the development of immunity to the parasites. Scarring may occur.

7.18.1 Clinical Finding

The sandfly bites occur on exposed areas of the skin and for this reason, the face is frequently affected, and consequently ulceration of the cheeks or eyelids may occur. The main ocular manifestations include the lesions on the eyelid which may lead to cicatricial ectropion and exposure keratopathy. Patients may develop nummular keratitis. The keratitis is due to the hypersensitivity to the parasite. Cicatricial and nummular keratitis have been observed in patients with cutaneous leishmaniasis. Intraretinal hemorrhages have been described by some authors following visceral leishmaniasis [70].

7.18.2 Laboratory Diagnosis

Microscopic examination of the skin scrapings from the base of the ulcer may reveal the presence of the *Leishmania* parasites. The slide may be stained with Giemsa and examined by light microscope.

7.18.3 Treatment

Treatment of cutaneous and mucocutaneous leishmaniasis is with sodium stibogluconate or meglumine antimoniate 20 mg/kg/day for 10 days; amphotericin B is the treatment of choice for visceral leishmaniasis [71]. Patients who have one single cutaneous lesion due to *Leishmania tropica* and the lesion is of no cosmetic damage may be treated with localized cryotherapy. On the other hand, these patients who developed generalized leishmaniasis may be given pentamidine isethionate with daily dose of 4 mg/kg body weight for a period of 2 weeks.

7.19 Keratitis Due to Onchocerciasis

Onchocerciasis is a disease caused by *Onchocerca volvulus*. This is a filarial parasite. Onchocerciasis is also known as African river blindness, and the vector is the blackfly *Simulium damnosum*, *yahense*, and other subspecies of the genus *Simulium*. The disease is common in sub-Saharan Africa and Latin America. Onchocerciasis is a common cause of infectious blindness worldwide [72]. The disease can be transmitted transplacentally from an infected mother to her fetus.

7.19.1 Clinical Findings

Infected individuals with *Onchocerca volvulus* develop subcutaneous nodules of the adult form of male and female *Onchocerca*, and the female produces millions of microfilaria, but the nodules are on the head, and the microfilariae migrate in the skin and may reach the eye. The microfilariae cause conjunctivitis and keratitis. The keratitis is usually nummular at the site of the death of the microfilariae resulting from localized inflammatory reaction which is well circumscribed. The microfilariae may reach the anterior chamber and can be seen easily with a slit lamp. The death of the microfilariae in the eye leads to an inflammatory reaction and may cause uveitis. In the cornea, it causes punctate keratitis with localized infiltration that appears as ill-defined (snowflakes) feathery round opacity measuring 0.5 mm or less. The inflammation may lead to sclerosing keratitis, anterior uveitis, secondary glaucoma, cataract, and the microfilaria may migrate to the posterior segment leading to chorioretinitis with optic atrophy with pigmented chorioretinal lesions [73].

7.19.2 Laboratory Diagnosis

Skin snip for specimens can be taken to identify the *Onchocerca volvulus*. Serological tests like ELISA and Western blot for antigen detection can also be used. PCR, ultrasound of the nodules, and sclerocorneal biopsy are also helpful.

7.19.3 Treatment

The treatment of choice for onchocerciasis is ivermectin 0.2 mg/kg orally once daily. Ivermectin has no effect on the adult worm and has narrow therapeutic window and is a good prophylactic agent for *Onchocerca volvulus* [74]. Other therapeutic modalities include suramin diethylcarbamazine, doxycycline, rifampin, and azithromycin. Excision of the nodules may help in decreasing the load of the microfilaria. Patients with *Onchocerca* keratitis may require topical use of corticosteroids in the form of fluorometholone 0.1 % eye drops 3 times daily and cycloplegics during the treatment with ivermectin. This will reduce the photophobia and corneal inflammation. The ocular pressure should be monitored. Patients with secondary glaucoma may be treated with topical beta-blockers and carbonic anhydrase inhibitors. PKP can be considered if vision is compromised from corneal scarring.

Compliance with Ethical Requirements

Conflict of Interest The authors declare that they have no conflict of interest.

Informed Consent No human studies were carried out by the authors for this article.

Animal Studies No animal studies were carried out by the authors for this article.

References

1. Cokingtin CD, Hyndiuk RA. Bacterial keratitis. In: Tabbara KF, Hyndiuk RA, editors. Infections of the eye. 2nd ed. Boston: Little, Brown and Company; 1996. p. 326.
2. Leibowitz HM. Clinical evaluation of ciprofloxacin 0.3 % ophthalmic solution for treatment of bacterial keratitis. Am J Ophthalmol. 1991;1123(4 Suppl):34S–47.
3. Yanoff M, Duker J. Ophthalmology. In: James J, editor. Augsburger. 3rd ed. Edinburgh: Mosby Elsevier; 2009. p. 274–88.
4. Lucht E, Brytting M, Bjerregaard L, Julander I, Linde A. Shedding of cytomegalovirus and herpesviruses 6, 7, and 8 in saliva of human immunodeficiency virus type 1-infected patients and healthy controls. Clin Infect Dis. 1998;27(1):137–41.
5. Hanshaw JB. Herpes virus hominis infections in the fetus and the newborn. Am J Dis Child. 1973;126:546.
6. Cook SD, Hill JH. Herpes simplex virus. Molecular biology and the possibility of corneal latency. Surv Ophthalmol. 1991;36(2):140–8.
7. Saini JS, Agarwal R. Clinical pattern of recurrent herpes simplex keratitis. Indian J Ophthalmol. 1999;47(11):11–4.
8. Hyndiuk RA, Glasser DB. Herpes simplex keratitis. In: Hyndiuk RA, Tabbara KF, editors. Infections of the eye. 2nd ed. Boston: Little, Brown and Company; 1996. p. 370–2.
9. Tabbara KF. Treatment of herpetic keratitis. Ophthalmology. 2005;112(9):1640.
10. Wilhelmus KR. The treatment of herpes simplex virus epithelial keratitis. Trans Am Ophthalmol Soc. 2000;98:505–32.
11. Knickelbein JE, Hendricks RL, Charukamnoetkanok P. Management of herpes simplex virus stromal keratitis: an evidence-based review. Surv Ophthalmol. 2009;54(2):226–34. doi:10.1016/j.survophthal.2008.12.004.
12. Wilhelmus KF, Gee L, Houck WW, Kurimij N, Jones DB, et al. Herpetic Eye Disease Study. A controlled trial of topical corticosteroids for herpes simplex stromal keratitis. Ophthalmology. 1994;101(12):1883–95.
13. Porter SM, Patterson A, Kho P. A comparison of local and systemic acyclovir in the management of herpetic disciform keratitis. Br J Ophthalmol. 1990;74(5):283–5.
14. Garcia DD, Farjo Q, Musch DC, Sugar A. Effect of prophylactic oral acyclovir after penetrating keratoplasty for herpes simplex keratitis. Cornea. 2007;26(8):930–4.
15. Tabbara KF, Al Balushi N. Topical ganciclovir in the treatment of acute herpetic keratitis. Clin Ophthalmol. 2010;4:905–12.
16. Sozen E, Avundeek AM, Akyd N. Comparison of efficacy of oral valacyclovir and topical acyclovir in the treatment of herpes simplex keratitis. A randomized clinical trial. Chemotherapy. 2006;52:29–31.
17. Borit J, Pentelei-Molnar J, Lazaro R. Varicella dendritic keratitis. Invest Ophthalmol Vis Sci. 1974;13(10):764–70.
18. Wilhelmus KR, Hamill MB, Jones DB. Varicella disciform stromal keratitis. Am J Ophthalmol. 1991;111(5):575–80.
19. Kennedy PG. Varicella-zoster virus latency in human ganglia. Rev Med Virol. 2002;12(5):327–34.
20. Pavan-Langston D. Herpes zoster ophthalmicus. Neurology. 1995;45(12 Suppl 8):S50–1.
21. Hutchinson J. Clinical report on herpes zoster frontalis ophthalmicus. Ophthal Hosp Rep. 1864;3(72):865–6; J R Lond Ophthal Hosp Lond. 1865;5:191.
22. Liesegang TG. Corneal complications from herpes zoster ophthalmicus. Ophthalmology. 1985;42(3):316–24.
23. Noseri A, Good WV, Cunningham T. Herpes zoster virus sclerokeratitis and uveitis in a child following varicella vaccination. Am J Ophthalmol. 2003;135(3):415–7.
24. Dworkin RH, Johnson RW. Recommendation for the management of herpes zoster. Clin Infect Dis. 2007;44:S1–26.

25. Wang AG, Liu ZH, Hsu WM, Lee AF, Yen MY. Optic neuritis in herpes zoster ophthalmicus. Jpn J Ophthalmol. 2000;44(5):550–4.
26. Lambiase A, Paolo R, Luigi A, Bionini S. Management of neurotrophic keratopathy. Curr Opin Ophthalmol. 1999;10(4):270–6.
27. Khokhar S, Natung T, Sony P, Sharma N, Agarwal N, Vajpayee RB. Amniotic membrane transplantation as refractory neutrophic corneal ulcers. Cornea. 2005;24(6):654–60.
28. Menke JJ, Heins JR. Treatment of postherpetic neuralgia. J Am Pharm Assoc (Wash). 1996;39(2):217–21.
29. Nalamanchu S, Morley-Foster P. Diagnosing and managing postherpetic neuralgia. Drugs Aging. 2012;29(11):863–9.
30. Oxman MN, et al., Shingles prevention study group. A vaccine to prevent herpes zoster and postherpetic neuralgia in older adults. N Engl J Med 2005;352: 2271–84. doi: 10.1056/NEJMoa051016
31. Matoba AY. Ocular disease associated with Epstein-Barr virus infection. Surv Ophthalmol. 1990;35(2):145–50.
32. Ongkosuwito JV, Ongkosuwito JV, Allegonda van der L, Bruinnenberg M, Wienssen van dorn M, Feron EJC, Bhyong C, de Keizer R, Klok A, Kijlstra A. Increased presence of EBV DNA in ocular fluid samples from HIV negative immunocompromised patients with uveitis. Br J Ophthalmol. 1998;82:245–51.
33. Chee SP, Bacsal K, Jap A, Se-Thoe SY, Cheng CL, Tan BH. Clinical features of cytomegalovirus anterior uveitis in immunocompetent patients. Am J Ophthalmol. 2008;145(5):834-40. doi: 10.1016/j.ajo.2007.12.015. Epub 2008 Feb 6.
34. Mietz H, Aisenbrey S, Bartz-Schmidt KU, Bamborschke S, Krieglstein GK. Ganciclovir for the treatment of anterior uveitis. Graefes Arch Clin Exp Ophthalmol. 2000;238(11):905–9.
35. Gupta S, Vemulakonda GA, Suhler EB, Yeh S, Albini TA, Mandelcorn E, Flaxel CJ. Cytomegalovirus retinitis in the absence of AIDS. Can J Ophthalmol. 2013;48(2):126–9.
36. Kappel PJ, Charonis AC, Holland GN, Narayanan R, Kulkarni AD, Yu F, Boyer DS. Outcomes associated with ganciclovir implants in patient with AIDS-related cytomegalovirus retinitis. Ophthalmology. 2006;113(4):683.e1–8.
37. Khairallah SH, Byrne KA, Tabbara KF. Fungal keratitis in Saudi Arabia. Doc Ophthalmol. 1992;79(3): 269–76.
38. Tanure MG, Cohen EJ, Sudesh S, Rapuano CG, Laibson PR. Spectrum of Fungal Keratitis at Wills Eye Hospital, Philadelphia, Pennsylvania. Cornea. 2000;19(3):307–12.
39. Tilak R, Singh A, Maurya OP, Chandra A, Tilak V, Gulati AK. Mycotic keratitis in India: a five year retrospective study. J Infect Dev Ctries. 2010;4(3): 171–4.
40. Thomas PA, Myatt AK. Characteristic clinical features as an aid to the diagnosis of suppurative keratitis caused by filamentous fungi. Br J Ophthalmol. 2005;89:1554–8.
41. Vaddavalli PK, Garg P, Sharma S, Sangwan VS, Rao GN, Thomas R. Role of confocal microscopy in the diagnosis of fungal and acanthamoeba keratitis. Ophthalmology. 2011;118(1):29–35. doi:10.1016/j.ophtha.2010.05.018.
42. Lalitha P, Prajna NV, Kabra A, Mahadevan K, Srinivasan M. Risk factors for treatment outcome in fungal keratitis. Ophthalmology. 2006;113(4):526–30.
43. Mellado F, Rojas T, Cumsille C. Fungal keratitis: review of diagnosis and treatment. Arq Bras Oftalmol. 2013;76(1):52–6. Article In Spanish.
44. Moraud K, Bartolleti AC, Bochot A, Barratt G, Brandely ML, Chost F. Liposomal amphotericin B eyedrops to treat fungal keratitis: physiochemical and formulation stability. Int J Pharm. 2007;344(1–2):150–3.
45. Behens-Baumann W, Kringe B, Ruchel B. Topical fluconazole for experimental Candida keratitis in rabbits. Br J Ophthalmol. 1990;74:40–2.
46. Isipradit S. Efficacy of fluconazole subconjunctival injection as adjunctive therapy for severe recalcitrant fungal corneal ulcer. J Med Assoc Thai. 2008;91(3):309–15.
47. Troke P, Obenga G, Gaujoux T, Goldschmidt P, Bienvenu AL, Cornet M, Grenouillet F, Pons D, Ranque S, Sitbon K, Chaumeil C, Borderie V, Lortholary O. The efficacy of voriconazole in 24 ocular fusarium infections. Infection. 2013;41(1):15–20.
48. Sponsel W, Chan N, Dang D, Paris G, Graybill J, Najvar LK, Zhou L, Lam KW, Glickman R, Scribbick P. Topical voriconazole as a novel treatment for fungal keratitis. Antimicrob Agents Chemother. 2006;50(1):262–8.
49. Sharma N, Agarwal P, Sinha R, Titiyal JS, Velpandian T, Vajpayee RB. Evaluation of intrastromal voriconazole injection in recalcitrant deep fungal keratitis: case series. Br J Ophthalmol. 2011;95(12):1735–7.
50. Xie L, Zgai H, Shi W. Penetrating keratoplasty for corneal perforations in fungal keratitis. Cornea. 2007;26(2):158–62.
51. Galperin G, Berra M, Tau J, Boscaro G, Zarate J, Berra A. Treatment of fungal keratitis from Fusarium infection by corneal cross-linking. Cornea. 2012;31(2):176–80.
52. Thebpatiphat N, Hammersmith KM, Rocha FN, Rapuano CJ, Ayres BD, Laibson PR, Eagle Jr RC, Cohen EJ. Acanthamoeba keratitis: a parasite on the rise. Cornea. 2007;26(6):701–6.
53. Radford CF, Bacon AS, Dart JK, Minassian DC. Risk factors for Acanthamoeba keratitis in contact lens users: a case study. BMJ. 1995;310(6994):1567–70.
54. Lindsay RG, Watters G, Johnson R, Ormonde SE, Snibson GR. Acanthamoeba keratitis and contact lens wear. Clin Exp Optom. 2007;90(5):351–60.
55. Sun X, Zhang Y, Li R, Wang Z, Luo S, Gao M, Deng S, Chen W, Jin X. Acanthamoeba keratitis: clinical characteristics and management. Ophthalmology. 2006;113(3):412–6.
56. Matin A, Jung S-Y. Interaction of Escherichia coli K1 and K5 with Acanthamoeba castellanii trophozoites and cysts. Korean J Parasitol. 2011;49(4):349–56.

57. Epstein RJ, Wilson LA, Visvesvara GS, Plourde Jr EG. Rapid diagnosis of Acanthamoeba keratitis from corneal scrapings using indirect fluorescent antibody staining. Arch Ophthalmol. 1986;104(9):1318–21.
58. Wilhelmus KR, Osato MS, Font RL, Robinson NM, Jones DB. Rapid diagnosis of Acanthamoeba keratitis using calcofluor white. Arch Ophthalmol. 1986;104(9):1309–12.
59. Parmar DN, Awwad ST, Petroll WM, Bowman RW, McCulley JP, Cavanagh HD. Tandem scanning confocal corneal microscopy in the diagnosis of suspected acanthamoeba keratitis. Ophthalmology. 2006;113(4):538–47.
60. Sharma S, Garg P, Rao GN. Patients characteristics, diagnosis and treatment of non-contact lens related Acanthamoeba keratitis. Br J Ophthalmol. 2000;84(10):1103–8.
61. Bang S, Edell E, Eghrari AO, Gottsch JD. Treatment with voriconazole in 3 eyes with resistant Acanthamoeba keratitis. Am J Ophthalmol. 2010;149(1):66–9.
62. Shadduck JA, Greeley E. Microsporidia and human infections. Clin Microbiol Rev. 1989;2(2):158–65.
63. Das S, Sharma S, Sahu SK, Nayak SS, Kar S. New microbial spectrum of epidemic keratoconjunctivitis: clinical and laboratory aspects of an outbreak. Br J Ophthalmol. 2008;92(6):861–2. No abstract available.
64. Joseph J, Vemuganti GK, Sharma S. Microsporidia: emerging ocular pathogens. Indian J Med Microbiol. 2005;23(2):80–91.
65. Cali A, Meisler DM, Lowder CY, Lembach R, Ayers L, Takvorian PM, Rutherford I, Longworth DL, McMahon J, Bryan RT. Corneal microsporidioses: characterization and identification. J Protozool. 1991;38(6):215–7.
66. Lowder CY, Meisler DM, McMahon JT, Longworth DL, Rutherford I. Microsporidia infection of the cornea in a man seropositive for human immunodeficiency virus. Am J Ophthalmol. 1990;109(2):242–4.
67. Rosberger DF, Serdarevic ON, Erlandson RA, Bryan RT, Schwartz DA, Visvesvara GS, Keenan PC. Successful treatment of microsporidial keratoconjunctivitis with topical fumagillin in a patient with AIDS. Cornea. 1993;12(3):261–5.
68. Khandelwal SS, Woodward MA, Hall T, Grossniklaus HE, Stulting RD. Treatment of microsporidia keratitis with topical voriconazole monotherapy. Arch Ophthalmol. 2011;129(4):509–10. doi:10.1001/archophthalmol.2011.54.
69. Chappuis F, Sundar S, Hailu A, Ghalib H, Rijal S, Peeling RW, Alvar J, Boelaert M. Visceral leishmaniasis: what are the needs for diagnosis, treatment and control? Nat Rev Microbiol. 2007;5(11):873–82.
70. Montero JA, Ruiz-Moreno JM, Sanchis E. Intraretinal hemorrhage associated with leishmaniasis. Ophthalmic Surg Lasers Imaging. 2003;34(3):212–4.
71. Thakur CP, Singh RK, Hassan SM, Kumar R, Narain S, Kumar A. Amphotericin B deoxycholate treatment of visceral leishmaniasis with newer modes of administration and precautions: a study of 938 cases. Trans R Soc Trop Med Hyg. 1999; 93(3):319–23.
72. WHO Library Cataloguing-in-Publication Data. Global Initiative for the Elimination of Avoidable Blindness: action plan 2006–2011. I.World Health Organization. ISBN 978 92 4 159588 9 (NLM classification: WW 140).
73. Kayembe DL, Kasonga DL, Kayembe PK, Mwanza JC, Boussinesq M. Profile of eye lesions and vision loss: a cross-sectional study in Lusambo, a forest-Savanna area hyperendemic for Onchocerciasis in the Democratic Republic of Congo. Trop Med Int Health. 2003;8(1):88–9.
74. Basáñez MG, Pion SD, Boakes E, Filipe JA, Churcher TS, Boussinesq M. Effect of single-dose ivermectin on Onchocerca volvulus: a systematic review and met-analysis. Lancet Infect Dis. 2008; 8(5):310–22.

Viral Anterior Uveitis

8

Samir S. Shoughy and Khalid F. Tabbara

8.1 Introduction

Anterior uveitis is the most common form of intraocular inflammation [1–3]. The disease is caused by immune-mediated, infectious, and undetermined disorders. Forty-eight percent of new cases of uveitis were idiopathic in a recent large epidemiological study [4]. With improvements in molecular diagnostic techniques, viruses are increasingly being identified as a cause of anterior uveitis. Viral anterior uveitis is the most common form of infectious anterior uveitis and accounts for more than 10 % of cases of anterior uveitis [5]. Viral etiology should be suspected in patients presenting with unilateral anterior uveitis and signs of diffuse, fine, stellate, or dendritiform keratic precipitates, ocular hypertension, and iris atrophy [6]. Although clinical features of viral anterior uveitis share common findings of elevated intraocular pressure, patchy or sectoral iris atrophy, and keratic precipitates that are distributed throughout the cornea, there are specific characteristic findings depending on the causative viral agent.

Viral anterior uveitis is caused mainly by viruses from the *Herpesviridae* family. Herpes viruses are commonly encountered causes of infections in immunocompetent and immunocompromised individuals. This family includes herpes simplex virus (HSV) types 1 and 2, varicella zoster virus (VZV), cytomegalovirus virus (CMV), Epstein–Barr virus (EBV), and human herpes virus (HHV) types 6, 7, and 8. The main viruses responsible for ocular inflammation are HSV type 1, VZV, and CMV. Epstein–Barr virus (EBV) and HSV type 2 have also been infrequently detected in ocular fluids of patients with anterior uveitis [7].

8.2 Herpes Simplex Virus and Varicella Zoster Virus

8.2.1 Clinical Findings

The clinical features of intraocular inflammation caused by herpes viruses share common characteristics, and hence it may not be possible to differentiate anterior uveitis caused by HSV and VZV. Patients may present with or without keratitis. Healed corneal scar may be seen in some patients with herpetic uveitis.

Herpetic anterior uveitis is almost always unilateral, and the course is acute and recurrent [8].

S.S. Shoughy, MD, FRCS (Glasg.)
The Eye Center and The Eye Foundation for Research in Ophthalmology, Riyadh, Saudi Arabia

K.F. Tabbara, MD, ABO, FRCOphth (✉)
Department of Ophthalmology, The Eye Center and The Eye Foundation for Research in Ophthalmology, Riyadh, Saudi Arabia

Department of Ophthalmology, College of Medicine, King Saud University, Riyadh, Saudi Arabia

The Wilmer Ophthalmological Institute of The Johns Hopkins University School of Medicine, Baltimore, MD, USA
e-mail: kftabbara@yahoo.com

K. Tabbara et al. (eds.), *Ocular Infections*, Essentials in Ophthalmology,
DOI 10.1007/978-3-662-43981-4_8,

Patients present with blurring of vision, redness, photophobia, and eye pain. The corneal signs include decreased corneal sensation and keratic precipitates which may appear fine stellate or mutton fat. In case of accompanying stromal or disciform keratitis, keratic precipitates tend to cluster on the endothelium in the region of active keratitis [9]. Anterior chamber reaction ranges from mild to severe flare and cells with hypopyon formation. Although hemorrhage does not occur commonly to be a characteristic feature of herpetic keratouveitis, hyphema may be observed [10]. The iris changes include posterior synechia and sectoral or diffuse iris atrophy. The increase in intraocular pressure which has been attributed to trabeculitis is temporary but may sometimes lead to glaucomatous damage to the optic nerve head [11].

Despite the clinical similarities between HSV and VZV anterior uveitis, some differentiating points do exist. The history or the presence of ipsilateral zoster dermatitis that involve a dermatome among the distribution of the ophthalmic nerve may suggest VZV. HSV may also lead to dermatitis consisting of grouped vesicles. The pattern of dendritic keratitis in case of corneal involvement may suggest the diagnosis. HSV dendrites have branches that terminate in end bulbs, while VZV pseudodendrites have heaped-up cells centrally that cause slight elevation with few end bulbs and small fine dendrites [12].

In a study by Miserocchi et al. [13], recurrence occurred in 70 % of eyes with HSV. Patients with HSV were more likely to have a recurrence and required more periocular steroids than VZV patients, whereas VZV had a more chronic course and presented with more posterior segment complications such as acute retinal necrosis (ARN). Fluorescein angiography of the iris may help in differentiating HSV from VZV. In VZV uveitis, the iris vessels are occluded at the site of atrophy, but in HSV uveitis, the iris circulation is intact.

8.2.2 Laboratory Diagnosis

In order to effectively manage patients with anterior uveitis, clear distinction between infectious and noninfectious etiologies should be done. Every effort should be made to identify the causative organism. This depends mainly on the clinical picture, and in cases of diagnostic uncertainty, laboratory investigations should be considered. Two types of tests are most commonly performed to detect the causative viral agent. The first one is detection of specific antibodies in ocular fluids. These antibodies which are found in the eye during an attack of uveitis can be either from blood due to disruption of the blood–aqueous barrier or due to intraocular synthesis by B cells [14]. Goldmann–Witmer coefficient is the method which is used in order to detect intraocular production of antibodies. The second method is to detect viral genome by using qualitative or quantitative PCR methods.

Combination of these two techniques gives better diagnostic yield. In certain instances like immunocompromised states, antibody testing is less reliable due to the presence of concomitant infections. PCR is a good alternative in these cases. On the other hand, the PCR may be positive only at repeat taps because of the limited viral load in a limited volume of aqueous [15].

8.2.3 Treatment

The goal of treatment of viral anterior uveitis is to suppress the inflammation and prevent complications. This can be achieved by using appropriate antiviral therapy, anti-inflammatory medications, and cycloplegics to prevent synechia formation during the acute phase of inflammation. Control of intraocular pressure with topical and systemic ocular antihypertensive agents is necessary to control the ocular hypertension, especially during the acute phase.

Systemic antivirals such as acyclovir, valacyclovir, or famciclovir are the mainstay of therapy in patients with severe uveitis [16]. Oral acyclovir is given at a dosage level of 400 mg five times daily for HSV and 800 mg five times daily for VZV. Valacyclovir which is a prodrug of acyclovir is given at a dose of 1,000 mg orally twice daily for HSV and 1 g three times daily for VZV [17]. Famciclovir 500 mg three times daily demonstrated efficacy similar to acyclovir 800 mg five times daily in the treatment of ophthalmic herpes zoster, but provides patients with a more convenient dosing regimen [18].

Oral acyclovir, 600–800 mg/day, has been found to diminish the number of recurrences in patients with herpetic anterior uveitis when given on a long-term basis [19]. Oral acyclovir has been shown also to reduce the incidence and severity of ocular complications, including anterior uveitis, when given for 10 days starting within 72 h of onset of skin lesions in patients with herpes zoster ophthalmicus [20].

Topical antiviral agents are usually ineffective in the treatment of anterior uveitis but may be indicated in patients with herpes simplex keratouveitis to prevent dendritic keratitis during topical corticosteroid treatment [21]. Acyclovir 3 % ointment four times daily was found to be effective in cases of herpetic iridocyclitis without active corneal inflammation, as it provides good ocular penetration [22]. Topical ganciclovir 0.15 % gel (Virgan®, Laboratoires Théa, Clermont-Ferrand, Cedex, France) may be given for patients with herpetic uveitis. Topical ganciclovir is given every 6 h for 1 month [23]. Oral acyclovir appears to provide benefit over acyclovir ointment because it does not blur vision.

Topical steroids are required to control the iridocyclitis. Steroids also acutely decrease intraocular pressure owing to their anti-inflammatory effects on the trabecular meshwork. Steroids are very difficult to discontinue in patients with herpes and require an extremely slow tapering process [11].

Topical cycloplegic is required to prevent posterior synechia formation and for inducing comfort. Topical and oral ocular antihypertensive agents are often necessary to control the ocular hypertension, especially during the first days of treatment. The ocular hypertension may become chronic owing to inflammation or the prolonged use of corticosteroids, and either long-term antihypertensive drops or a filtering procedure may be required.

8.3 Cytomegalovirus

Cytomegalovirus (CMV) is a member of the herpes virus family. Following primary infection, CMV establishes latent infection. The seroprevalence of CMV antibodies ranges from 52 to 87 % in two different studies [24, 25].

Anterior uveitis caused by CMV may occur in immunocompetent patients. Anterior segment ocular involvement in immunocompetent individuals may occur as a unilateral anterior uveitis which may have either an acute recurrent course (resembling Posner–Schlossman syndrome), a chronic persistent course (resembling Fuchs uveitis syndrome), or as corneal endotheliitis [26].

8.3.1 Clinical Findings

Eyes with CMV anterior uveitis share common features such as elevated intraocular pressure, diffuse iris atrophy, and absence of both posterior synechia and posterior segment involvement. Despite these common features, there are some important differences between the acute and the chronic form [27, 28].

8.3.1.1 Acute Anterior Uveitis

Acute anterior uveitis presents with recurrent episodes of mild iritis and a few fine keratic precipitates (KPs), which are usually white and fine-to-medium sized, a grade of less than 2+ (16–25 cells) for anterior chamber (AC) cells, and epithelial edema secondary to elevated intraocular pressure [28, 29]. Iris atrophy may occur, and it is either patchy or diffuse and is present in 15 % of eyes. The eye may be quiet with normal intraocular pressure between attacks [29].

8.3.1.2 Chronic Anterior Uveitis

The keratic precipitates in eyes with chronic uveitis are more numerous and diffusely distributed. There is usually a mixture of different-sized keratic precipitates occasionally, even of mutton-fat appearance. The anterior chamber cellular reaction, again, is generally mild, with 2+ cells or less. Elevated intraocular pressure is a prominent feature [29]. Patients with chronic uveitis tend to be older than those with acute recurrent uveitis; the intraocular pressure elevation is lower than eyes with acute recurrent uveitis. Diffuse iris atrophy and cataracts are more common in eyes with chronic persistent disease [29].

8.3.1.3 Corneal Endotheliitis

Unlike eyes with anterior uveitis, the KPs in eyes with corneal endotheliitis tend to be pigmented and are often arranged in a linear or coin-shaped pattern. The linear KPs tend to occur at the leading edge of the stromal edema. The coin-shaped KPs are usually medium sized and arranged in a circular pattern around an area of corneal edema [30].

8.3.2 Laboratory Findings

There are no specific clinical features for the diagnosis of CMV infection. The diagnosis can only be confirmed on aqueous sampling for evidence of intraocular CMV. CMV in the anterior chamber can be detected by PCR or detection of intraocular production of CMV-specific antibodies. Combination of both these techniques will improve the yield of tests. In some cases, the detection of the viral genome by PCR may be difficult because of the limited viral load in a small specimen or due to a short-lived release of the virus [7, 31].

8.3.3 Treatment

Topical ganciclovir was originally developed for the treatment of herpetic keratitis, but it has been found to achieve high concentrations in the cornea, iris tissue, and aqueous, especially with the 0.2 % gel [32]. Ganciclovir 0.15 % gel is available as Virgan (Laboratoires Théa, Clermont-Ferrand, Cedex, France). Ganciclovir or valganciclovir has been the first line of treatment of CMV anterior segment infection. Various routes for administration of ganciclovir exist including topical, systemic administration, and intraocular treatment using intravitreal implants or intravitreal injections [33].

Chee and Jap [33] reported that long-term topical ganciclovir 0.15 % application resulted in a lower recurrence rate and less severe adverse effects as compared to systemic ganciclovir or device implantation. Therefore, they suggested topical ganciclovir therapy in CMV anterior uveitis. Ganciclovir gel has a relatively low response rate [33]. Although the response to systemic antiviral therapy is high (up to 75 % of affected patients), the relapse rate has also been high, and a prolonged period of treatment may be required [33]. Intravitreal ganciclovir injection as a loading dose with or without subsequent oral valganciclovir in patients with CMV anterior uveitis was found to control the inflammation and IOP [34].

As in HSV and HZV anterior uveitis, topical steroids may be needed to control the inflammation. Ocular antihypertensive medications or even filtering surgery may be needed to control the elevated intraocular pressure.

8.4 Epstein–Barr Virus

Epstein–Barr virus (EBV) is a member of the herpes virus group. It is ubiquitous virus and the majority of the adult population are infected. Individuals are usually infected through saliva during adolescence. EBV infection leads to infectious mononucleosis. Patients may develop pharyngitis, fever, skin rash, and lymphadenopathy. The role of EBV in the pathogenesis of ocular disease is still controversial. It has been associated with a variety of ocular inflammatory diseases, such as conjunctivitis, keratitis, uveitis, choroiditis, and retinitis [35].

The clinical features include a prodrome of flulike illness. The disease is characterized by severe acute anterior uveitis with fibrinous exudates which may become granulomatous in the chronic stage. The vitreous shows little inflammation. Fundus findings show hyperemia and edema of the disk, sunset glow fundus which may simulate Harada disease in the adults, and retinal pigment epithelial disorders [36, 37].

8.4.1 Laboratory Testing

The high incidence of elevated antibody titers to Epstein–Barr virus in patients with uveitis suggests that uveitis might be a disease accompanied by EBV reactivation. Again combination of both

PCR and detection of local antibody production in the ocular fluids will enhance the diagnostic yield [35, 38].

8.4.2 Treatment

No efficient therapy against EBV has been documented. Based on its antiviral and immunomodulatory effects, interferon alpha may represent a new therapeutic approach for these patients [39].

8.5 Rubella Virus

The rubella virus is an enveloped RNA virus which is classified as a *Rubivirus* in the *Togaviridae* family. Rubella is an acute disease characterized by a generalized erythematous maculopapular rash, generalized lymphadenopathy, and low-grade fever.

The anterior uveitis caused by rubella virus induces a distinct clinical spectrum of ocular symptoms similar to Fuchs uveitis syndrome (FUS), which suggests that rubella virus might be involved in the pathogenesis of FUS [40, 41].

As mentioned earlier, chronic anterior uveitis caused by CMV was found also to induce a clinical picture similar to FUS. Interestingly, the cases of FUS that were reported from Europe were strongly associated with rubella and those from Asia were associated with CMV [28, 29].

8.6 Fuchs Uveitis Syndrome

Fuchs uveitis syndrome is a chronic persistent cause of anterior uveitis. It occurs more commonly in the third and fourth decades of life with an equal gender distribution. Patients may complain of floaters or blurring of vision. The diagnosis may be delayed due to the mild nature of the inflammation, and vision may be decreased from cataract. The keratic precipitates are diffuse, fine, stellate, and white; the iris shows diffuse atrophy and heterochromia. The iris and trabecular meshwork show abnormal vessels that may sometimes lead to a hyphema. Synechia formation is uncommon. Vitritis and sectoral peripheral retinal vascular leakage with disk hyperfluorescence may be seen [42]. Cataract, mainly posterior subcapsular, and glaucoma may occur in longstanding cases [43].

Rubella can induce uveitis during childhood in the unvaccinated children [44]. Maternal rubella is now rare in many developed countries because of rubella vaccination programs. However, in areas where the vaccine is not available, congenital rubella syndrome (CRS) remains a major cause of developmental anomalies, particularly blindness and deafness [45].

8.6.1 Laboratory Testing

Intraocular production of antibodies against the rubella virus may be determined in the aqueous. The Goldmann–Witmer ratio can be detected in almost 90 % of patients with FUS. Rubella virus can be also detected by polymerase chain reaction [46, 47].

8.6.2 Treatment

No specific antiviral treatment is available to modulate the clinical course of anterior uveitis due to rubella. Treatment is symptomatic. Topical steroids may be used to control the intraocular inflammation. The risk of developing cataract and secondary glaucoma should be considered due to the chronic nature of the inflammation. Topical nonsteroidal anti-inflammatory drugs are good alternatives in cases that require extended periods of treatment. The long-term prognosis is good, and patients usually maintain a visual acuity of 20/40 or better [43].

8.7 Chikungunya Virus

Chikungunya is an RNA virus belonging to family *Togaviridae*, genus *Alphavirus*. Chikungunya (CHIK) fever is a re-emerging viral disease characterized by abrupt onset of fever with severe arthralgia followed by constitutional symptoms and rash lasting for 1–7 days. The disease is almost self-limiting and rarely fatal [48]. The disease is prevalent in eastern Africa.

The main ocular manifestations of chikungunya virus infection include granulomatous or nongranulomatous anterior uveitis, episcleritis, optic neuritis, retrobulbar neuritis, and retinitis. The visual prognosis is generally good, with most patients recovering good vision [49, 50].

Interestingly, chikungunya virus has been reported in association with a case of bilateral Fuchs heterochromic iridocyclitis [51].

8.8 Parechovirus

Human parechoviruses have been recently associated with anterior uveitis. They belong to the genus *Parechovirus* within the family of *Picornaviridae*. Systemically, they may cause gastroenteritis, encephalitis, and flaccid paralysis in young children, but rarely in adults. Human parechoviruses cause unilateral anterior uveitis with corneal involvement and cells in the anterior chamber [52].

Compliance with Ethical Requirements

Conflict of Interest The authors declare that they have no conflict of interest.

Informed Consent No human studies were carried out by the authors for this article.

Animal Studies No animal studies were carried out by the authors for this article.

References

1. Islam SM, Tabbara KF. Causes of uveitis at The Eye Center in Saudi Arabia: a retrospective review. Ophthalmic Epidemiol. 2002;9:239–49.
2. Yang P, Zhang Z, Zhou H, Li B, Huang X, Gao Y, et al. Clinical patterns and characteristics of uveitis in a tertiary center for uveitis in China. Curr Eye Res. 2005;30:943–8.
3. Khairallah M, Yahia SB, Ladjimi A, Messaoud R, Zaouali S, Attia S, et al. Pattern of uveitis in a referral centre in Tunisia, North Africa. Eye. 2007;21:33–9.
4. Kim EC, Margolis TP. Hypertensive iridocyclitis. Br J Ophthalmol. 2006;90(7):812–3.
5. Garweg JG. Diagnostics of virus-induced anterior uveitis 2011 Acta Ophthalmologica. Article first published online: 11 AUG 2011 doi:10.1111/j.1755-3768.2011.4445.x.
6. Tugal-Tutkun I, Otük-Yasar B, Altinkurt E. Clinical features and prognosis of herpetic anterior uveitis: a retrospective study of 111 cases. Int Ophthalmol. 2010;30:559–65.
7. De Groot-Mijnes JD, Rothova A, Van Loon AM, Schuller M, Ten Dam-Van Loon NH, De Boer JH, Schuurman R, Weersink AJ. Polymerase chain reaction and Goldmann-Witmer coefficient analysis are complimentary for the diagnosis of infectious uveitis. Am J Ophthalmol. 2006;141(2):313–8.
8. Wensing B, Relvas LM, Caspers LE, et al. Comparison of rubella virus- and herpes virus-associated anterior uveitis: clinical manifestations and visual prognosis. Ophthalmology. 2011;118:1905–10.
9. Cunningham Jr ET. Diagnosing and treating herpetic anterior uveitis. Ophthalmology. 2000;107:2129–30.
10. Kimura SJ. Herpes simplex uveitis: a clinical and experimental study. Trans Am Ophthalmol Soc. 1962;60:441–70.
11. Falcon MG, Williams HP. Herpes simplex keratouveitis and glaucoma. Trans Opthalmol Soc U K. 1978;98:101–4.
12. Piebanga LW, Laibson PR. Dendritic lesions in herpes zoster ophthalmicus. Arch Ophthalmol. 1973;90:268.
13. Miserocchi E, Waheed NK, Dios E, et al. Visual outcome in herpes simplex virus and varicella zoster virus uveitis: a clinical evaluation and comparison. Ophthalmology. 2002;109:1532–7.
14. de Boer JH, Luyendijk L, Rothova A, Kijlstra A. Analysis of ocular fluids for local antibody production in uveitis. Br J Ophthalmol. 1995;79:610–6.
15. Matos K, Muccioli C, Belfort Junior R, Rizzo LV. Correlation between clinical diagnosis and PCR analysis of serum, aqueous, and vitreous samples in patients with inflammatory eye disease. Arq Bras Oftalmol. 2007;70(1):109–14.
16. Siverio Júnior CD, Imai Y, Cunningham Jr ET. Diagnosis and management of herpetic anterior uveitis. Int Ophthalmol Clin. 2002;42:43–8.
17. Colin J, Prisant O, Cochener B, et al. Comparison of the efficacy and safety of valacyclovir and acyclovir for the treatment of herpes zoster ophthalmicus. Ophthalmology. 2000;107:1507–11.
18. Tyring S, Engst R, Corriveau C, Robillard N, Trottier S, Van Slycken S, Crann RA, Locke LA, Saltzman R, Palestine AG. Famciclovir for ophthalmic zoster: a randomised aciclovir controlled study. Br J Ophthalmol. 2001;85(5):576–81.
19. Rodriguez A, Power WJ, Neves RA, et al. Recurrence rate of herpetic uveitis in patients on long-term oral acyclovir. Doc Ophthalmol. 1995;90:331–40.
20. Cobo ML, Foulks GN, Liesegang T, et al. Oral acyclovir in the treatment of acute herpes zoster ophthalmicus. Ophthalmology. 1986;93:763–70.
21. Parrish CM. Herpes simplex virus eye disease. In: Focal points: clinical modules for ophthalmologists,

vol. 101. San Fancisco: American Academy of Ophthalmology; 1997. p. 1871–82.
22. Wilhelmus KR, Falcon MG, Jones BR. Herpetic iridocyclitis. Int Ophthalmol. 1981;4:143–50.
23. Tabbara KF, Al Balushi N. Topical ganciclovir in the treatment of acute herpetic keratitis. Clin Ophthalmol. 2010;4:905–12.
24. Wong A, Tan KH, Tee CS, Yeo GS. Seroprevalence of cytomegalovirus, toxoplasma and parvovirus in pregnancy. Singapore Med J. 2000;41(4):151–5.
25. Gratacap-Cavallier B, Bosson JL, Morand P, et al. Cytomegalovirus seroprevalence in French pregnant women: parity and place of birth as major predictive factors. Eur J Epidemiol. 1998;14(2):147–52.
26. Hwang YS, Shen CR, Chang SH, Lai CC, Liu CL, Chen KJ, Lin KK, Chen TL, Hsiao CH. The validity of clinical feature profiles for cytomegaloviral anterior segment infection. Graefes Arch Clin Exp Ophthalmol. 2011;249(1):103–10.
27. de Schryver I, Rozenberg F, Cassoux N, et al. Diagnosis and treatment of cytomegalovirus iridocyclitis without retinal necrosis. Br J Ophthalmol. 2006; 90(7):852–5.
28. Chee SP1, Bacsal K, Jap A, Se-Thoe SY, Cheng CL, Tan BH. Clinical features of cytomegalovirus anterior uveitis in immunocompetent patients. Am J Ophthalmol. 2008 May;145(5):834-40. doi:10.1016/j.ajo.2007.12.015. Epub 2008 Feb 6.
29. Chee SP, Jap A. Presumed Fuchs heterochromic iridocyclitis and Posner-Schlossman syndrome: comparison of cytomegalovirus-positive and negative eyes. Am J Ophthalmol. 2008;146(6):883–9.
30. Koizumi N, Suzuki T, Uno T, et al. Cytomegalovirus as an etiologic factor in corneal endotheliitis. Ophthalmology. 2008;115(2):292–7.
31. Doornenbal P, Seerp Baarsma G, Quint WG, Kijlstra A, Rothbarth PH, Niesters HG. Diagnostic assays in cytomegalovirus retinitis: detection of herpesvirus by simultaneous application of the polymerase chain reaction and local antibody analysis on ocular fluid. Br J Ophthalmol. 1996;80(3):235–40.
32. Castela N, Vermerie N, Chast F, et al. Ganciclovir ophthalmic gel in herpes simplex virus rabbit keratitis: intraocular penetration and efficacy. J Ocul Pharmacol. 1994;10(2):439–51.
33. Chee SP, Jap A. Cytomegalovirus anterior uveitis: outcome of treatment. Br J Ophthalmol. 2010;94: 1648–52.
34. Hwang YS, Lin KK, Lee JS, Chang SH, Chen KJ, Lai CC, Huang JC, Kuo YH, Hsiao CH. Intravitreal loading injection of ganciclovir with or without adjunctive oral valganciclovir for cytomegalovirus anterior uveitis. Graefes Arch Clin Exp Ophthalmol. 2010;248(2):263–9.
35. Ongkosuwito J, Van der Lelij A, Bruinenberg M, Wienesen-van Doorn M, Feron E, Hoyng C, de Keizer RJW, Klok A, Kijlstra A. Increased presence of Epstein-Barr virus DNA in ocular fluid samples from HIV negative immunocompromised patients with uveitis. Br J Ophthalmol. 1998;82(3):245–51.
36. Sakai J, Usui M, Usui N. The possible association of Epstein-Barr virus and uveitis. Nihon Ganka Gakkai Zasshi. 1990;94(5):496–507.
37. Usui M, Sakai J. Three cases of EB virus-associated uveitis. Int Ophthalmol. 1990;14(5–6):371–6.
38. Touge C, Agawa H, Sairenji T, Inoue Y. High incidence of elevated antibody titers to Epstein-Barr virus in patients with uveitis. Arch Virol. 2006;151(5):895–903.
39. Lemaitre C, Bodaghi B, Murat F, Fardeau C, Cassoux N, Rosenberg F, LeHoang P. EBV–associated uveitis diagnosed by polymerase chain reaction (PCR): report of 3 cases. Invest Ophthalmol Vis Sci. 2004;45: E-Abstract 1670.
40. de Visser L, Braakenburg A, Rothova A, de Boer JH. Rubella virus-associated uveitis: clinical manifestations and visual prognosis. Am J Ophthalmol. 2008;146(2):292–7.
41. Suzuki J, Goto H, Komase K, Abo H, Fujii K, Otsuki N, Okamoto K. Rubella virus as a possible etiological agent of Fuchs heterochromic iridocyclitis. Graefes Arch Clin Exp Ophthalmol. 2010;248(10):1487–91.
42. Bouchenaki N, Herbort CP. Fluorescein angiographic findings and clinical features in Fuchs' uveitis. Int Ophthalmol. 2010;30:511–9.
43. Bonfioli AA, Curi AL, Orefice F. Fuchs' heterochromic cyclitis. Semin Ophthalmol. 2005;20(3):143–6.
44. Siemerink MJ, Sijssens KM, de Groot-Mijnes JD, de Boer JH. Rubella virus-associated uveitis in a nonvaccinated child. Am J Ophthalmol. 2007;143(5):899–900.
45. Banatvala JE, Brown DW. Rubella. Lancet. 2004;363(9415):1127–37.
46. Stunf S, Petrovec M, Žigon N, Hawlina M, Kraut A, de Groot-Mijnes JD, Valentinčič NV. High concordance of intraocular antibody synthesis against the rubella virus and Fuchs heterochromic uveitis syndrome in Slovenia. Mol Vis. 2012;18:2909–14.
47. Quentin CD, Reiber H. Fuchs' heterochromic cyclitis: rubella virus antibodies and genome in aqueous humor. Am J Ophthalmol. 2004;138:46–54.
48. Chhabra M, Mittal V, Bhattacharya D, Rana U, Lal S. Chikungunya fever: a re-emerging viral infection. Indian J Med Microbiol. 2008;26(1):5–12.
49. Lalitha P, Rathinam S, Banushree K, Maheshkumar S, Vijayakumar R, Sathe P. Ocular involvement associated with an epidemic outbreak of chikungunya virus infection. Am J Ophthalmol. 2007;144(4):552–6.
50. Mahendradas P, Ranganna SK, Shetty R, Balu R, Narayana KM, Babu RB, Shetty BK. Ocular manifestations associated with chikungunya. Ophthalmology. 2008;115(2):287–91.
51. Mahendradas P, Shetty R, Malathi J, Madhavan HN. Chikungunya virus iridocyclitis in Fuchs' heterochromic iridocyclitis. Indian J Ophthalmol. 2010;58(6):545–7.
52. de Groot-Mijnes JD, de Visser L, Zuurveen S, Martinus RA, Völker R, ten Dam-van Loon NH, de Boer JH, Postma G, de Groot RJ, van Loon AM, Rothova A. Identification of new pathogens in the intraocular fluid of patients with uveitis. Am J Ophthalmol. 2010;150(5):628–36.

Infections of the Posterior Segment: Ocular Tuberculosis

9

Ahmed M. Abu El-Asrar, Marwan Abouammoh, and Hani S. Al-Mezaine

9.1 Introduction

Tuberculosis (TB) is a slowly progressive chronic, granulomatous infection caused by *Mycobacterium tuberculosis* [1]. This acid-fast bacillus usually affects the lungs, but can also affect other organs and systems like the cardiovascular system, gastrointestinal system, musculoskeletal system, genitourinary tract, central nervous system, skin, and eyes [2, 3].

Epidemiologic data for ocular tuberculosis are unreliable. This is due to the lack of standardized diagnostic criteria and the difficulty in confirming the diagnosis by laboratory methods. Among all causes of uveitis, incidence of ocular tuberculosis ranges from as low as 1.1–10.5 % [4–24]. In a series of 351 patients admitted to King Abdulaziz University Hospital in Riyadh, Saudi Arabia, with the diagnosis of panuveitis or posterior uveitis, 28.2 % of the patients were diagnosed to have presumed tuberculous uveitis [25].

A.M. Abu El-Asrar, MD, PhD (✉)
M. Abouammoh, MD • H.S. Al-Mezaine, MD
Department of Ophthalmology,
College of Medicine, King Saud University,
KAUH, Old Airport Road, Box 245,
Riyadh 11411, Saudi Arabia
e-mail: abuasrar@ksu.edu.sa;
mabouammoh@ksu.edu.sa; halmezaine@ksu.edu.sa

9.2 Clinical Features

Clinically, intraocular TB can be due to direct infection or indirect immune-mediated hypersensitivity response to mycobacterial antigens when there is no defined active systemic lesion elsewhere or the lesion is thought to be inactive [26–30]. Intraocular TB is a great mimicker of various uveitis entities. The clinical manifestations of intraocular TB include acute anterior uveitis, chronic granulomatous anterior uveitis which may be associated with iris or angle granulomas, mutton-fat keratic precipitates and posterior synechiae (Figs. 9.1, 9.2, and 9.3), intermediate uveitis, vitritis, macular edema (Fig. 9.3), retinal vasculitis (Figs. 9.4, 9.5, and 9.6), neuroretinitis, solitary or multiple choroidal tubercles, multifocal

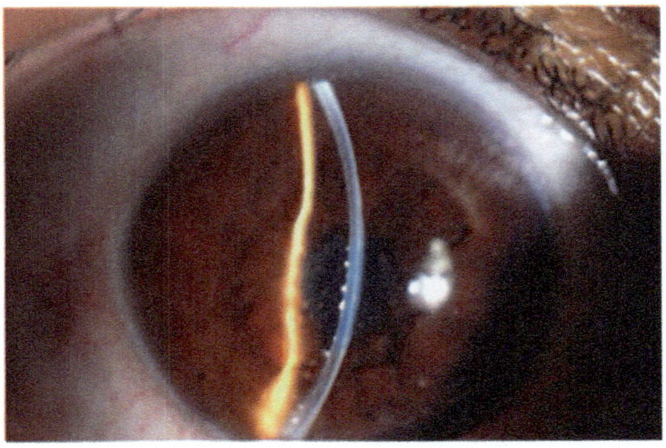

Fig. 9.1 Slit-lamp biomicroscopy of a 42-year-old woman with strongly positive tuberculin skin test (24 mm induration) shows mutton-fat keratic precipitates and posterior synechiae

K. Tabbara et al. (eds.), *Ocular Infections*, Essentials in Ophthalmology,
DOI 10.1007/978-3-662-43981-4_9, © Springer-Verlag Berlin Heidelberg 2014

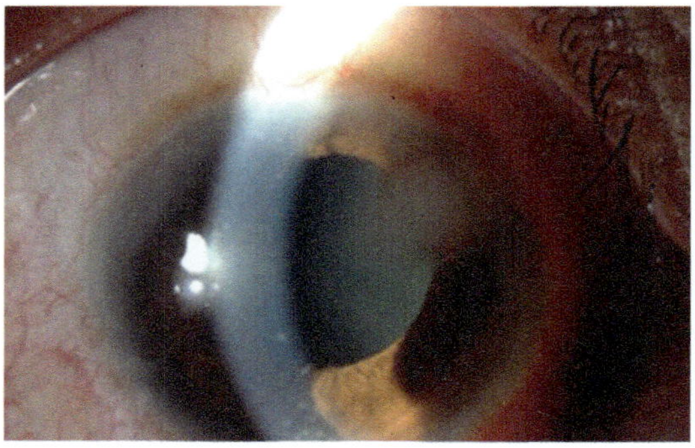

Fig. 9.2 Slit-lamp biomicroscopy of a 24-year-old woman with strongly positive tuberculin skin test (28 mm induration) shows interstitial keratitis and mutton-fat keratic precipitates

choroiditis (Figs. 9.7 and 9.8), choroidal granulomas (Fig. 9.9), serpiginous-like choroiditis (Fig. 9.10), subretinal abscess, endophthalmitis, and panophthalmitis [26–45].

Choroidal tubercles and tuberculomas (large, solitary masses) are reported to be the most common intraocular manifestations of TB. The presence of choroidal tubercles is indicative of hematogenous seeding of bacilli [27]. There may be an overlying exudative retinal detachment. The differential diagnosis includes sarcoid granulomas, syphilitic gummas, and metastatic tumors. Choroidal TB might also present as multifocal progressive choroiditis, which shows progression to confluent, diffuse choroiditis with an active edge or diffuse choroiditis with amoeboid pattern and a leading edge. These morphologic presentations resemble serpiginous choroiditis [34, 38, 45].

Tuberculous retinal vasculitis is typically an obliterative periphlebitis affecting the retina in multiple quadrants, starting at or anterior to the equator and progressing posteriorly. Occasionally, it can begin close to the optic nerve head, mimicking a vein occlusion. Ophthalmoscopic findings vary and depend on the stage of the disease. Initially, it presents as active retinal periphlebitis with thick exudates around the retinal veins associated with retinal hemorrhages and hemorrhagic infarction of the retina. Active retinal periphlebitis is associated with mild degree of cellular infiltrate in the anterior chamber and mild vitreous infiltrate. Healed periphlebitis results in sclerosed venules and abnormal vascular anastomosis. The periphlebitis may cause nonperfusion of a substantial portion of the retina that may lead to proliferative vascular retinopathy with sequelae such as recurrent vitreous hemorrhage, traction retinal detachment, rubeosis iridis, and neovascular glaucoma [26, 31, 36]. Several studies reported that clinical signs significantly associated with presumed tuberculous uveitis include extensive posterior synechiae, retinal vasculitis with or without choroiditis, severe vitritis, and serpiginous-like choroiditis [46, 47]. Of these various intraocular changes, the most common clinical presentation appears to be panuveitis and posterior uveitis [43].

9.3 Diagnosis

In recent years, ocular involvement due to TB has reemerged associated with an increasing prevalence of TB. A high index of clinical suspicion is essential for the early diagnosis of tuberculous uveitis. Late diagnosis and delay in management can result in loss of the eye and can even be life threatening in severe conditions. The diagnosis should be considered by the ophthalmologist when unexplained chronic uveitis with the characteristic clinical signs occur that promptly recurs upon tapering corticosteroid and/or immunosuppressive therapy. Tuberculous retinal vasculitis should be suspected in the presence of florid retinal periphlebitis with marked capillary closure with a relatively mild degree of vitreous cellular infiltrate, particularly in patients of Asiatic origin: genetic predisposition may account for the propensity to develop retinal vasculitis in these patients [26]. Most patients with ocular involvement have no history of pulmonary or other systemic forms [26, 27, 35, 40, 43], making a definitive diagnosis difficult. Therefore, tuberculous uveitis is frequently misdiagnosed, and the disease is recognizable after a very long diagnostic delay [40]. The absence of clinically evident pulmonary TB does not rule out the possibility of ocular TB, as about 60 % of patients with extrapulmonary TB have no evidence of pulmonary TB [48].

The diagnosis of ocular involvement with TB is considered in the setting of (1) isolation of *M. tuberculosis* from ocular fluid or tissue specimen by a microbiologic or histopathologic study. However, the process is prolonged as it may take several weeks before culture results become available for starting specific therapy. Moreover, obtaining biopsy specimens from intraocular tissues for making a confirmatory histopathological diagnosis is difficult with potential morbidity associated with obtaining the biopsy material from the eye, (2) as presumed ocular disease suggestive of TB with proven active systemic disease, or (3) as presumed ocular disease without

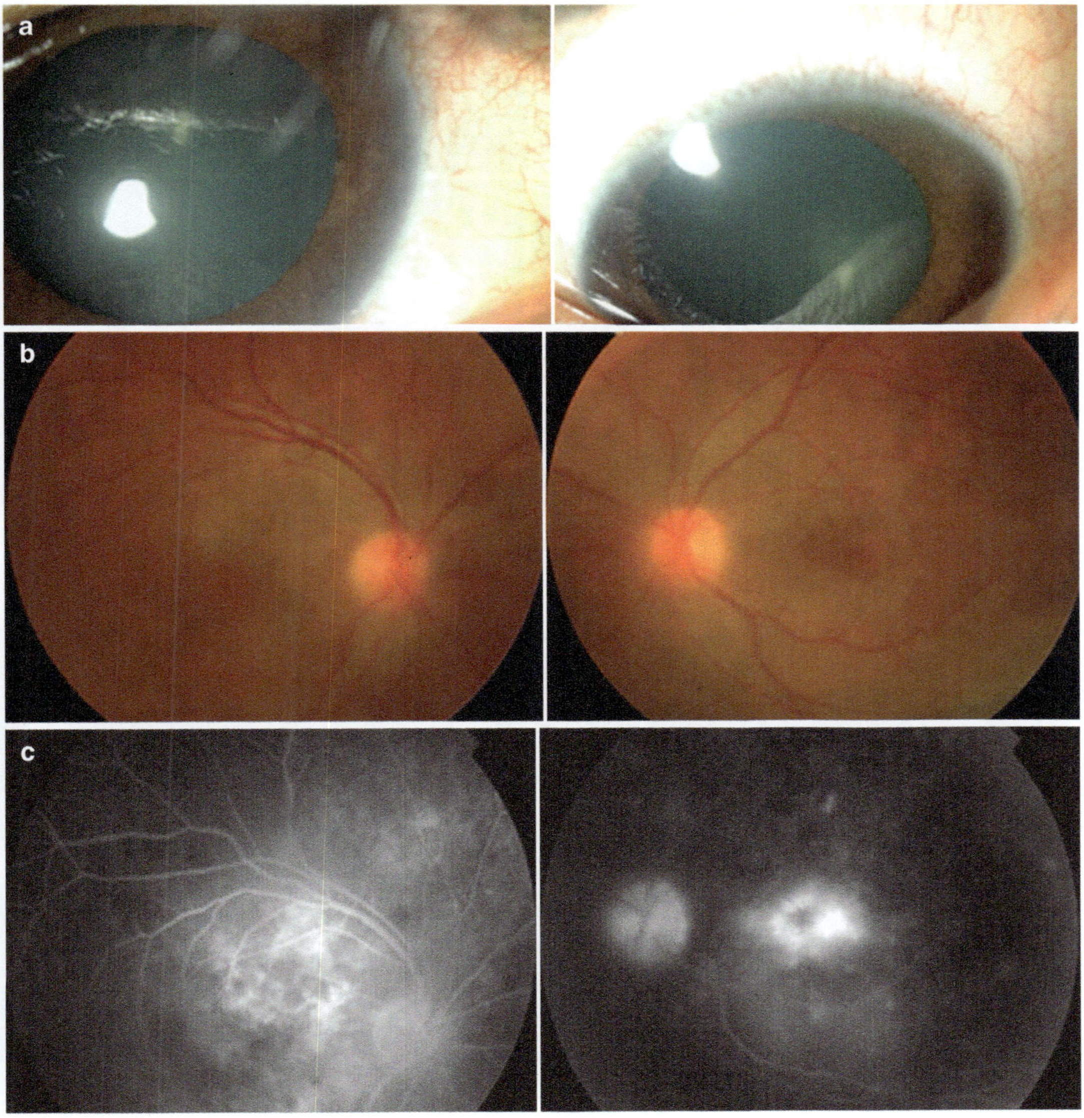

Fig. 9.3 A 32-year-old man with strongly positive tuberculin skin test (24 mm induration). Slit-lamp biomicroscopy shows bilateral iris nodules (**a**). Fundus photographs show disk swelling and hyperemia (**b**). Fluorescein angiography shows leakage from the optic nerve head and retinal vessels and cystoid macular edema (**c**). Indocyanine green angiography shows choroidal hypofluorescent areas (**d**). Optical coherence tomography shows cystoid macular edema. Visual acuity was 20/100 (**e**). Two months after starting antituberculous therapy and systemic corticosteroids, optical coherence tomography displays reduction of macular edema. Visual acuity improved to 20/30 (**f**)

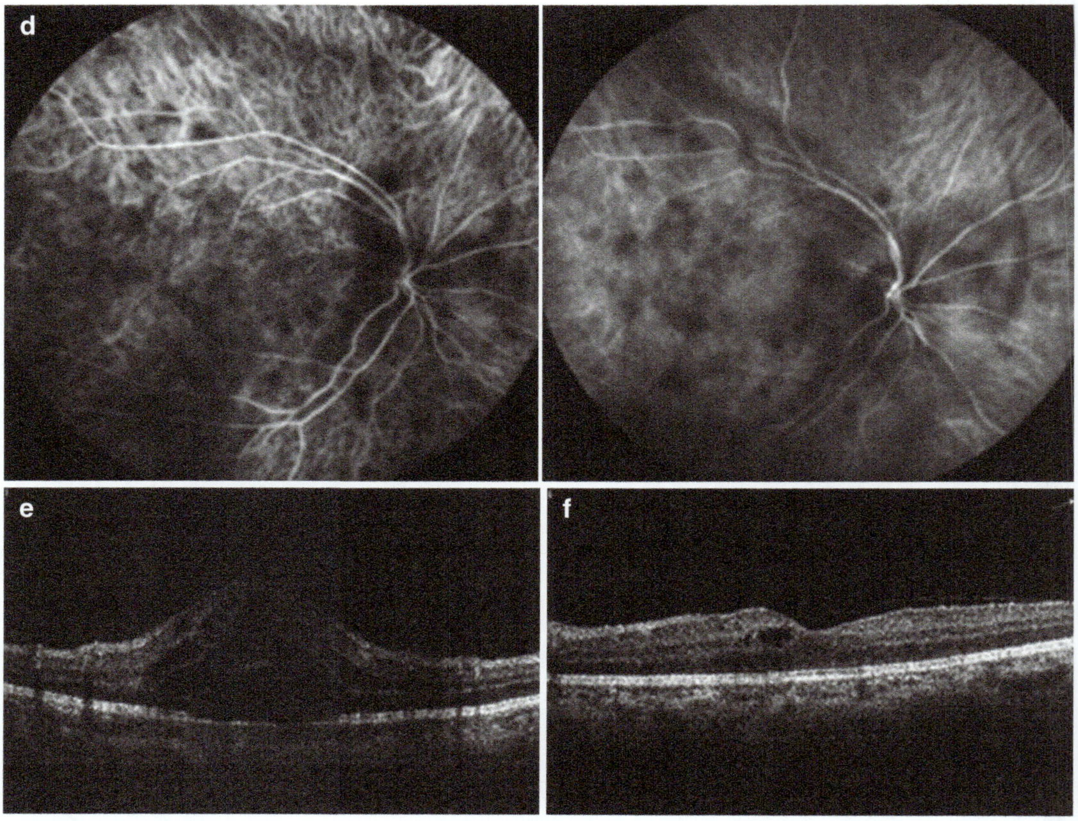

Fig. 9.3 (continued)

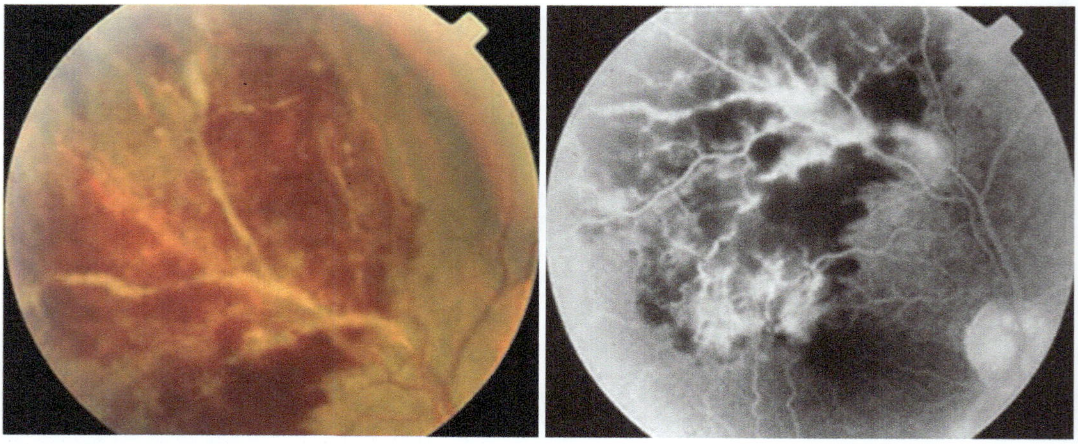

Fig. 9.4 Right eye of a 29-year-old man with strongly positive tuberculin skin test (24 mm induration) shows thick perivenous sheathing with intraretinal hemorrhage (*left*). Fluorescein angiography shows leakage from the retinal veins (*right*)

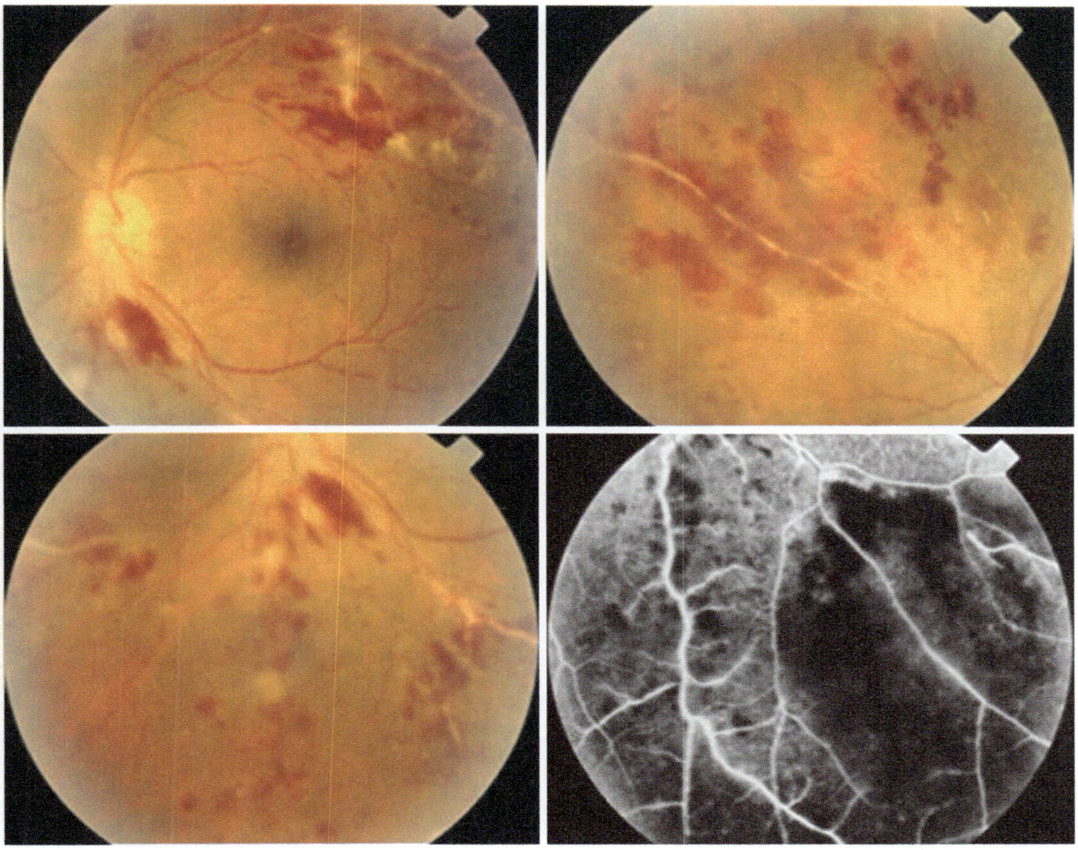

Fig. 9.5 Left eye of a 27-year-old man with strongly positive tuberculin skin test (16 mm induration) shows thick perivenous sheathing and intraretinal hemorrhages. Fluorescein angiography shows leakage from the retinal veins and retinal nonperfusion (*bottom left*)

evidence of active systemic disease [26]. In the last two situations, the diagnosis of ocular TB remains largely presumptive. Because of the difficulty in obtaining microbiologic evidence, in nearly all reported cases, the diagnosis of intraocular TB was only presumptive [26, 29, 30, 32–37, 40, 42].

In most studies, the diagnostic criteria for presumed tuberculous uveitis were [26, 29, 30, 32–37, 40, 43]:

1. Ocular findings consistent with possible intraocular TB with no other cause of uveitis suggested by history of symptoms or ancillary testing
2. Strongly positive tuberculin skin test results (≥15 mm area of induration/necrosis)
3. Response to antituberculous therapy with absence of recurrences

Tuberculin skin test remains a vital part of systemic workup for uveitis patients as it provides supportive information when clinical signs and symptoms suggest TB. The test is carried out by injecting 5 tuberculin units intradermally to raise a wheal of 6–10 mm in diameter. Any induration is measured after 48–72 h. An induration of less than 5 mm is considered a negative result. The specificity of the tuberculin skin test for *M. tuberculosis*

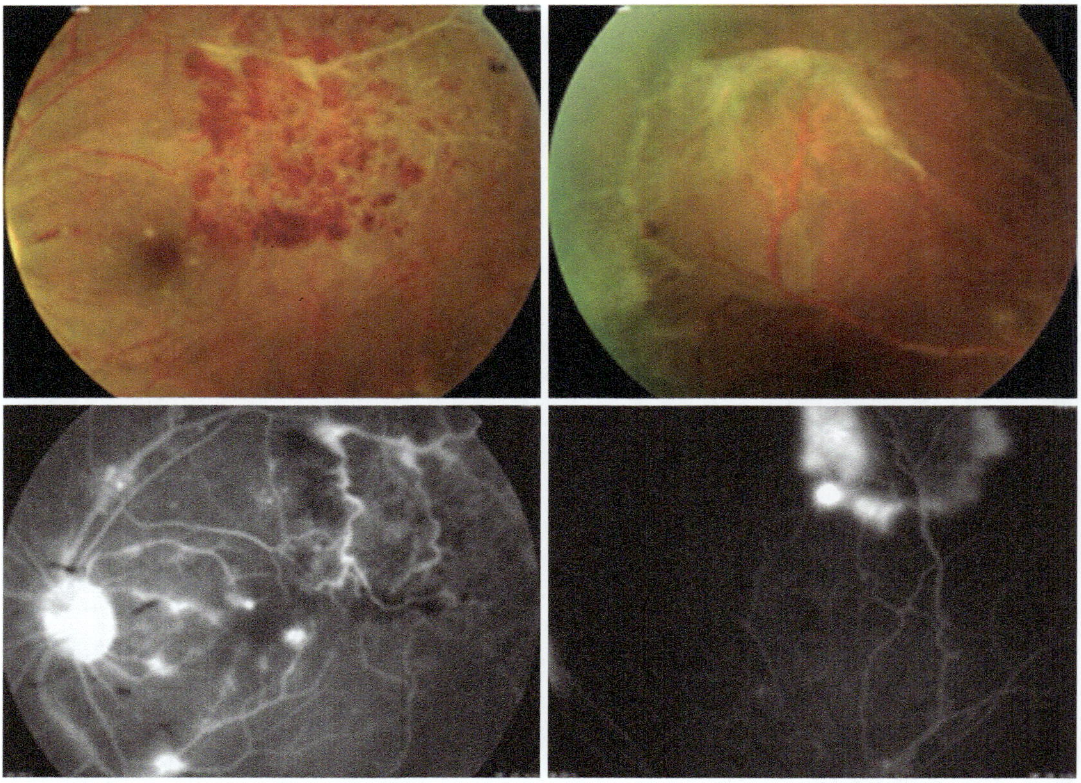

Fig. 9.6 Left eye of a 22-year-old man with strongly positive tuberculin skin test (22 mm induration) shows perivenous sheathing and intraretinal hemorrhages (*top left*) and peripheral sclerosed vessels and fibrovascular proliferation (*top right*). Fluorescein angiography shows leakage from the retinal vessels (*bottom left*), peripheral retinal nonperfusion, and leakage from the peripheral neovessels (*bottom right*)

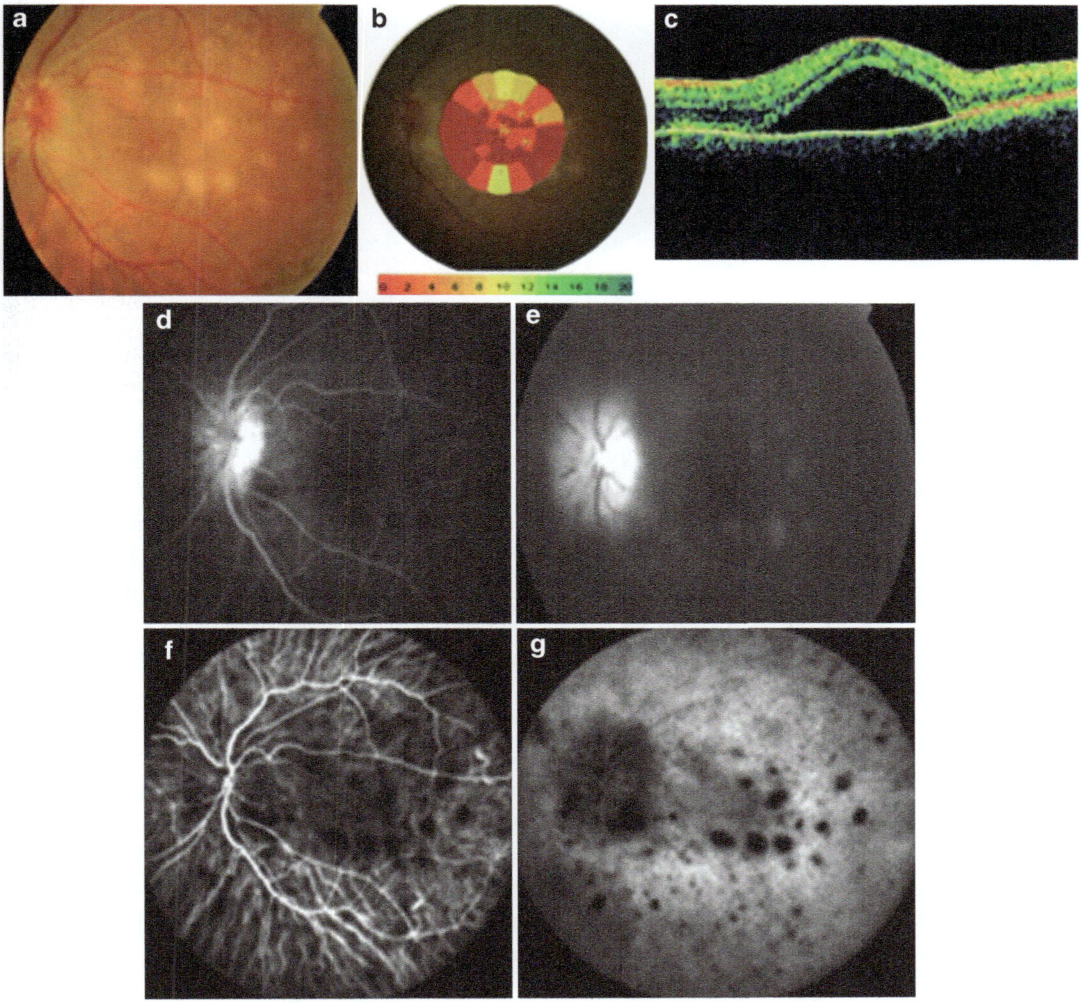

Fig. 9.7 Left eye of a 50-year-old woman with strongly positive tuberculin skin test (26 mm induration) shows multifocal choroiditis and disk swelling and hyperemia. Visual acuity was 20/100 (**a**). MP-1 microperimetry shows reduced sensitivity. The mean central retinal sensitivity was 1.1 decibels (dB). Color-coded, numeric scale shows the threshold in 2 dB steps from 0 to 20 dB. Normal sensitivity is indicated by green color and decreased sensitivity is indicated by red color (**b**). Optical coherence tomography shows exudative retinal detachment (**c**). On fluorescein angiography, the lesions are hypofluorescent in the early phase (**d**) and hyperfluorescent in the late phase (**e**). The optic nerve head shows leakage and staining. Indocyanine green angiography shows that the lesions are hypofluorescent throughout (**f**, **g**). Note that the lesions on indocyanine green angiography are more numerous than on fluorescein angiography. Six months after starting antituberculous therapy and systemic corticosteroids, visual acuity improved to 20/30. Fundus photography shows resolution of the lesions (**h**). The mean central retinal sensitivity improved to 11.1 dB (**i**). Optical coherence tomography displays resolution of exudative retinal detachment (**j**)

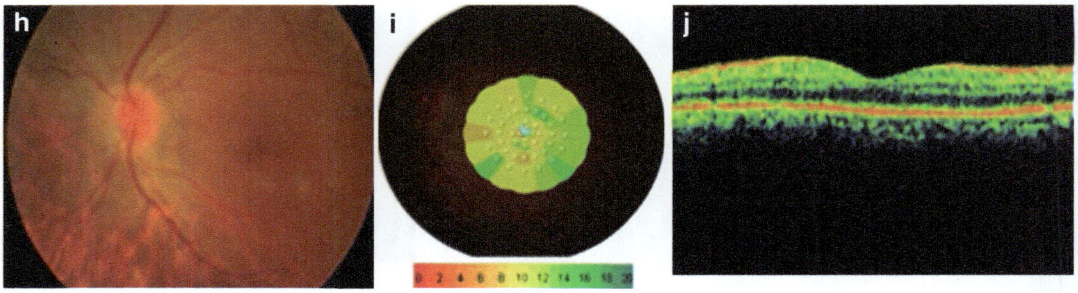

Fig. 9.7 (continued)

increases with larger skin reactions (Fig. 9.11) and with a history of exposure to an active case of TB [27]. It is important to note that the effect of neonatal vaccination with bacilli Calmette-Guérin (BCG) on tuberculin skin test declines over the first 7 years of life. In addition, it was demonstrated that an induration greater than 14 mm is unlikely to be due to prior BCG vaccination [49].

Interferon (IFN)-γ release assays are considered highly specific for *M. tuberculosis* because they are not confounded by prior vaccination for TB. A recent study [50] raised concerns about the sensitivity of QuantiFERON-TB Gold assay (QuantiFERON-TB Gold In-Tube, Cellestis, Carnegie, Australia) for detection of latent TB infection. In addition, another study demonstrated that there was no statistically significant difference in specificity between QuantiFERON-TB Gold assay and tuberculin skin test and that QuantiFERON-TB Gold assay may be less sensitive than the tuberculin skin test using a 15-mm induration cutoff value [51]. Kurup et al. [52] reported no demonstrable advantage of QuantiFERON-TB Gold test over tuberculin skin test for detection of latent TB infection in patients with granulomatous uveitis. Recently, Ang et al. [53] demonstrated that QuantiFERON-TB Gold assay was not superior to tuberculin skin test in sensitivity as a screening test or first-line study in TB-related uveitis. Similarly, Babu et al. [54] showed that QuantiFERON-TB Gold test is not specific for intraocular TB. In addition, Gineys et al. [55] showed a significantly higher median QuantiFERON-TB Gold value in a group of tuberculous uveitis patients with a successful therapeutic response to full antituberculous treatment compared to the group with treatment failure. A recent study showed that TB history or contact in the past and associated retinal vasculitis were significantly associated with tuberculosis-related uveitis. Sensitivity and specificity of the tuberculin skin test and QuantiFERON-TB Gold assay did not differ significantly with fair agreement [56].

Polymerase chain reaction (PCR) is a molecular technique used to detect mycobacterial DNA in clinical specimens. The false-positive PCR results and the low specificity of PCR might challenge the understanding of PCR results [57]. Aqueous, vitreous, and epiretinal membranes from patients with presumed TB uveitis are

Fig. 9.8 A 30-year-old woman with strongly positive tuberculin skin test (30 mm induration). Fundus photographs show multifocal choroiditis. Visual acuity was 20/80 in the right eye and 20/30 in the left eye (**a**). Fluorescein angiography shows that the lesions are hypofluorescent in the early phase and hyperfluorescent in the late phase (**b**). Indocyanine green angiography shows that the lesions are hypofluorescent throughout (**c**). Note that the lesions on indocyanine green angiography are more numerous than on fluorescein angiography. At presentation, the mean central retinal sensitivity was 3.5 dB in the right eye and 8.0 dB in the left eye (**d**). Two months after starting antituberculous therapy and systemic corticosteroids, the mean central retinal sensitivity improved to 7.3 dB in the right eye and 13 dB in the left eye. Visual acuity improved to 20/20 in both eyes (**e**)

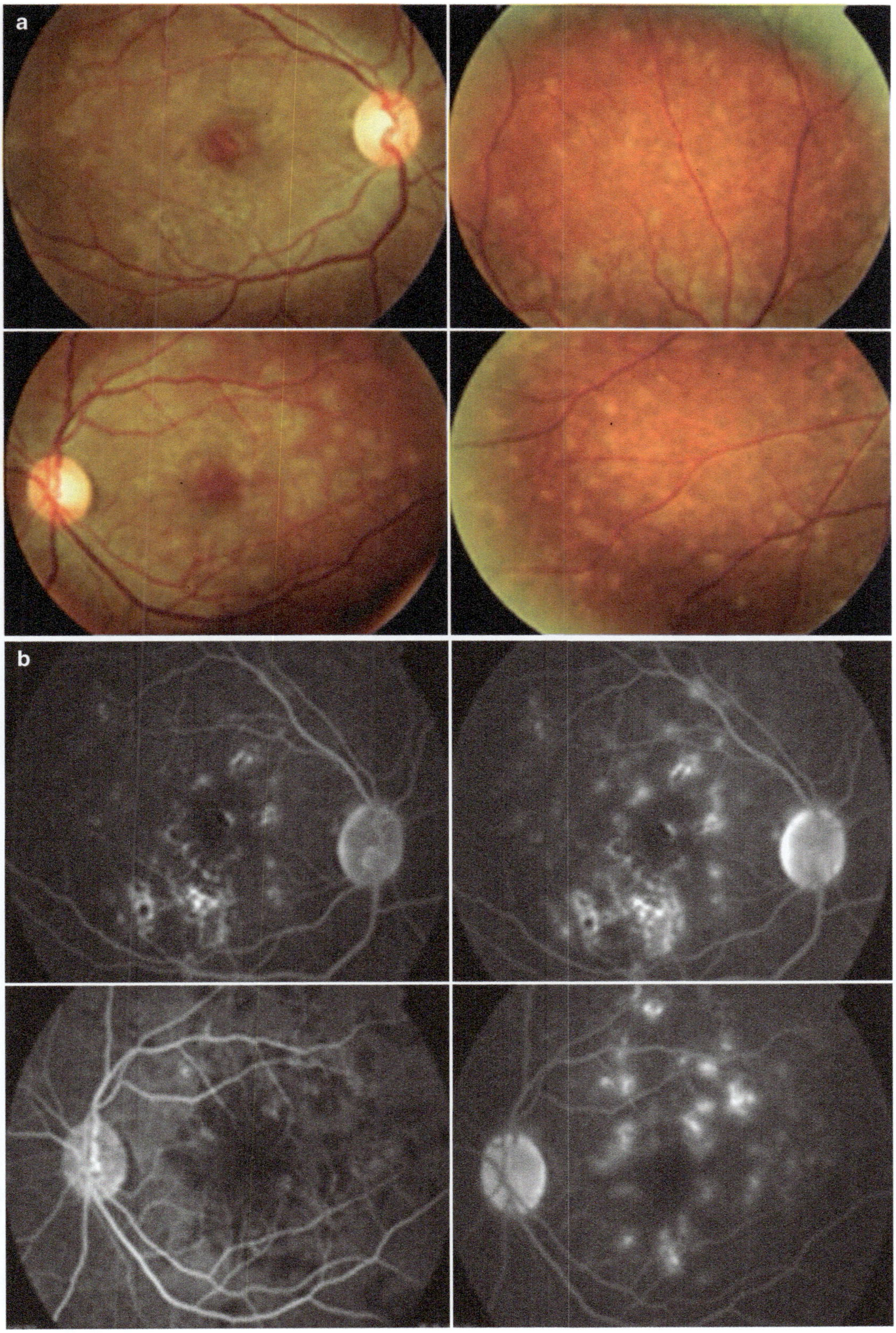
a
b

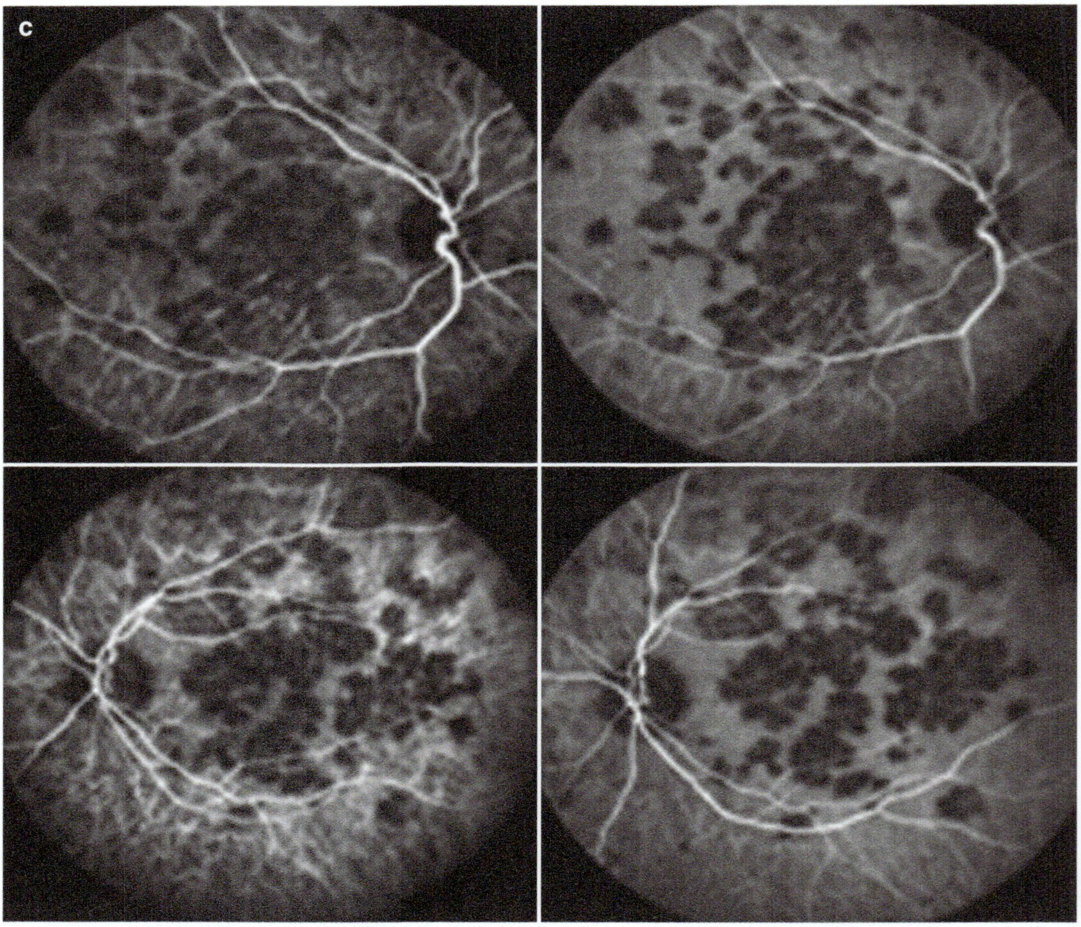

Fig. 9.8 (continued)

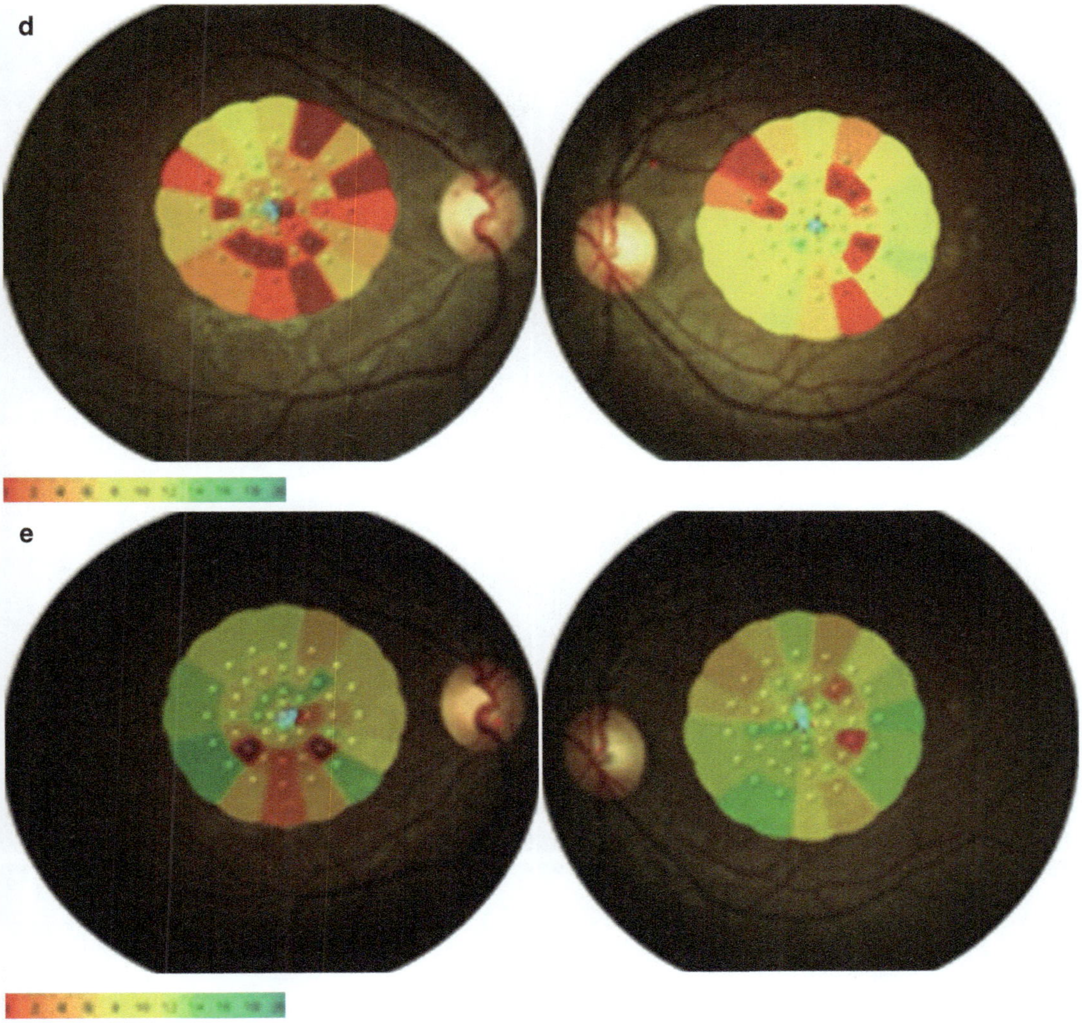

Fig. 9.8 (continued)

used as specimens for PCR. However, sensitivity was reported to be low [33]. Enzyme-linked immunosorbent assay detection of IgG antibodies against purified cord factor prepared from *M. tuberculosis* may be useful to support the diagnosis of presumed tuberculous uveitis [30]. Chest computed tomography (CT) is more sensitive in detecting presence, dimensions, and activity of tuberculous mediastinal lymphadenopathy which routine chest x-rays cannot detect in patients with presumed TB uveitis [58]. Recently, it was demonstrated that the use of positron emission tomography/CT is useful to identify lesions appropriate for biopsy and helps to establish the diagnosis [59].

9.4 Treatment

Our recommended therapy for tuberculous uveitis consists of isoniazid 5 mg/kg/day, rifampicin 450 mg/day if body weight is <50 kg and 600 mg if the weight is greater than 50 kg, ethambutol 15 mg/kg/day, and pyrazinamide 25–30 mg/kg/day initially for 2 months. Thereafter, rifampicin and isoniazid are used for another 7 months. Oral prednisone is added at a dose of 1 mg/kg/day until a clinical response is seen, then a slow reduction is established [60]. This treatment is effective in inducing resolution of inflammation without any recurrence after stopping antituberculous therapy and

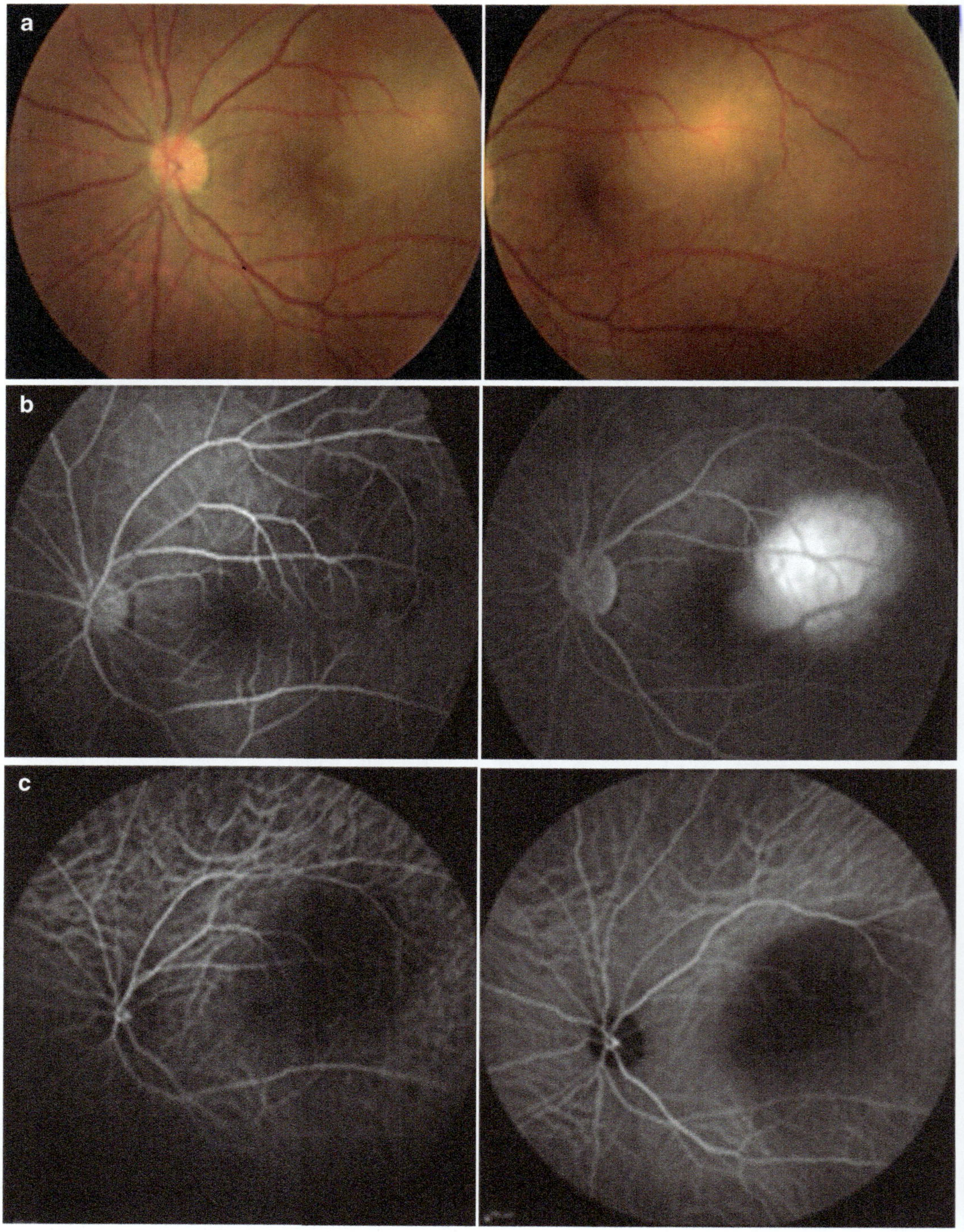

Fig. 9.9 Left eye of a 37-year-old man with strongly positive tuberculin skin test (18 mm induration). Visual acuity was measured by counting fingers at 3 ft. Fundus photographs shows subretinal amelanotic choroidal mass with exudative retinal detachment (**a**). Fluorescein angiography shows that the lesion is hypofluorescent in the early phase and hyperfluorescent in the late phase (**b**). Indocyanine green angiography shows that the lesion is hypofluorescent throughout (**c**). Optical coherence tomography shows exudative retinal detachment (**d**). Ultrasonography shows a solid elevated mass lesion on B-scan and a low internal reflectivity on A-scan (**e**). Two months after starting antituberculous therapy and systemic corticosteroids. Visual acuity improved to 20/25. Fundus photography shows resolution of the granuloma and chorioretinal scar. Optical coherence tomography displays resolution of exudative retinal detachment (**f**)

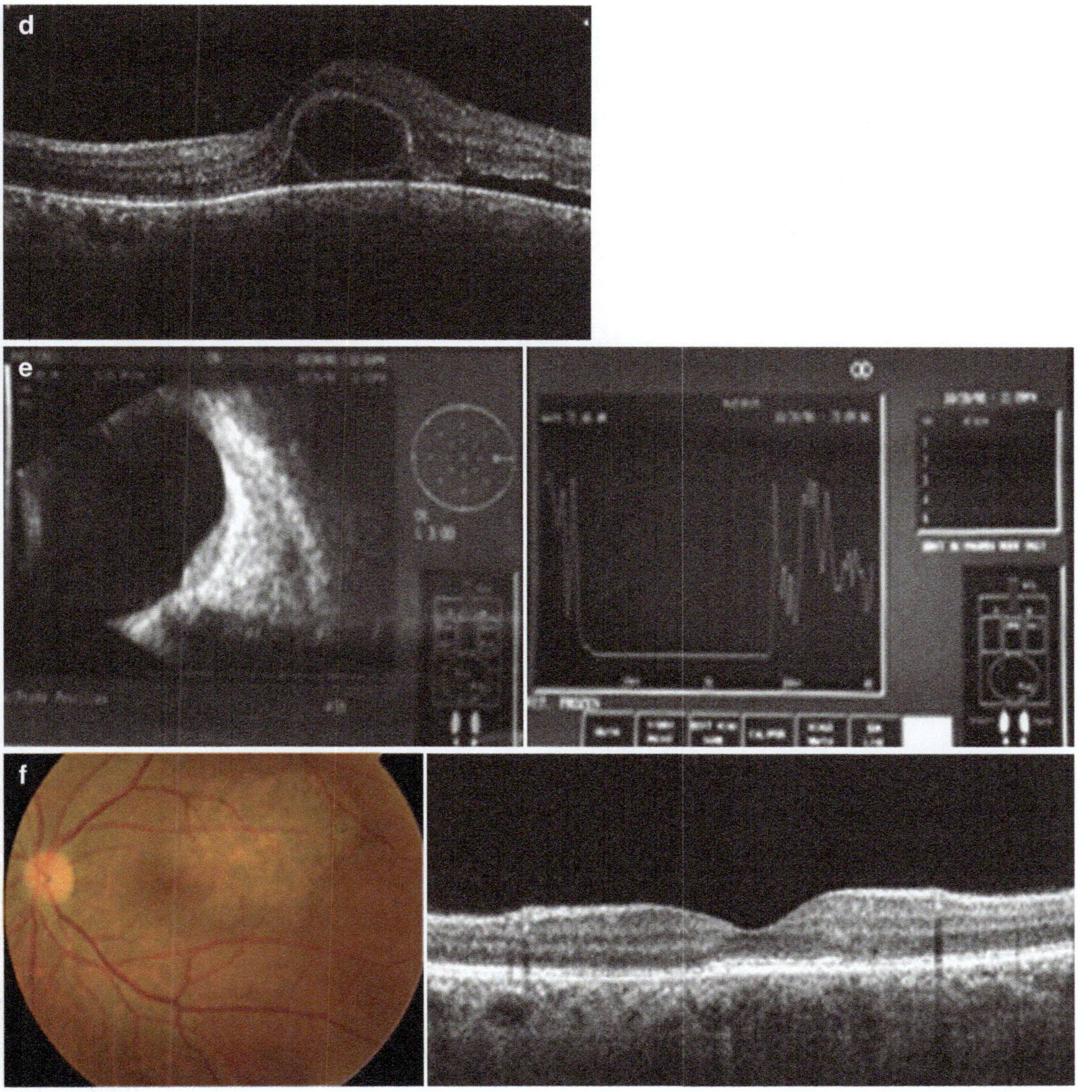

Fig. 9.9 (continued)

systemic corticosteroids. In addition, this treatment regimen induced a significant reduction in central macular thickness associated with significant improvement in visual acuity in eyes with macular edema (Fig. 9.3) [43]. We recently showed that antituberculous therapy combined with systemic corticosteroids improves central retinal sensitivity and fixation characteristics in patients with presumed tuberculous choroiditis (Figs. 9.7 and 9.8) [61].

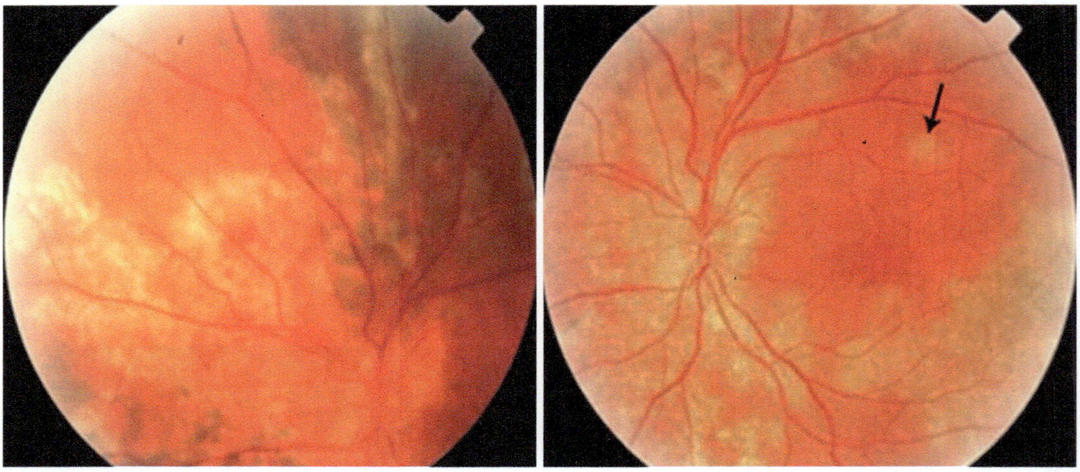

Fig. 9.10 Left eye of the a 45-year-old man with strongly positive tuberculin skin test (25 mm induration) shows widespread serpiginous-like areas of hyperpigmentary and hypopigmentary changes, which extended from the peripapillary region to mid-peripheral retina. Note the presence of active lesions in the macular area (*arrow*)

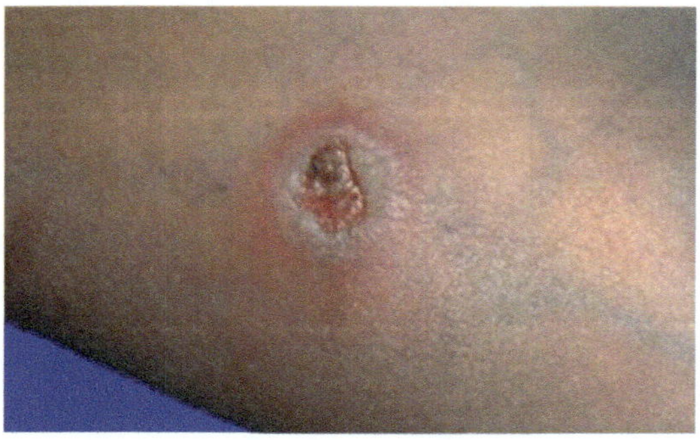

Fig. 9.11 A 30-year-old woman with presumed tuberculous uveitis with strongly positive tuberculin skin test (32 mm induration)

Compliance with Ethical Requirements

Conflict of Interest The authors declare that they have no conflict of interest.

Informed Consent No human studies were carried out by the authors for this article.

Animal Studies No animal studies were carried out by the authors for this article.

References

1. Centers for Disease Control and Prevention. Case definitions for infectious conditions under public health surveillance. MMWR Recomm Rep. 1997; 46:1–55.
2. Glassroth J, Robins AG, Snider DE. Tuberculosis in the 1980s. N Engl J Med. 1980;302:1441–50.
3. Baydur A. The spectrum of extrapulmonary tuberculosis. West J Med. 1977;126:253–62.
4. Kazokoglu H, Onal S, Tugal-Tutkun I, Mirza E, Akova Y, Ozyazgan Y, Soylu M, Batioglu F, Apaydin C. Demographic and clinical features of uveitis in tertiary centers in Turkey. Ophthalmic Epidemiol. 2008;15:285–93.
5. Pathanapitoon K, Kunavisarut P, Ausayakhun S, Sirirungsi W, Rothova A. Uveitis in a tertiary ophthalmology centre in Thailand. Br J Ophthalmol. 2008;92: 474–8.
6. Khairallah M, Yahia SB, Ladjimi A, Messaoud R, Zaouali S, Attia S, Jenzeri S, Jelliti B. Pattern of uveitis in a referral centre in Tunisia, North Africa. Eye. 2007;21:33–9.
7. Rathinam SR, Namperumalsamy P. Global variation and pattern changes in epidemiology of uveitis. Indian J Ophthalmol. 2007;55:173–83.
8. Yang P, Zhang Z, Zhou H, Li B, Huang X, Gao Y, Zhu L, Ren Y, Klooster J, Kijlstra A. Clinical patterns and characteristics of uveitis in a tertiary canter for uveitis in China. Curr Eye Res. 2005;30(11):943–8.
9. Sengun A, Karadag R, Karakurt A, Saricaoglu MS, Abdik O, Hasiripi H. Causes of uveitis in a referral hospital in Ankara, Turkey. Ocul Immunol Inflamm. 2005;13:45–50.
10. Soheilian M, Heidari K, Yazdani S, Shahsavari M, Ahmadieh H, Dehghan M. Patterns of uveitis in a tertiary eye care center in Iran. Ocul Immunol Inflamm. 2004;12:297–310.
11. Singh R, Gupta V, Gupta A. Pattern of uveitis in a referral eye clinic in north India. Indian J Ophthalmol. 2004;52:121–5.
12. Wakabayashi T, Morimura Y, Miyamoto Y, Okada AA. Changing pattern of intraocular inflammatory disease in Japan. Ocul Immunol Inflamm. 2003;11:277–86.

13. Islam SM, Tabbara KF. Causes of uveitis at The Eye Center in Saudi Arabia: a retrospective review. Ophthalmic Epidemiol. 2002;9:239–49.
14. Mercanti A, Parolini B, Bonora A, Lequaglie Q, Tomazzoli L. Epidemiology of endogenous uveitis in north-eastern Italy. Analysis of 655 new cases. Acta Ophthalmol Scand. 2001;79:64–8.
15. KaimboWaKimbo D, Bifuko A, Dernouchamps JP, Missotten L. Chronic uveitis in Kinshasa (D R Congo). Bull Soc Belge Ophthalmol. 1998;270:95–100.
16. Kotake S, Furudate N, Sasamoto Y, Yoshikawa K, Goda C, Matsuda H. Characteristics of endogenous uveitis in Hokkaido, Japan. Graefes Arch Clin Exp Ophthalmol. 1997;235:5–9.
17. Merrill PT, Kim J, Cox TA, Betor CC, McCallum RM, Jaffe GJ. Uveitis in southeastern United States. Curr Eye Res. 1997;16:865–74.
18. Rodriguez A, Calonge M, Pedroza-Seres M, Akova YA, Messmer EM, D'Amico DJ, Foster CS. Referral pattern of uveitis in tertiary eye care center. Arch Ophthalmol. 1996;114:593–9.
19. Thean LH, Thompson J, Rosenthal AR. A uveitis register at the Leicester Royal Infirmary. Ophthalmic Epidemiol. 1996;3:151–8.
20. Smit RL, Baarsma GS, de Vries J. Classification of 750 consecutive uveitis patients in the Rotterdam Eye Hospital. Int Ophthalmol. 1993;17:71–6.
21. Rothova A, Buitenhuis HJ, Meenken C, Brinkman CJ, Linssen A, Alberts C, Luyendijk L, Kijlstra A. Uveitis and systemic disease. Br J Ophthalmol. 1992;76:137–41.
22. Weiner A, BenEzra D. Clinical patterns and associated conditions in chronic uveitis. Am J Ophthalmol. 1991;112:151–8.
23. Palmares J, Coutinho MF, Castro-Correia J. Uveitis in northern Portugal. Curr Eye Res. 1990;9(Suppl):31–4.
24. Henderly DE, Genstler AJ, Smith RE, Rao NA. Changing pattern of uveitis. Am J Ophthalmol. 1987;103:131–6.
25. Almezaine HS, Kangave D, Abu El-Asrar AM. Patterns of uveitis in patients admitted to a university hospital in Riyadh Saudi Arabia. Ocul Immunol Inflamm. 2010;18:424–31.
26. Rosen PH, Spalton DJ, Graham EM. Intraocular tuberculosis. Eye. 1990;4:486–92.
27. Helm CJ, Holland GN. Ocular tuberculosis. Surv Ophthalmol. 1993;38:229–56.
28. Biswas J, Madhavan HN, Gopal L, Badrinath SS. Intraocular tuberculosis. Clinocopathologic study of five cases. Retina. 1995;15:461–8.
29. Sheu SJ, Shyu JS, Chen LM, Chen YY, Chirn SC, Wang JS. Ocular manifestations of tuberculosis. Ophthalmology. 2001;108:1580–5.
30. Sakai J-I, Matsuzawa S, Usui M, Yano I. New diagnostic approach for ocular tuberculosis by ELISA using the cord factor as antigen. Br J Ophthalmol. 2001;85:130–3.
31. Gupta A, Gupta V, Arora S, Dogra MR, Bambery P. PCR-positive tubercular retinal vasculitis. Clinical characteristics and management. Retina. 2001;21: 435–44.
32. Morimura Y, Okada AA, Kawahara S, Miyamoto Y, Kawai S, Hirakata A, Hida T. Tuberculin skin testing in uveitis patients and treatment of presumed intraocular tuberculosis in Japan. Ophthalmology. 2002;109:851–7.
33. Gupta V, Arora S, Gupta A, Ram J, Bambery P, Sehgal S. Management of presumed intraocular tuberculosis: possible role of the polymerase chain reaction. Acta Ophthalmol Scand. 1998;35:237–9.
34. Gupta V, Gupta A, Arora S, Bambery P, Dogra MR, Agarwal A. Presumed tubercular serpiginous-like choroiditis. Clinical presentation and management. Ophthalmology. 2003;110:1744–9.
35. Sarvananthan N, Wiselka M, Bibby K. Intraocular tuberculosis without detectable systemic infection. Arch Ophthalmol. 1998;116:1386–8.
36. Abu El-Asrar AM, Al-Kharashi SA. Full panretinal photocoagulation and early vitrectomy improve prognosis of retinal vasculitis associated with tuberculoprotein hypersensitivity (Eales' disease). Br J Ophthalmol. 2002;86:1248–51.
37. Wolfensberger TJ, Piguet B, Herbort CP. Indocyanine green angiographic features in tuberculouschorioretinitis. Am J Ophthalmol. 1999;127:350–3.
38. Mackensen F, Becker MD, Wiehler U, Max R, Dalpke A, Zimmermann S. QuantiFERON TB-Gold – a new test strengthening long-suspected tuberculous involvement in serpiginous-like choroiditis. Am J Ophthalmol. 2008;146:761–6.
39. Gupta V, Gupta A, Rao NA. Intraocular tuberculosis – an update. Surv Ophthalmol. 2007;52:561–87.
40. Cimino L, Herbort CP, Aldigeri R, Salvarani C, Boiardi L. Tuberculous uveitis, a resurgent and undiagnosed disease. Int Ophthalmol. 2009;29:67–74.
41. Bansal R, Gupta A, Gupta V, Dogra MR, Bambery P, Arora SK. Role of anti-tubercular therapy in uveitis with latent/manifest tuberculosis. Am J Ophthalmol. 2008;146:772–9.
42. Tabbara KF. Tuberculosis. Curr Opin Ophthalmol. 2007;18:493–501.
43. Al-Mezaine HS, Al-Muammar A, Kangave D, Abu El-Asrar AM. Clinical and optical coherence tomographic findings and outcome of treatment in patients with presumed tuberculous uveitis. Int Ophthalmol. 2008;28:413–23.
44. Demirci H, Shields CL, Shields JA, Eagle Jr RC. Ocular tuberculosis masquerading as ocular tumors. Surv Ophthalmol. 2004;49:78–89.
45. Bansal R, Gupta A, Gupta V, Dogra MR, Sharma A, Bambery P. Tubercular serpiginous-like choroiditis presenting as multifocal serpiginoidchoroiditis. Ophthalmology. 2012;119:2334–42.
46. Gupta A, Bansal R, Gupta V, Sharma A, Bambery P. Ocular signs predictive of tubercular uveitis. Am J Ophthalmol. 2010;149:562–70.
47. Ang M, Hedayatfar A, Zhang R, Chee SP. Clinical signs of uveitis associated with latent tuberculosis. Clin Experiment Ophthalmol. 2012;40:689–96.
48. Alvarez S, McCabe WR. Extrapulmonary tuberculosis revisited: a review of experience at Boston City and other hospitals. Medicine (Baltimore). 1984;63:25–55.

49. Rowland K, Guthmann R, Jamieson B, Malloy B. Clinical inquiries. How should we manage a patient with positive PPD and prior BCG vaccination? J Fam Pract. 2006;55:718–20.
50. Pollock NR, Campos-Neto A, Kashino S, Napolitano D, Behar SM, Shin D, Sloutsky A, Joshi S, Guillet J, Wong M, Mardell E. Discordant Quanti FERON-TB Gold test results among US healthcare workers with increased risk of latent tuberculosis infection: a problem or solution? Infect Control Hosp Epidemiol. 2008;29:878–86.
51. Mazurek GH, Zajdowicz MJ, Hankinson AL, Costigan DJ, Toney SR, Rothel JS, Daniels LJ, Pascual FB, Shang N, Keep LW, LoBue PA. Detection of *Mycobacterium tuberculosis* infection in United States navy recruits using the tuberculin skin test or whole-blood interferon-gamma release assays. Clin Infect Dis. 2007;45:826–36.
52. Kurup SK, Buggage RR, Clarke GL, Ursea R, Lim WK, Nussenblatt RB. Gamma interferon assay as an alternative to PPD skin testing in selected patients with granulomatous intraocular inflammatory disease. Can J Ophthalmol. 2006;41:737–40.
53. Ang M, Htoon HM, Chee SP. Diagnosis of tuberculous uveitis: clinical application of an interferon-gamma release assay. Ophthalmology. 2009;116(7):1391–6.
54. Babu K, Satish V, Satish S, et al. Utility of QuantiFERON TB gold test in a South Indian patient population of ocular inflammation. Indian J Ophthalmol. 2009;57:427–30.
55. Gineys R, Bodaghi B, Carcelain G, et al. QuantiFERON-TB gold cut-off value: implications for the management of tuberculosis-related ocular inflammation. Am J Ophthalmol. 2011;152(3):433–40.
56. Llorenç V, González-Martin J, Keller J, Rey A, Pelegrín L, Mesquida M, Adán A. Indirect supportive evidence for diagnosis of tuberculosis-related uveitis: from the tuberculin skin test to the new interferon gamma release assays. Acta Ophthalmol. 2013;91:e99–107.
57. Honoré-Bouakline S, Vincensini JP, Giacuzzo V, Lagrange PH, Hermann JL. Rapid diagnosis of extrapulmonary tuberculosis by PCR: impact of sample preparation and DNA extraction. J Clin Microbiol. 2003;41:2323–9.
58. Mehta S. Role of computed chest tomography (CT scan) in tuberculous retinal vasculitis. Ocul Immunol Inflamm. 2002;10:151–5.
59. Doycheva D, Deuter C, Hetzel J, et al. The use of positron emission tomography/CT in the diagnosis of tuberculosis-associated uveitis. Br J Ophthalmol. 2011;95:1290–4.
60. Abu El-Asrar AM, Abouammoh M, Al-Mezaine HS. Tuberculous uveitis. Int Ophthalmol Clin. 2010;50:19–39.
61. Abu El-Asrar AM, Almezaine HS. Anti-tuberculoustherapy combined with systemic corticosteroids improves retinal sensitivity in patients with active presumed tuberculous choroiditis. Int Ophthalmol. 2010;30:567–76.

Infections of the Posterior Segment: Ocular Syphilis

10

Sonia Zaouali, Rim Kahloun, and Moncef Khairallah

10.1 Introduction

Syphilis is a multisystem chronic bacterial infection caused by the gram-negative spirochete *Treponema pallidum*. The disease is most often transmitted during sexual contact. Congenital syphilis is transmitted through the placenta infection after the tenth week of pregnancy. Despite effective antibiotic treatment, the incidence of syphilis infection around the world is on the rise, with over 90 % of which are reported in developing nations, mostly in sub-Saharan Africa and Asia [1]. In the developed world, there have been alarming increases in the rates of syphilis infection in recent years, and this may be related to the post-AIDS/HAART era, with a growing pool of HIV-positive patients [2–4]. In fact, concurrent HIV infection is shown to be a risk factor for syphilis, with infection rates five to seven times higher in HIV-positive patients compared with the rate in the general population [5]. The most common ocular finding of syphilis is uveitis, occurring in 2.5–5 % of patients with tertiary syphilis and in 1–2 % of all uveitis cases [6]. Uveitis can occur at all stages of the infection including primary syphilis [7].

S. Zaouali, MD • R. Kahloun, MD
M. Khairallah, MD (✉)
Department of Ophthalmology, Fattouma Bourguiba University Hospital, Monastir, Tunisia

Faculty of Medicine, University of Monastir, Monastir, Tunisia
e-mail: moncef.khairallah@rns.tn

10.2 Clinical Features

10.2.1 Acquired Syphilis

The natural history of untreated acquired syphilis has been divided into four stages: primary, secondary, latent, and tertiary syphilis. Primary syphilis follows an incubation period of approximately 3 weeks and is characterized by a chancre, which is a painless, solitary lesion that originates at the site of inoculation, resolving spontaneously within 12 weeks regardless of treatment [8]. The central nervous system may be seeded with treponemes during this period, although there is an absence of neurologic findings. Secondary syphilis occurs 6–8 weeks later and is heralded by the appearance of lymphadenopathy and a generalized maculopapular rash that may be prominent on the palms and soles. This is followed by a latent period ranging from 1 year to decades [8]. Approximately one-third of untreated patients develop tertiary syphilis, which can be divided into a more benign localized granulomatous reaction, the gumma, and a severe diffuse inflammation involving primarily the cardiovascular and central nervous systems.

Ocular syphilis may present in a wide variety of inflammatory manifestations, reflecting its status as “the Great Imitator.” The ocular

K. Tabbara et al. (eds.), *Ocular Infections*, Essentials in Ophthalmology,
DOI 10.1007/978-3-662-43981-4_10, © Springer-Verlag Berlin Heidelberg 2014

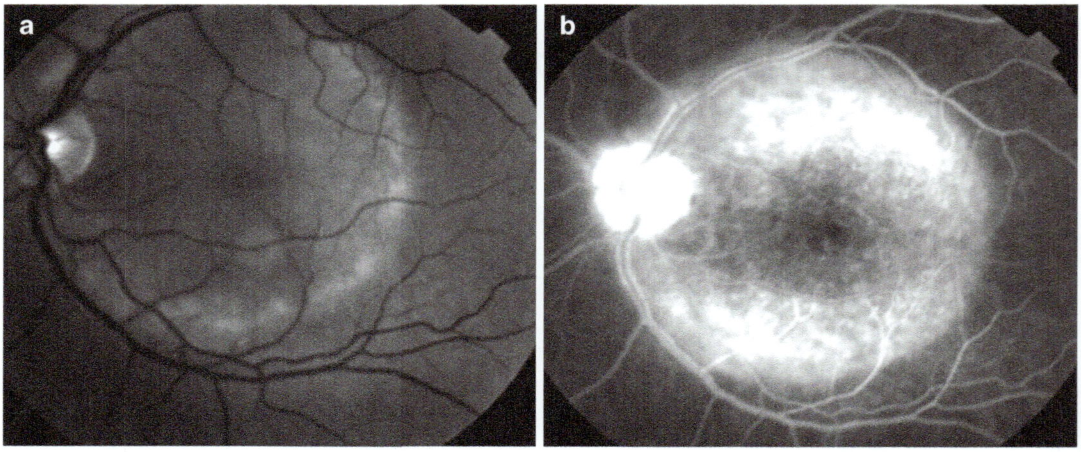

Fig. 10.1 (**a**) Red-free photograph of the left eye reveals an active, nonelevated, placoid, outer retinal lesion in the macula. (**b**) Late-phase fluorescein angiogram shows a geographic hyperfluorescent area and optic disk leakage (Courtesy, Bahram Bodaghi)

inflammation may be unilateral or bilateral and may affect both the anterior and posterior segments. Anterior uveitis may be nongranulomatous or granulomatous and may be associated with iris roseola, vascularized papules, large red nodules, and gummata. Other findings include episcleritis, scleritis, interstitial keratitis, posterior synechiae, lens dislocation, and iris atrophy [9–11].

Posterior segment findings of acquired syphilis include vitritis, chorioretinitis, focal or multifocal retinitis, necrotizing retinitis, retinal vasculitis, exudative retinal detachment, and optic neuropathy [8–10, 12–15].

A syphilitic posterior placoid chorioretinitis has been described, with clinical appearance and angiographic characteristics that are thought to be pathognomonic of secondary syphilis [16, 17]. Solitary or multifocal, macular or papillary, placoid, yellowish-gray lesions at the level of the retinal pigment epithelium (RPE), often with accompanying vitritis, display corresponding early hypofluorescence and late staining, along with retinal perivenous staining on fluorescein angiography (FA) (Fig. 10.1) [16, 17]. Indocyanine green angiography may show late-phase scattered hyperfluorescent spots [18].

Patients with acute syphilitic posterior placoid chorioretinitis show characteristic outer retinal abnormalities on SD OCT imaging including disruption of the inner segment/outer segment band, nodular thickening of the RPE with loss of the linear outer segment/RPE junction, and, in some cases, loss of the external limiting membrane, accumulation of subretinal fluid, and punctate hyperreflectivity in the choroid [19, 20].

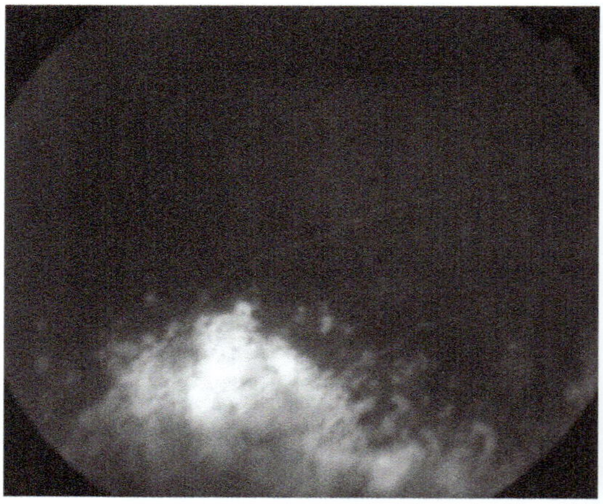

Fig. 10.2 Late-phase fluorescein angiogram shows multiple peripheral hyperfluorescent areas of retinitis. (Courtesy, Bahram Bodaghi)

Syphilitic uveitis can also manifest as retinitis without choroidal involvement, involving the posterior pole or the periphery (Fig. 10.2). The retinitis may be associated with vasculitis, papillitis, and vitritis with minimal if any anterior segment inflammation [14]. In addition to vessel wall staining and vascular and optic nerve leakage, FA may reveal intraretinal lesions in the areas of retinitis. Punctate retinitis with inner retinal and preretinal white dots is a possible feature of ocular syphilis [12, 15, 21].

Syphilis can present as a necrotizing retinitis in the midperiphery and peripheral retina and may resemble acute retinal necrosis or progressive outer retinal necrosis [22].

Isolated retinal vasculitis that affects the retinal arterioles, capillaries, and larger arteries or veins, or both, is another feature of syphilitic intraocular inflammation that may best be appreciated on FA. Focal retinal vasculitis may masquerade as a branch retinal vein occlusion.

Neuro-ophthalmic manifestations of syphilis include the Argyll Robertson pupil, ocular motor nerve palsies, isolated papillitis, optic neuropathy, neuroretinitis, and retrobulbar optic neuritis, which all appear most often in patients with tertiary syphilis or in neurosyphilis. Progressively visual loss secondary to optic atrophy can be seen as a manifestation of tertiary syphilis [6].

Ocular involvement in syphilis patients with HIV infection in the HAART era is more frequently bilateral and seems to involve the posterior segment more often with high frequencies of posterior uveitis, posterior placoid chorioretinitis, necrotizing retinitis, and optic nerve involvement [7, 10, 23–26].

10.2.2 Congenital Syphilis

Ocular inflammatory signs of syphilis may present at birth or decades later and include uveitis, interstitial keratitis, optic neuritis, glaucoma, and congenital cataract. A multifocal chorioretinitis and, less commonly, retinal vasculitis are the most frequent uveitic manifestations of early congenital infection [8]. Consequently, a bilateral "salt and pepper" fundus may develop, affecting the peripheral retina, posterior pole, or a single quadrant. These changes are not progressive, and the patient may have normal vision. A less commonly described funduscopic variation is that of a bilateral secondary degeneration of the RPE, which may mimic retinitis pigmentosa with narrowing of the retinal and choroidal vessels, optic disk pallor with sharp margins, and morphologically variable deposits of pigment [8].

10.3 Laboratory Investigations

The diagnosis of syphilitic uveitis is usually based on history and clinical presentation and is supported by a combination of *Treponema-specific* tests, such as the Venereal Disease Research Laboratory (VDRL) and rapid plasma reagin (RPR), and nontreponemal tests, such as the fluorescent treponemal antibody-absorption test (FTA-ABS) and *T. pallidum* particle agglutination test (TP-PA) [10].

False-positive nontreponemal and treponemal test results may be seen in case of systemic lupus erythematosus, leprosy, advanced age, intravenous drug abuse, bacterial endocarditis, tuberculosis, vaccinations, infectious mononucleosis, HIV infection, atypical pneumonia, malaria, pregnancy, rickettsial infections, and other spirochetal infections [10]. Subsequently, the use of only one serological test is insufficient in making the diagnosis. Patients should be initially tested using one of the nontreponemal tests, with the treponemal tests used to confirm a positive result.

RT-PCR for *Treponema pallidum* in aqueous humor or vitreous may be useful to confirm syphilitic uveitis [27, 28].

Testing for HIV should be performed in all patients with syphilis, given the high frequency of coinfection [7, 23].

10.4 Differential Diagnosis

Syphilis is one of the great masqueraders of medicine and should be always considered in the differential diagnosis of any intraocular inflammatory disease [6].

10.5 Treatment

Patients with syphilitic uveitis should be considered as having a CNS disease, requiring neurologic dosing regimens regardless of immune status. The recommended treatment is 18–24 million units (MU) of aqueous crystalline penicillin G per day, administered as 3–4 MU intravenously (IV) every 4 h or as a continuous infusion for 10–14 days [10]. Alternatively, ocular syphilis may be treated with 2.4 MU/day of intramuscular procaine penicillin plus probenecid 500 mg four times a day, both for 10–14 days. In the late stage, this may be followed by intramuscular benzathine penicillin G 2.4 MU weekly for up to 3 weeks [9, 10].

The recommended treatment regimen for congenital syphilis in infants during the first months of life is intravenous crystalline penicillin G at 100.000–150.000 units/kg/day, administered as 50.000 units/kg/day every 12 h during the first 7 days of life and every 8 h thereafter, for a total of 10 days [8]. Alternatively, intramuscular procaine penicillin G, 50.000 U/kg in a single daily dose for 10 days may be used.

Alternative treatments in penicillin-allergic patients who show no signs of neurosyphilis and who are HIV negative include doxycycline and tetracycline [9]. Ceftriaxone 2 g IV or IM daily for 10–14 days have been reported to be an effective alternative in patients with ocular syphilis who are penicillin allergic and HIV coinfected [9, 10].

Patients should be monitored for the development of the Jarisch-Herxheimer reaction, a hypersensitivity response of the host to treponemal antigens that are released in large numbers as spirochetes are killed during the first 24 h of treatment [9, 10, 29]. Patients present with constitutional symptoms but may also experience a concomitant increase in the severity of ocular inflammation that may require local and/or systemic corticosteroids.

Topical steroids may be used as an adjunctive treatment in case of keratitis, scleritis, or anterior uveitis. Periocular and/or systemic corticosteroids, appropriately covered with antibiotic therapy, may be useful adjuncts for treating the posterior segment inflammation [30]. Finally, the sexual contacts of the patient must be identified and treated, as a high percentage of these individuals are at risk for developing and transmitting this disease.

Compliance with Ethical Requirements

Conflict of Interest The authors declare that they have no conflict of interest.

Informed Consent No human studies were carried out by the authors for this article.

Animal Studies No animal studies were carried out by the authors for this article.

References

1. Hook 3rd EW, Peeling RW. Syphilis control: a continuing challenge. N Engl J Med. 2004;351:122–4.
2. Doris JP, Saha K, Jones NP, Sukthankar A. Ocular syphilis: the new epidemic. Eye (Lond). 2006;20: 703–5.
3. Chao JR, Khurana RN, Fawzi AA, Reddy HS, Rao NA. Syphilis: reemergence of an old adversary. Ophthalmology. 2006;113:2074–9.
4. Fonollosa A, Giralt J, Pelegrín L, Sánchez-Dalmau B, Segura A, García-Arumí J, Adan A. Ocular syphilis–back again: understanding recent increases in the incidence of ocular syphilitic disease. Ocul Immunol Inflamm. 2009;17:207–12.
5. Heffelfinger JD, Swint EB, Berman SM, Weinstock HS. Trends in primary and secondary syphilis among men who have sex with men in the United States. Am J Public Health. 2007;97:1076–83.
6. Aldave AJ, King JA, Cunningham Jr ET. Ocular syphilis. Curr Opin Ophthalmol. 2001;12:433–41.
7. Browning DJ. Posterior segment manifestations of active ocular syphilis, their response to a neurosyphilis regimen of penicillin therapy, and the influence of human immunodeficiency virus status on response. Ophthalmology. 2000;107:2015–23.
8. Margo CE, Hamed LM. Ocular syphilis. Surv Ophthalmol. 1992;37:203–20.
9. Kiss S, Damico FM, Young LH. Ocular manifestations and treatment of syphilis. Semin Ophthalmol. 2005;20:161–7.
10. Gaudio PA. Update on ocular syphilis. Curr Opin Ophthalmol. 2006;17:562–6.
11. Anshu A, Cheng CL, Chee SP. Syphilitic uveitis: an Asian perspective. Br J Ophthalmol. 2008;92: 594–7.
12. Fu EX, Geraets RL, Dodds EM, Echandi LV, Colombero D, McDonald HR, Jumper JM, Cunningham Jr ET. Superficial retinal precipitates in patients with syphilitic retinitis. Retina. 2010;30:1135–43.
13. Yang P, Zhang N, Li F, Chen Y, Kijlstra A. Ocular manifestations of syphilitic uveitis in Chinese patients. Retina. 2012;32:1906–14.
14. Wickremasinghe S, Ling C, Stawell R, Yeoh J, Hall A, Zamir E. Syphilitic punctate inner retinitis in immunocompetent gay men. Ophthalmology. 2009; 116:1195–200.
15. Puech C, Gennai S, Pavese P, Pelloux I, Maurin M, Romanet JP, Chiquet C. Ocular manifestations of syphilis: recent cases over a 2.5-year period. Graefes Arch Clin Exp Ophthalmol. 2010;248:1623–9.

16. Gass JDM, Braunstein RA, Chenoweth RG. Acute syphilitic posterior placoid chorioretinitis. Ophthalmology. 1990;97:1288–97.
17. Eandi CM, Neri P, Adelman RA, Yannuzzi LA, Jr Cunningham ET, International Syphilis Study Group. Acute syphilitic posterior placoid chorioretinitis: report of a case series and comprehensive review of the literature. Retina. 2012;32:1915–41.
18. Mora P, Borruat FX, Guex-Crosier Y. Indocyanine green angiography anomalies in ocular syphilis. Retina. 2005;25:171–81.
19. Pichi F, Ciardella AP, Cunningham Jr ET, Morara M, Veronese C, Jumper JM, Albini TA, Sarraf D, McCannel C, Voleti V, Choudhry N, Bertelli E, Giuliari GP, Souied E, Amer R, Regine F, Ricci F, Neri P, Nucci P. Spectral domain optical coherence tomography findings in patients with acute syphilitic posterior placoid chorioretinopathy. Retina. 2014;34: 373–84.
20. Brito P, Penas S, Carneiro A, Palmares J, Reis FF. Spectral-domain optical coherence tomography features of acute syphilitic posterior placoid chorioretinitis: the role of autoimmune response in pathogenesis. Case Rep Ophthalmol. 2011;2:39–44.
21. Reddy S, Cunningham Jr ET, Spaide RF. Syphilitic retinitis with focal inflammatory accumulations. Ophthalmic Surg Lasers Imaging. 2006;37:429–31.
22. Mendelsohn AD, Jampol LM. Syphilitic retinitis. A cause of necrotizing retinitis. Retina. 1984;4:221–4.
23. Tucker JD, Li JZ, Robbins GK, Davis BT, Lobo AM, Kunkel J, Papaliodis GN, Durand ML, Felsenstein D. Ocular syphilis among HIV-infected patients: a systematic analysis of the literature. Sex Transm Infect. 2011;87:4–8.
24. Tran TH, Cassoux N, Bodaghi B, Fardeau C, Caumes E, Lehoang P. Syphilitic uveitis in patients infected with human immunodeficiency virus. Graefes Arch Clin Exp Ophthalmol. 2005;243:863–9.
25. Li SY, Birnbaum AD, Tessler HH, Goldstein DA. Posterior syphilitic uveitis: clinical characteristics, co-infection with HIV, response to treatment. Jpn J Ophthalmol. 2011;55:486–94.
26. Amaratunge BC, Camuglia JE, Hall AJ. Syphilitic uveitis: a review of clinical manifestations and treatment outcomes of syphilitic uveitis in human immunodeficiency virus-positive and negative patients. Clin Experiment Ophthalmol. 2010;38: 68–74.
27. Cornut PL, Sobas CR, Perard L, De Bats F, Salord H, Manificat HJ, Denis P, Burillon C. Detection of Treponema pallidum in aqueous humor by real-time polymerase chain reaction. Ocul Immunol Inflamm. 2011;19:127–8.
28. Müller M, Ewert I, Hansmann F, Tiemann C, Hagedorn HJ, Solbach W, Roider J, Nölle B, Laqua H, Hoerauf H. Detection of Treponema pallidum in the vitreous by PCR. Br J Ophthalmol. 2007;91: 592–5.
29. Fathilah J, Choo MM. The Jarisch-Herxheimer reaction in ocular syphilis. Med J Malaysia. 2003;58: 437–9.
30. Solebo AL, Westcott M. Corticosteroids in ocular syphilis. Ophthalmology. 2007;114:1593.

11 Infections of the Posterior Segment: Other Bacterial Infections

Bechir Jelliti, Imen Khairallah-Ksiaa, and Riadh Messaoud

11.1 Introduction

Although tuberculosis and syphilis are the most important bacterial causes of uveitis, other bacterial diseases including cat-scratch disease, Lyme disease, and Whipple's disease have been associated with ocular posterior segment manifestations, including retinitis, choroiditis, retinal vasculitis, and optic neuropathy. Diagnosis of any of these infectious diseases is primarily based on epidemiological data, history, systemic symptoms, and pattern of ocular involvement. Laboratory diagnosis relies on cytology, serology, and/or PCR. Management involves systemic antibiotic therapy with or without the use of corticosteroids.

11.2 Cat-Scratch Disease

Cat-scratch disease (CSD) is a worldwide distributed self-limited, systemic illness caused by the gram-negative bacillus, *Bartonella henselae*. The disease entity was first described in 1950 by Debré et al., but the causative agent was discovered only in 1983. An array of ocular manifestations, dominated by neuroretinitis, has been described in association with CSD [1].

11.2.1 Epidemiology

CSD is a worldwide-distributed feline-associated zoonotic disease. In the USA there are an estimated 22.000 new cases of CSD per year, and in the Netherlands the incidence of CSD was estimated to be 2.000 cases per year [1]. Children and young adults are reported to be at increased risk for systemic *B. henselae* infection, which appears to have a seasonal pattern, occurring predominantly in the fall and winter [2]. HIV positivity may be a risk factor for *Bartonella* infection [1]. Ocular involvement occurs in 5–10 % of patients with cat-scratch disease [3].

11.2.2 Life Cycle and Pathogenesis

Cats are the primary mammalian reservoir of *B. henselae*, and the cat flea is an important vector for the transmission of the organism among cats. The disease is transmitted to humans by the scratches, licks, and bites of domestic cats, particularly kittens [1].

The eye can be involved either with the primary inoculation complex, resulting in Parinaud oculoglandular syndrome, or by hematogenous

B. Jelliti, MD • I. Khairallah-Ksiaa, MD
R. Messaoud, MD (✉)
Department of Ophthalmology, Fattouma Bourguiba University Hospital, Monastir, Tunisia

Faculty of Medicine, University of Monastir, Monastir, Tunisia
e-mail: messaoud_riadh@yahoo.fr

K. Tabbara et al. (eds.), *Ocular Infections*, Essentials in Ophthalmology,
DOI 10.1007/978-3-662-43981-4_11, © Springer-Verlag Berlin Heidelberg 2014

spread, leading to an array of ocular and neuro-ophthalmic manifestations [1, 2].

11.2.3 Clinical Features

11.2.3.1 Systemic Features

CSD is commonly diagnosed in children and young adults. The infected individual often develops a local minor lesion at the inoculation site, followed by tender regional lymphadenopathy and flu-like syndrome that resolves over several weeks [3]. However, in a small percentage of patients, particularly within the immunocompromised population, there may be extranodal dissemination with severe systemic complications, including encephalitis, pneumonia, osteomyelitis, and hepatosplenic disease [3].

11.2.3.2 Ocular Features

Adnexal and anterior segment involvement in CSD may include Parinaud oculoglandular syndrome, which is the most common ocular manifestation of CSD [2]. It is characterized by the association of regional lymphadenopathy with infection of the conjunctiva, eyelid, or adjacent skin [8]. CSD has been occasionally associated with conjunctival involvement simulating rhabdomyosarcoma, orbital abscess, stromal keratitis, anterior uveitis, and neovascular glaucoma.

CSD is the most common recognized cause of neuroretinitis [5–7]. The ocular condition is usually unilateral, although bilateral cases have also been reported. The onset of visual symptoms usually follows the inoculation by approximately 4 weeks and the systemic symptoms by 2–3 weeks. The most common complaint is decreased vision, with visual acuity ranging from 20/20 to light perception. A relative afferent pupillary defect, dyschromatopsia, and a visual field defect are usually seen. Mild anterior chamber and vitreous inflammation is also common. Fundus examination typically shows optic disk edema associated with a partial or complete macular star (Fig. 11.1). The optic disk edema occurs approximately 1 week prior to the development of stellate maculopathy, which therefore may be absent at the time of initial presentation. The optic nerve involvement leads to peripapillary retinal thickening and, frequently, an exudative retinal detachment [4]. Intraretinal hemorrhages or telangiectatic vessels may be seen [5]. Fluorescein angiography shows leakage from the optic disk with no evidence of capillary abnormality in the macular area [6]. Indocyanine green angiography also may show optic disk hyperfluorescence. Optical coherence tomography may be helpful in detecting serous detachment.

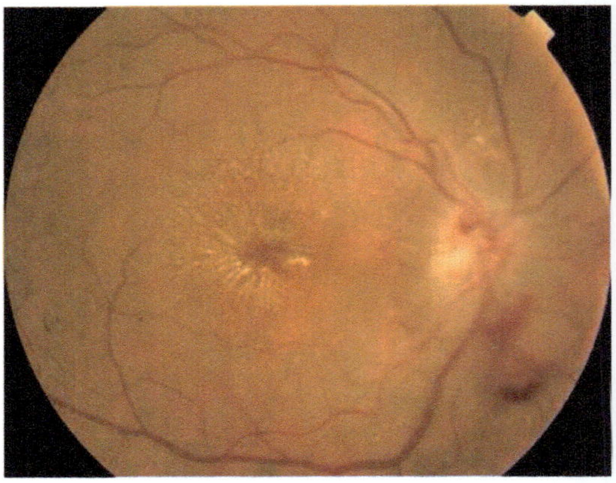

Fig. 11.1 Fundus photograph of the right eye of a patient with cat-scratch disease shows optic disk edema with telangiectasis, a complete macular star, and retinal and preretinal hemorrhages

Neuroretinitis usually has a self-limited course. Most patients recover excellent visual acuity over a period of several weeks to months [7]. The macular star usually resolves in approximately 8–12 weeks, but it may be present for up to 1 year. A few patients may be left with mild pallor of the optic disk [8]. Retinal pigment epithelial changes also may develop after resolution of a prominent macular star. Cat-scratch disease may occasionally present with a large inflammatory mass or exudate of the optic nerve head [9].

One or more white areas of inner retinitis or chorioretinitis, typically juxtavascular in location, may accompany neuroretinitis [7, 10] or occur in the absence of obvious optic disk involvement [7, 11, 12]. These retinal lesions were found to be more common than neuroretinitis by some authors [11]. They may be associated with an angiomatous-like proliferation of retinal capillaries, which is more clearly characterized by fluorescein angiography [13, 14]. The inner white retinal lesions in the posterior fundus may simulate cotton-wool ischemic spots, but their distribution in the fundus is not necessarily associated with the distribution of a first-order arteriole as is the case with cotton-wool spots. Branch retinal arteriolar occlusion [10, 11, 15] or branch retinal venous occlusion [8, 15] may be associated with an area of focal retinitis. A case of central retinal artery and vein occlusion has been reported [16].

Less common chorioretinal manifestations of CSD include large inflammatory retinal mass in the posterior pole [9], subretinal mass associated with an abnormal vascular network [16], intermediate uveitis with retinal vasculitis [17], unilateral panuveitis with clinical and fluorescein angiographic features simulating Vogt-Koyanagi-Harada disease [18], isolated serous macular detachment [19], serous macular detachment simulating central serous chorioretinopathy [20], macular hole [21], and vitreous hemorrhage [22].

11.2.4 Laboratory Investigations

The earliest test for the diagnosis is a positive skin test in response to CSD antigen. This test is likely to remain positive for life. Another possibility for the diagnosis is the detection of histopathological changes in a lymph node or conjunctival biopsy (the Warthin-Starry silver impregnation stain). The blood culture isolation of *B. henselae* is difficult, expensive, and requires 12–45 days. Thanks to the development of serological tests, the diagnosis of CSD is now much easier [23]. An indirect fluorescent antibody (IFA) test was developed to detect the humoral response to the organism. The sensitivity and specificity of this assay appear to be 90 % or better for immunocompetent patients [24]. Enzyme-linked immunoassays (EIA) and Western blot procedures were later developed, and EIA was shown to have IgG sensitivity of 86–95 % and specificity of 96 % compared with IFA [25]. A single positive indirect fluorescent antibody or enzyme immunoassay titer for IgG or IgM is sufficient to confirm the diagnosis of CSD. Positive IgM test is related to acute disease, but production of IgM is ephemeral. IgG titers less than 1:64 suggest the patient does not have Bartonella infection. Titers between 1:64 and 1:256 characterize possible infection, and the test should be repeated in 10–14 days. Titers greater than 1:256 suggest active or recent infection [1].

More recently, a polymerase chain reaction-based assay for the detection of *B. henselae* 16S ribosomal RNA gene in a very small sample of serum or other body fluids has been employed for diagnosis purposes [26].

11.2.5 Differential Diagnosis

Differential diagnosis of neuroretinitis includes several infectious and inflammatory diseases, including syphilis, Lyme disease, tuberculosis, sarcoidosis, diffuse unilateral subacute neuroretinitis (DUSN), toxoplasmosis, toxocariasis, leptospirosis, salmonella, chickenpox, herpes simplex, ehrlichiosis, rickettsioses, and recurrent idiopathic neuroretinitis [2]. Other causes of optic disk edema and macular star include systemic hypertension, diabetes mellitus, increased intracranial pressure, branch retinal vein occlusion, and anterior ischemic optic neuropathy.

11.2.6 Treatment

Till now, there are no guidelines for the treatment of CSD or its ocular complications. For most immunocompetent patients the disease has a self-limited course. Many physicians do not treat mild to moderate systemic CSD. They treat severe ocular or systemic complications of *B. henselae* infection in immunocompetent patients and all immunocompromised patients. They often use doxycycline, erythromycin, ciprofloxacin, azithromycin, trimethoprim-sulfamethoxazole, rifampin, or intramuscular gentamicin [23, 27].

A typical regimen for immunocompetent patients older than age 8 consists of doxycycline, 100 mg orally twice daily for 2–4 weeks. In case of severe infection, doxycycline may be given intravenously or used in combination with rifampin, 300 mg orally twice daily. Among immunocompromised individuals, treatment duration is extended to 4 months. Children with CSD may be treated with azithromycin. Paradoxical response to treatment has been reported in ocular bartonellosis [28]. The role of oral corticosteroids in the management of ocular CSD is unknown.

To prevent CSD, it is recommended to wash and disinfect any wounds immediately after a cat scratch or bite, and avoid contact with stray felines. Immunocompromised patients should be especially careful to avoid scratches and to control flea infestation. Long-term use of doxycycline or a macrolide antibiotic such as erythromycin may be useful for preventing recurrences in HIV-positive patients [2].

11.3 Lyme Disease

Lyme disease or Lyme borreliosis is an emerging tick-borne infection caused by a group of related spirochetes [29].

11.3.1 Epidemiology

Lyme disease is a worldwide-distributed infection. In North America, the only species of Lyme Borrelia known to cause human disease is *Borrelia burgdorferi*. In Europe, at least five species of Lyme Borrelia (*B. afzelii*, *B. garinii*, *B. burgdorferi*, *B. spielmanii*, and *B. bavariensis*) can cause the disease [29].

Lyme disease affects men slightly more often than women and has a bimodal age distribution, with peaks in children aged 5–14 years and in adults aged 30–59 years. Most cases occur between May and September.

11.3.2 Life Cycle and Pathogenesis

Animal reservoirs include deer, horses, cows, rodents, birds, cats, and dogs. The spirochete is transmitted to humans through the bite of infected ticks. The main vector of Lyme Borrelia in Europe is *Ixodes ricinus*, whereas *Ixodes persulcatus* is the main vector in Asia. *Ixodes scapularis* is the main vector in northeastern and upper midwestern USA, and *Ixodes pacificus* is the vector in western USA [29]. The pathogenesis of ocular involvement remains controversial, but the symptoms are believed to be due to direct ocular infection and a delayed hypersensitivity mechanism.

11.3.3 Clinical Features

11.3.3.1 Systemic Features

The clinical manifestations of Lyme disease have been divided into three stages: early, disseminated, and persistent or late stages [29, 30]. Early stage is characterized by erythema migrans that occurs 7–10 days following the bite, fever, and lymphadenopathy. Disseminated stage occurs few days to several months after the bite and may manifest with erythema chronica migrans, lymphocytoma, arthritis, and cardiac and neurologic manifestations. In late stage, patients may develop arthritis of major joints, progressive encephalomyelitis, and skin disorders.

11.3.3.2 Ocular Features

Ocular inflammation is uncommon and occurs mainly in the second and late stages of the disease. It may manifest as anterior uveitis, intermediate uveitis, posterior uveitis, or panuveitis [30–40]. Intermediate uveitis with associated granulomatous anterior chamber reaction and papillitis is the most common clinical presentation (Fig. 11.2). Retinal vasculitis may result in macular edema, vascular occlusion, and cotton-wool spots [41, 42]. A distinct clinical entity of peripheral multifocal choroiditis has been described in patients with Lyme disease. It is characterized by multiple, small, round, punched-out lesions associated with vitritis similar to those seen with sarcoidosis [31, 43]. Choroidal involvement may lead to retinal pigment epithelial clumping resembling the inflammatory changes seen with syphilis or rubella.

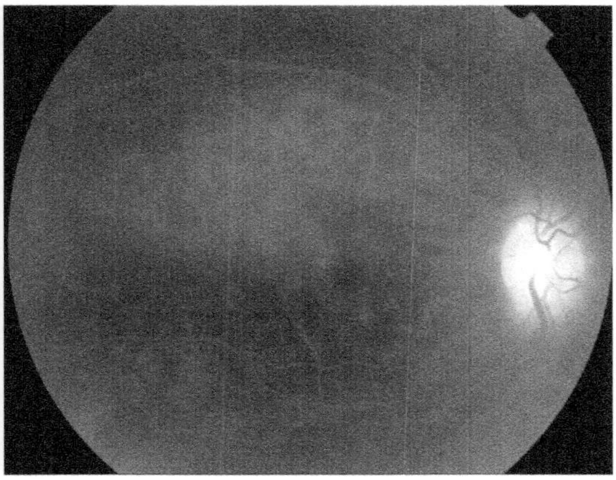

Fig. 11.2 Intermediate uveitis in a patient with Lyme disease with vitritis, retinal vasculitis, optic disk hyperfluorescence, and macular edema

Optic nerve involvement includes papillitis, optic neuritis, neuroretinitis, and papilledema associated with meningitis [44–46]. Neuro-ophthalmic manifestations include multiple cranial nerve involvement (II, III, IV, V, VI, and, most commonly, VII) unilaterally or bilaterally, either sequentially or simultaneously [30]. Horner syndrome, tonic pupil, and mydriasis have also been reported [30].

Other ophthalmic manifestations of Lyme disease may include conjunctivitis, episcleritis, interstitial and ulcerative keratitis, posterior scleritis, dacryoadenitis, and orbital myositis [30, 31, 47, 48].

11.3.4 Laboratory Investigations

The diagnosis of Lyme disease is based on epidemiological data, medical history, clinical ocular and systemic presentation, and serology. However, false-positive serological tests may lead to incorrect diagnosis in the presence of conditions such as infectious mononucleosis, rheumatoid disease, autoimmune diseases, and other spirochetal infections. A testing approach using ELISA for IgM and IgG, followed by Western blot testing, is recommended [49].

PCR-based assays have been successfully used to amplify both genomic and plasmid *B. burgdorferi* DNA from a variety of tissues including ocular fluids, with the highest yields being obtained from the skin [32].

11.3.5 Differential Diagnosis

The differential diagnosis of uveitis associated with Lyme disease includes syphilis, tuberculosis, rubella, cat-scratch disease, sarcoidosis, leptospirosis, rickettsioses, and Whipple's disease [30].

11.3.6 Treatment

Treatment of Lyme disease is based on combination of antibiotics and corticosteroids. The most commonly used antibiotics are amoxicillin, doxycycline, cefotaxime, and cefuroxime. Intraocular inflammation associated with Lyme disease may be treated with oral doxycycline 200 mg/day or intravenous ceftriaxone at the dose of 2 g IV qd in adults for at least 3 weeks [37]. New ketolide antibiotics such as telithromycin and cethromycin are very effective against Borrelia organisms with high plasma and tissue concentrations following oral administration and hold promise as alternative treatments for Lyme disease [50].

Anterior segment inflammation may be treated with topical corticosteroids and mydriatics.

One case of macular edema associated with Lyme disease treated with intravitreal triamcinolone has been reported [42].

A Jarisch-Herxheimer reaction with transient worsening of ocular symptoms after treatment has been reported in Lyme disease [31, 32].

Prevention strategies for Lyme disease include avoiding tick-infested habitats, use of tick repellents, wearing protective outer garments, prompt removal of attached ticks, and reducing tick populations.

Doxycycline chemoprophylaxis can reduce the chance of developing Lyme borreliosis after removal of an *I. scapularis* or an *I. persulcatus* tick. One 200 mg dose of doxycycline within 72 h of tick removal should be considered for individuals in highly endemic areas [29].

A trial on new vaccine against Lyme disease showed promising results [51].

11.4 Whipple's Disease

Whipple's disease is a rare, chronic, multisystem disease, caused by the gram-positive bacillus, *Tropheryma whipplei*. It was first described by George Hoyt Whipple in 1907 [52].

11.4.1 Epidemiology

Whipple's disease is most common in middle-aged white men. The sex ratio is three males to one female, mostly of Caucasian origin. Mean age at diagnosis is 48–54 years for male patients and a few years older for female patients [53].

11.4.2 Clinical Features

Systemic involvement in Whipple's disease includes migratory arthritis and gastrointestinal symptoms, including diarrhea, steatorrhea, and malabsorption [53]. Intestinal loss of protein results in pitting edema and weight loss. Cardiomyopathy and valvular disease can also occur. Central nervous system involvement occurs in 10 % of cases and may result in seizures, dementia, and coma [54].

Ocular involvement is rare in patients with Whipple's disease and may occur alone or with gastrointestinal, neurologic, or other systemic manifestations. It occurs in less than 5 % of cases, usually late in the course of the disease [55]. However, in up to one third of the patients, ocular involvement may be the only clinical manifestation of disease before performing systemic investigations [56, 57].

A broad spectrum of ocular manifestations in Whipple's disease has been reported including uveitis, retinitis, choroiditis, retinal vasculitis, retinal hemorrhages, and cystoid macular edema [55–65]. Patients can present with bilateral panuveitis and retinal vasculitis. Both granulomatous or nongranulomatous anterior uveitis and moderate to severe vitritis may be present. Diffuse chorioretinal inflammation and diffuse retinal vasculitis may occur. Retinal vascular occlusions, retinal hemorrhages, and vitreous hemorrhage may result from the vasculitis. Optic disk edema

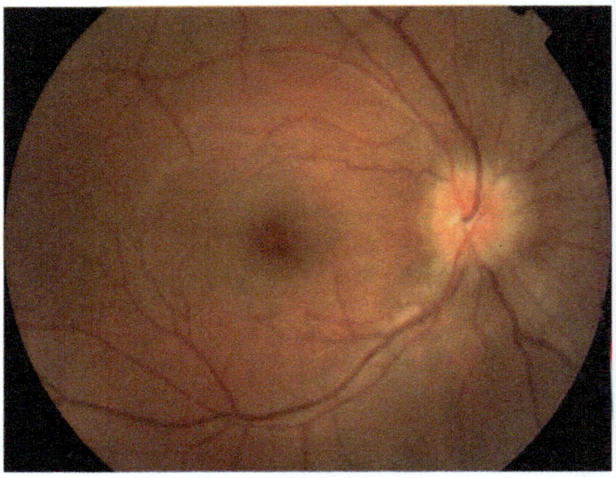

Fig. 11.3 Optic disk edema in a patient with Whipple's disease

(Fig. 11.3) and, later, optic atrophy may occur. Other neuro-ophthalmic manifestations can include cranial nerve palsies, nystagmus, ophthalmoplegia, ptosis, and convergence paresis associated with oculomasticatory myokymia. Some patients develop progressive supranuclear palsy-like condition.

11.4.3 Laboratory Investigations

Diagnosis of ocular Whipple's disease is challenging, especially in the absence of gastrointestinal involvement. Cytologic diagnosis, based on the observation of periodic acid-Schiff (PAS)-positive macrophages in biopsy of the duodenal mucosa, is still used routinely. It remains highly sensitive but is nonspecific. Electron microscopy can demonstrate the presence of degenerated bacillary microorganisms in the vitreous or gastrointestinal tract.

PCR analysis of peripheral blood and vitreous or cerebrospinal fluid may show *T. whipplei* DNA and confirm the diagnosis [64]. Culturing of *T. whipplei* is difficult, but possible [65].

11.4.4 Differential Diagnosis

The differential diagnosis of uveitis associated with Whipple's disease includes sarcoidosis, tuberculosis, Behçet's disease, systemic lupus erythematosus, periarteritis nodosa, histoplasmosis, multifocal choroiditis, intraocular lymphoma, amyloidosis, Lyme disease, and *Mycobacterium avium-intracellulare* infection [55, 56].

11.4.5 Treatment

Different antibiotic regimens have been proposed including chloramphenicol, rifampin, penicillin, cephalosporin, streptomycin, tetracyclines, or sulfonamides such as trimethoprim-sulfamethoxazole (TMP-SMX) [56]. Oral TMP (160 mg) and SMX (800 mg) twice daily, associated with rifampin (600 mg/day), for at least 1 year is the treatment of choice in CNS or ocular Whipple's disease. Folate supplementation is required during treatment with TMP-SMX. A low-dose antibiotic regimen (TMP 160 mg/day and SMX 800 mg/day once daily) for more than 1 year to prevent relapse, neurologic involvement, and death is recommended [56]. The optimal duration of treatment remains to be defined.

Third-generation cephalosporins are effective in the treatment of Whipple's disease resistant to TMP-SMX. Corticosteroids are usually not required to control intraocular inflammation during antibiotic treatment.

Compliance with Ethical Requirements

Conflict of Interest The authors declare that they have no conflict of interest.

Informed Consent No human studies were carried out by the authors for this article.

Animal Studies No animal studies were carried out by the authors for this article.

References

1. Biancardi AL, Curi AL. Cat scratch disease. Ocul Immunol Inflamm. 2014;22:148–54.
2. Cunningham ET, Koehler JE. Ocular bartonellosis. Am J Ophthalmol. 2000;130:340–9.
3. Carithers HA. Cat scratch disease: an overview based on a study of 1,200 patients. Am J Dis Child. 1985;139:1124–33.
4. Wade NK, Levi L, Jones MR, Bhisitkul R, Fine L, Cunningham Jr ET. Optic disk edema associated with peripapillary serous retinal detachment: an early sign of systemic *Bartonella henselae* infection. Am J Ophthalmol. 2000;130:327–34.
5. Bar S, Segal M, Shapira R, Savir H. Neuroretinitis associated with cat scratch disease. Am J Ophthalmol. 1990;110:703–5.
6. Lombardo J. Cat-scratch neuroretinitis. J Am Optom Assoc. 1999;70:525–30.
7. Reed JB, Scales KD, Wong MT, Lattuada Jr CP, Dolan MJ, Schwab IR. *Bartonella henselae* neuroretinitis in cat scratch disease: diagnosis, management, and sequelae. Ophthalmology. 1998;105:459–66.
8. Ormerod LD, Dailey JP. Ocular manifestations of cat scratch disease. Curr Opin Ophthalmol. 1999;10: 209–16.
9. Cunningham Jr ET, McDonald HR, Schatz H, Johnson RN, Ai E, Grand MG. Inflammatory mass of the optic nerve head associated with systemic *Bartonella henselae* infection. Arch Ophthalmol. 1997;115: 1596–7.
10. Ormerod LD, Skolnick KA, Menosky MM, Pavan PR, Pon DM. Retinal and choroidal manifestations of cat-scratch disease. Ophthalmology. 1998;105: 1024–31.
11. Solley WA, Martin DF, Newman NJ, King R, Callanan DG, Zacchei T, Wallace RT, Parks DJ, Bridges W, Sternberg Jr P. Cat scratch disease: posterior segment manifestations. Ophthalmology. 1999;106:1546–53.
12. Zacchei AC, Newman NJ, Sternberg P. Serous retinal detachment of the macula associated with cat scratch disease. Am J Ophthalmol. 1995;120:796–7.
13. Gray AV, Reed JB, Wendel RT, Morse LS. Bartonella henselae infection associated with peripapillary angioma, branch retinal artery occlusion, and severe vision loss. Am J Ophthalmol. 1999;127:223–4.
14. Fish RH, Hogan RN, Nightingale SD, Anand R. Peripapillary angiomatosis associated with cat-scratch neuroretinitis. Arch Ophthalmol. 1992;110:323.
15. Cohen SM, Davis JL, Gass JDM. Branch retinal arterial occlusions in multifocal retinitis with optic nerve edema. Arch Ophthalmol. 1995;113:1271–6.
16. Curi AL, Machado DO, Heringer G, Campos WR, Orefice F. Ocular manifestation of cat-scratch disease in HIV positive patients. Am J Ophthalmol. 2006;14:400–1.
17. Soheilian M, Markomichelakis N, Foster CS. Intermediate uveitis and retinal vasculitis as manifestations of cat scratch disease. Am J Ophthalmol. 1996;122:582–4.
18. Khurana RN, Albini T, Green RL, Rao NA, Lim JI. *Bartonella henselae* infection presenting as a unilateral panuveitis simulating Vogt-Koyanagi-Harada syndrome. Am J Ophthalmol. 2004;138:1063–5.
19. Asensio-Sánchez VM, Rodríguez-Delgado B, García-Herrero E, Cabo-Vaquera V, García-Loygorri C. Serous macular detachment as an atypical sign in

cat scratch disease. Arch Soc Esp Oftalmol. 2006;81:717–9.
20. Matsuo T, Kato M. Submacular exudates with serous retinal detachment caused by cat scratch disease. Ocul Immunol Inflamm. 2002;10:147–50.
21. Albini TA, Lakhanpal RR, Foroozan R, Holz ER. Macular hole in cat scratch disease. Am J Ophthalmol. 2005;140:149–51.
22. Degueldre F, Bonnet S. Cause of unusual unilateral vitreous hemorrhage: neuroretinitis of Cat-Scratch disease. Presentation of a case. Bull Soc Belge Ophtalmol. 2002;285:37–40.
23. Spach DH, Koehler JE. *Bartonella*-associated infections. Infect Dis Clin North Am. 1998;12:137–55.
24. Dalton MJ, Robinson LE, Cooper J, Regnery RL, Olson JG, Childs JE. The use of *Bartonella* antigens for serologic diagnosis of cat-scratch disease at a national referral center. Arch Intern Med. 1995;155: 1670–6.
25. Barka NE, Hadfield T, Patnaik M, Schwartzman WA, Peter JB. EIA for detection of *Rochalimaea henselae-reactive* IgG, IgM, and IgA antibodies in patients with suspected cat-scratch disease (letter). J Infect Dis. 1993;167:1503.
26. Relman DA, Loutit JS, Schmidt TM, Falkow S, Tompkins LS. The agent of bacillary angiomatosis. An approach to the identification of uncultured pathogens. N Engl J Med. 1990;323:1573–80.
27. Margileth AM. Antibiotic therapy for cat-scratch disease: clinical study of therapeutic outcome in 268 patients and a review of the literature. Pediatr Infect Dis J. 1992;11:474–8.
28. Zimran E, Shilo S, Florescu T, Dotan S, Balag S, Mevorach D, Shibolet O, Amer R. Paradoxical response in ocular bartonellosis. J Ophthalmic Inflamm Infect. 2012;2:53–6.
29. Stanek G, Wormser GP, Gray J, Strle F. Lyme borreliosis. Lancet. 2012;379(9814):461–73.
30. Winterkorn JM. Lyme disease: neurologic and ophthalmic manifestations. Surv Ophthalmol. 1990;35: 191–204.
31. Mikkila HO, SeppaHi II, Viljanen MK, Peltomaa MP, Karma A. The expanding clinical spectrum of ocular Lyme borreliosis. Ophthalmology. 2000;107:581–7.
32. Karma A, Mikkilä H. Ocular manifestations and treatment of Lyme disease. Curr Opin Ophthalmol. 1996;7:7–12.
33. Mora P, Carta A. Ocular manifestations of Lyme borreliosis in Europe. Int J Med Sci. 2009;6:124–5.
34. Copeland Jr RA. Lyme uveitis. Int Ophthalmol Clin. 1990;30:291–3.
35. Karma A, Seppälä I, Mikkilä H, Kaakkola S, Viljanen M, Tarkkanen A. Diagnosis and clinical characteristics of ocular Lyme borrelioses. Am J Ophthalmol. 1995;119:127–35.
36. Copeland RA, Nozik RA, Shimokaji G. Uveitis in Lyme disease. Ophthalmology. 1989;107(Suppl):127.
37. Bodaghi B. Ocular manifestations of Lyme disease. Med Mal Infect. 2007;37:518–22.
38. Sauer A, Hansmann Y, Jaulhac B, Bourcier T, Speeg-Schatz C. Ocular Lyme disease occurring during childhood: five case reports. J Fr Ophtalmol. 2012;35:17–22.
39. Breeveled J, Rothova A, Kuiper H. Intermediate uveitis and Lyme Borreliosis. Br J Ophthalmol. 1992;76:181–2.
40. Huppertza HI, Munchmeier D, Lieb W. Ocular manifestations in children and adolescents with Lyme arthritis. Br J Ophthalmol. 1999;83:1149–52.
41. Klaeger AJ, Herbort CP. Cotton wool spots as possible indicators of retinal vascular pathology in ocular lyme borreliosis? Int Ophthalmol. 2010;30:599–602.
42. Reibaldi M, Faro S, Motta L, Longo A. Intravitreal triamcinolone for macular edema in Lyme disease. Graefes Arch Clin Exp Ophthalmol. 2008;246:457–8.
43. Lardeoye CWTA, Van der Lelji A, de Loos WS, Treffers WF, Rothova A. Peripheral multifocal chorioretinitis. A distinct clinical entity? Ophthalmology. 1997;104:1820–6.
44. Träisk F, Lindquist L. Optic nerve involvement in Lyme disease. Curr Opin Ophthalmol. 2012;23: 485–90.
45. Babu K, Murthy PR. Neuroretinitis as a Manifestation of Lyme disease in South India: a case report. Ocul Immunol Inflamm. 2010;18:97–8.
46. McVeigh K, Vakros G. Case report: papillitis as the sole ocular sign in Lyme disease. Clin Ophthalmol. 2012;6:1093–7.
47. Krist D, Wenkel H. Posterior scleritis associated with Borrelia burgdorferi (Lyme disease) infection. Ophthalmology. 2002;109:143–5.
48. Nieto JC, Kim N, Lucarelli MJ. Dacryoadenitis and orbital myositis associated with lyme disease. Arch Ophthalmol. 2008;126:1165–6.
49. Johnson BJ, Robbins KE, Bailey RE, Cao BL, Sviat SL, Craven RB, Mayer LW, Dennis DT. Serodiagnosis of Lyme disease: accuracy of a two-step approach using a flagella-based ELISA and immunoblotting. J Infect Dis. 1996;174:346–53.
50. Hunfeld KP, Wichelhaus TA, Rödel R, Acker G, Brade V, Kraiczy P. Comparison of in vitro activities of ketolides, macrolides, and an azalide against the spirochete Borrelia burgdorferi. Antimicrob Agents Chemother. 2004;48:344–7.
51. Wressnigg N, Pöllabauer EM, Aichinger G, Portsmouth D, Löw-Baselli A, Fritsch S, Livey I, Crowe BA, Schwendinger M, Brühl P, Pilz A, Dvorak T, Singer J, Firth C, Luft B, Schmitt B, Zeitlinger M, Müller M, Kollaritsch H, Paulke-Korinek M, Esen M, Kremsner PG, Ehrlich HJ, Barrett PN. Safety and immunogenicity of a novel multivalent OspA vaccine against Lyme borreliosis in healthy adults: a double-blind, randomised, dose-escalation phase 1/2 trial. Lancet Infect Dis. 2013;13:680–9.
52. Whipple GH. A hitherto undescribed disease characterized anatomically by deposits of fat and fatty acids in the intestinal and mesenteric lymphatic tissues. Bull Johns Hopkins Hosp. 1907;18:382–91.
53. Durand DV, Lecomte C, Cathebras P, Rousset H, Godeau P. SNFMI Research Group on Whipple

Disease. Whipple disease: clinical review of 52 cases. Medicine (Baltimore). 1997;76:170–84.

54. Fenollar F, Puechal X, Raoul D. Whipple's disease. N Engl J Med. 2007;356:55–66.
55. Chan RY, Yannuzzi LA, Foster CS. Ocular Whipple's disease: earlier definitive diagnosis. Ophthalmology. 2001;108:2225–31.
56. Touitou V, Fenollar F, Cassoux N, Merle-Beral H, LeHoang P, Amoura Z, Drancourt M, Bodaghi B. Ocular Whipple's disease: therapeutic strategy and long-term follow-up. Ophthalmology. 2012;119:1465–9.
57. Nishimura JK, Cook Jr BE, Pach JM. Whipple disease presenting as posterior uveitis without prominent gastrointestinal symptoms. Am J Ophthalmol. 1998;126:130–2.
58. Lee AG. Ocular whipple's disease. Ophthalmology. 2002;109:1952–3, author reply 1953.
59. Williams JG, Edward DP, Tessler HH, Persing DH, Mitchell PS, Goldstein DA. Ocular manifestations of Whipple disease: an atypical presentation. Arch Ophthalmol. 1998;116:1232–4.
60. Razonable RR, Pulido JS, Deziel PJ, Dev S, Salomão DR, Walker RC. Chorioretinitis and vitreitis due to Tropheryma whipplei after transplantation: case report and review. Transpl Infect Dis. 2008;10:413–8.
61. Avila MP, Jalkh AE, Feldman E, Trempe CL, Schepens CL. Manifestations of Whipple's disease in the posterior segment of the eye. Arch Ophthalmol. 1984;102:384–90.
62. Selsky EJ, Knox DL, Maumenee AE, Green WR. Ocular involvement in Whipple's disease. Retina. 1984;4:103–6.
63. Lee AG. Whipple disease with supranuclear ophthalmoplegia diagnosed by polymerase chain reaction of cerebrospinal fluid. J Neuroophthalmol. 2002;22:18–21.
64. Ramzan NN, Loftus Jr E, Burgart LJ, Rooney M, Batts KP, Wiesner RH, Fredricks DN, Relman DA, Persing DH. Diagnosis and monitoring of Whipple disease by polymerase chain reaction. Ann Intern Med. 1997;126:520–7.
65. Raoult D, Fenollar F, Birg ML. Culture of *T. whipplei* from the stool of a patient with Whipple's disease [letter]. N Engl J Med. 2006;355:1503–5.

12 Infections of the Posterior Segment: Parasitic and Fungal Infections

Moncef Khairallah and Rim Kahloun

12.1 Introduction

Parasitic and fungal infections of the eye are major, worldwide distributed causes of infectious posterior uveitis that may lead to blindness. The causative agents include several species of Protozoa and Helminths that have a natural predilection for the eye. These parasitic infections may be transmitted by vectors, food consumption, or acquired indirectly from the environment. Ocular involvement can be due to damage directly caused by the infectious pathogen, indirect pathology caused by toxic products, or the immune response incited by infections or ectopic parasitism. Epidemiologic data, clinical features, diagnostic tools, and management of the clinically important species of parasites involved in posterior uveitis including toxoplasmosis and toxocariasis are reviewed in this chapter. Presumed ocular histoplasmosis syndrome, which is considered to be of fungal origin, also will be discussed.

M. Khairallah, MD (✉) • R. Kahloun, MD
Department of Ophthalmology, Fattouma Bourguiba University Hospital, Monastir, Tunisia

Faculty of Medicine, University of Monastir, Monastir, Tunisia
e-mail: moncef.khairallah@rns.tn

12.1.1 Toxoplasmosis

Toxoplasmosis is a worldwide distributed infection caused by the intracellular parasite *Toxoplasma gondii*. The parasite was first discovered in Tunis in 1908 by Charles Nicolle and Louis Manceaux [1].

12.1.1.1 Epidemiology

Toxoplasmosis is the most common cause of infectious retinochoroiditis (RC) in both adults and children, accounting for 20–60 % of all posterior uveitis cases [2]. Toxoplasmosis occurs worldwide, but its incidence is higher in tropical areas as compared to Europe and Northern America, and is quite rare in China. The prevalence increases with age and decreases with increasing latitude [3]. Ocular disease is more severe in South America than in other continents due to the presence of extremely virulent genotypes of the parasite [2, 4].

12.1.1.2 Life Cycle and Pathogenesis

Toxoplasma gondii is a single-cell obligate intracellular protozoan parasite that exists in three major forms: the oocyst or soil form (10–12 μm), the tachyzoite or infectious form (4–8 μm), and the tissue cyst or latent form (10–200 μm), which contains as many as 3.000 bradyzoites.

Cats are the definitive hosts of *T gondii*, and humans and a variety of other animals serve as

K. Tabbara et al. (eds.), *Ocular Infections*, Essentials in Ophthalmology,
DOI 10.1007/978-3-662-43981-4_12, © Springer-Verlag Berlin Heidelberg 2014

intermediate hosts [5]. Human infection by *T gondii* may be either acquired or congenital. The principal modes of transmission include ingestion of undercooked infected meat, contaminated water, fruits, or vegetables or unpasteurized milk from infected animal, inadvertent contact with soil, transplacental transmission, blood transfusion or organ transplantation, and rarely introduction of tachyzoites through a break in the skin.

Following ingestion, the organisms will spread by hematogenous dissemination reaching muscles, brain, and retina with formation of tissue cysts containing bradyzoites which will transform into tachyzoites upon cyst rupture and will invade new cells. A possible infection route from the brain to the eye via the optic nerve has been suggested [5]. Although toxoplasmosis after infancy was considered to be exclusively the result of reactivation of congenital disease, acquired infection is now thought to play an important role in the development of ocular toxoplasmosis in children and adults [6].

12.1.1.3 Clinical Features

Main presenting symptoms include unilateral blurring or loss of vision, central scotoma, and floaters. An associated mild to moderate granulomatous anterior uveitis is frequently observed and can be hypertensive in nature in 30 % of cases [7].

Moderate or severe vitreous inflammatory reaction, usually more intense near the active RC lesion, is present in almost all cases. In some cases, vitritis is so severe that visualization of the fundus is very difficult, giving the classic "headlight in the fog" appearance.

Active toxoplasmic RC typically presents as a unilateral, single gray-white retinochoroidal lesion, with indistinct borders due to surrounding retinal edema, near or adjacent to a pigmented and/or atrophic scar indicative of previous toxoplasmic infection [8, 9] (Fig. 12.1). However, 25–35 % of eyes with active toxoplasmic RC do not exhibit associated old scar (Fig. 12.2). RC lesions may have various sizes and may occur in the posterior pole, sparing or involving the center, in periphery, or occasionally immediately adjacent to or directly involving the optic disk. Various associated fundus changes may occur including focal or diffuse retinal vein sheathing, retinal arterial involvement especially in the form of Kyrieleis arteriolitis, retinal hemorrhages, macular edema, serous retinal detachment (SRD), and optic disk hyperemia.

The course of toxoplasmic RC is self-limiting in immunocompetent patients. The inflammation gradually resolves in 6–8 weeks, and a chorioretinal scar replaces the active lesion [7].

Ocular toxoplasmosis is a progressive and recurrent disease, with new lesions occurring at the margins of old scars as well as elsewhere in the fundus. Recurrences are totally unpredictable and may occur years after the original lesion resolved. Recurrence rates of 40–79 % have been reported [10].

The classic presentation of congenital toxoplasmosis is RC with a predilection for the posterior pole and macula (Fig. 12.3). Congenital toxoplasmosis may be bilateral in approximately 85 % of affected individuals [11–13] (Fig. 12.3).

RC developing in immunocompromised and older patients may present with atypical findings, including large, multiple, and/or bilateral lesions, with or without associated chorioretinal scars.

Other atypical presentations of toxoplasmic RC include punctate outer or inner retinal toxoplasmosis, neuroretinitis, optic neuritis, intraocular inflammation without RC, unilateral pigmentary retinopathy simulating retinitis pigmentosa, scleritis, and a presentation in association with Fuchs uveitis syndrome [14].

Early and late complications of ocular toxoplasmosis include retinal vascular occlusions (Fig. 12.4), SRD, choroidal ischemia, cataract, posterior synechiae, significant vitreous opacification and organization, rhegmatogenous or tractional retinal detachment, preretinal neovascularization, vitreous hemorrhage, choroidal neovascularization (CNV), epiretinal membrane (ERM), subretinal fibrosis, vasoproliferative tumor, optic atrophy, glaucoma, and phthisis bulbi [9, 10, 15].

12.1.1.4 Imaging

Fluorescein angiography (FA) shows early hypofluorescence of active focus of RC, followed by

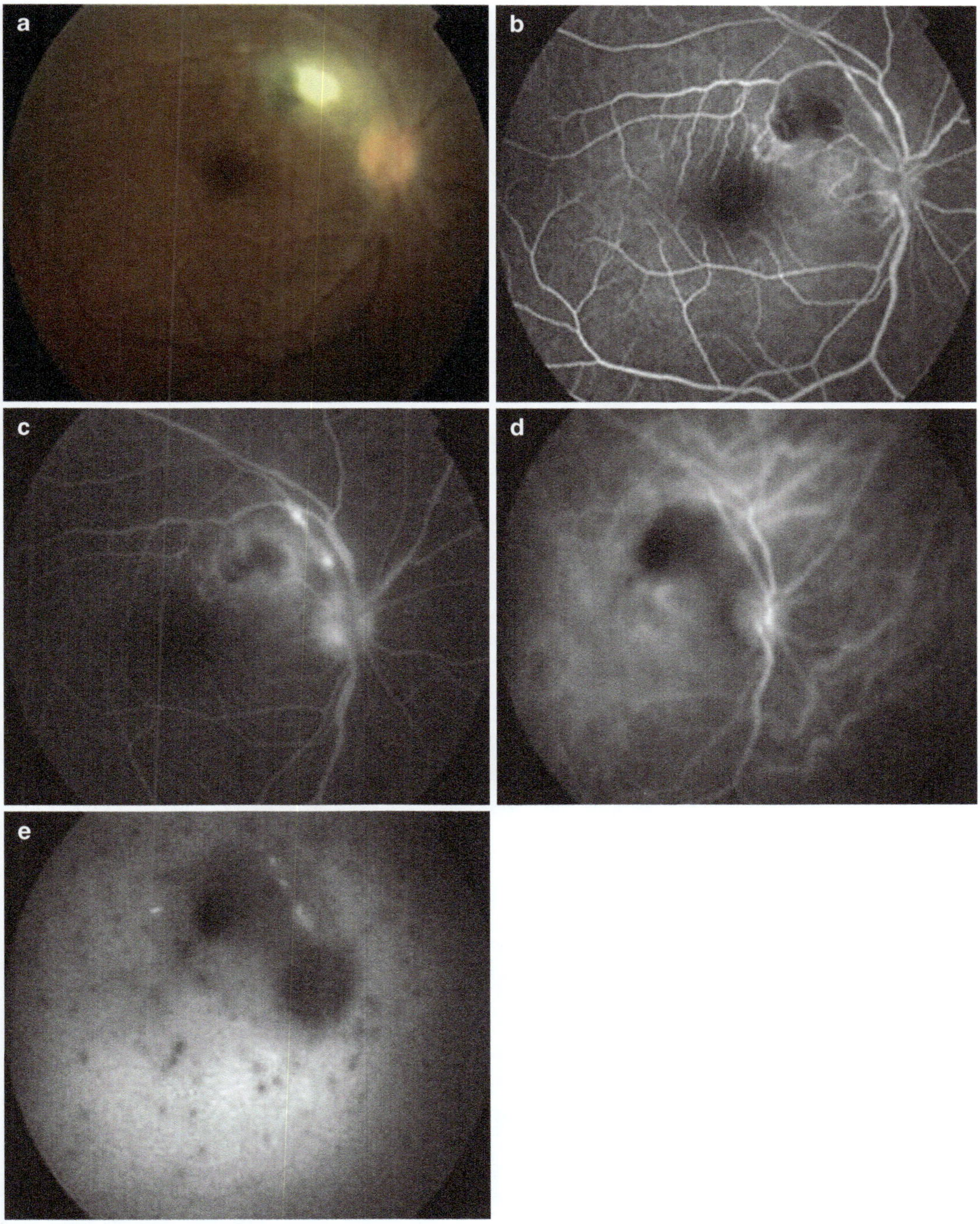

Fig. 12.1 (**a**) Fundus photograph shows an active focus of toxoplasmic retinochoroiditis adjacent to an old pigmented scar located at the superotemporal the superior vascular arcade in the vicinity of the optic disk. (**b**) Early-phase fluorescein angiogram shows hypofluorescence of both active and old focus. (**c**) Late-phase fluorescein angiogram shows peripheral hyperfluorescence and persistent central hypofluorescence of the active lesion with vascular leakage and optic disk hyperfluorescence. (**d**) Early-phase indocyanine green angiogram shows hypofluorescence of the retinochoroiditis focus. (**e**) Late-phase indocyanine green angiogram shows persistence of hypofluorescence of the retinochoroiditis focus with multiple satellite dark dots and retinal vascular staining. (**f**) Optical coherence tomography reveals a subclinical serous retinal detachment (*arrow*) with foveal involvement

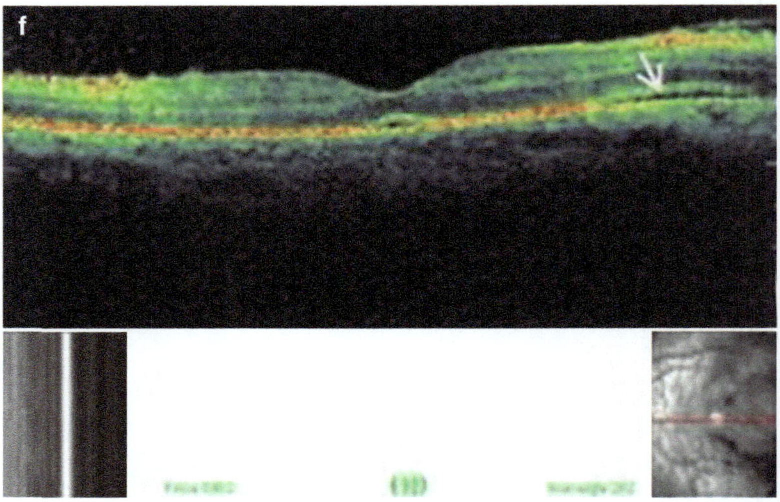

Fig. 12.1 (continued)

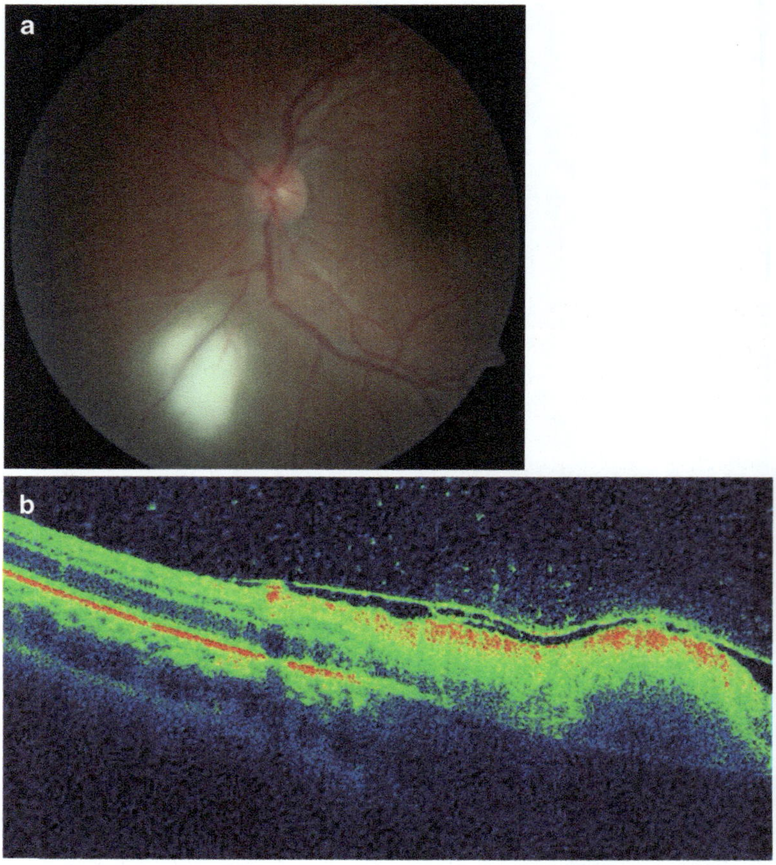

Fig. 12.2 (**a**) Fundus photograph shows an active focus of toxoplasmic retinochoroiditis without old scar. (**b**) Optical coherence tomography shows increased retinal reflectivity and thickening of the active lesion, retinal pigment epithelial and choriocapillaris band shadowing, posterior hyaloid thickening and detachment, and vitreous hyperreflective dots

gradual staining starting from the lesion borders (Fig. 12.1). This imaging modality is useful in the detection and evaluation of associated retinochoroidal vascular changes including focal or diffuse retinal vascular leakage, macular edema, retinal or choroidal vascular occlusion, optic disk leakage, CNV, and retinochoroidal anastomosis [7, 8].

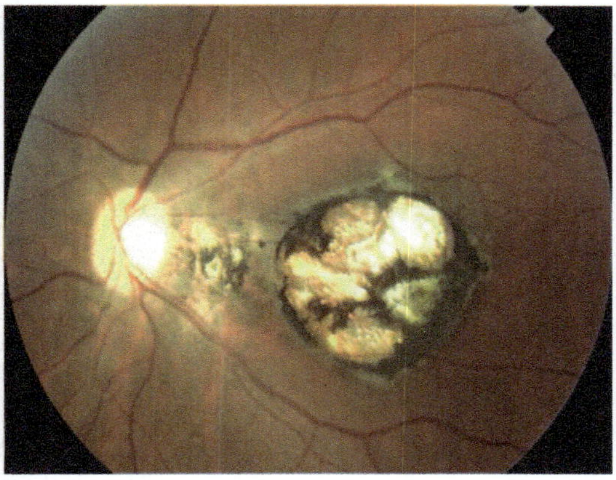

Fig. 12.3 Fundus photograph shows congenital toxoplasmosis involving the macula

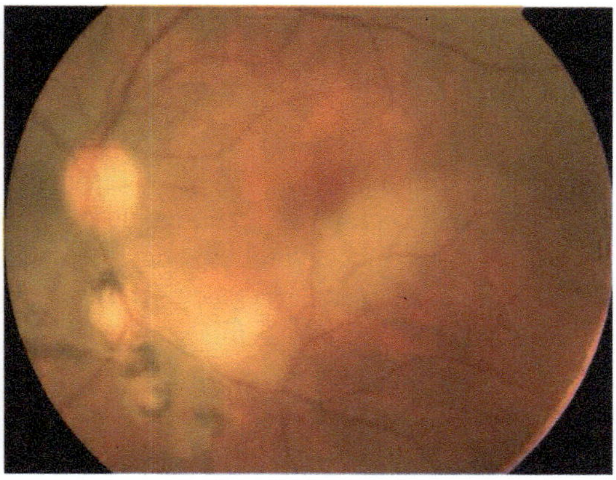

Fig. 12.4 Color fundus photograph of the left eye of a patient with ocular toxoplasmosis shows an active focus of retinochorioretinitis adjacent to old pigmented scars infero-temporally and an area of retinal whitening along the inferior temporal arcade consistent with a diagnosis of branch retinal artery occlusion

Indocyanine green angiography (ICGA) shows hypofluorescence of the main focus of RC at all phases of the angiogram (Fig. 12.1) [16]. ICGA also shows in up to 75 % of cases multiple hypofluorescent satellite dark dots, possibly due to choriocapillaris hypoperfusion, that disappear after therapy in the majority of cases (Fig. 12.1). More pronounced choroidal ischemia could be confirmed by ICGA in a subset of patients of patients with toxoplasmic RC [17, 18].

Optical coherence tomography (OCT) is a noninvasive test that is useful in evaluating and monitoring active toxoplasmic RC and associated changes. Findings include increased retinal reflectivity and thickening of the active lesion, retinal pigment epithelial and choriocapillaris band shadowing, posterior hyaloid thickening and detachment, vitreoschisis, vitreous hyperreflective dots, ERM, and SRD (Figs. 12.1 and 12.2). Disorganization of the retinal layers reflectivity with interruption of the inner/outer segment (IS/OS) junction due to scar formation may be observed [18–22]. Imaging of congenital toxoplasmosis macular scars reveals retinal thinning, retinal pigment epithelial hyper-reflectivity, excavation, intraretinal cysts, and fibrosis [23].

Ultrasonography is useful when view of the fundus is limited by posterior synechiae or vitreous opacity. The most frequent findings include intravitreal opacities, thickening of posterior hyaloids, partial or complete posterior vitreous detachment, focal retinochoroidal thickening, and tractional and rhegmatogenous retinal detachment.

Visual field testing reveals absolute defects breaking out to the periphery when scars occur within one disk diameter to the optic disk [24] or in case of retinal vascular occlusion [15].

12.1.1.5 Laboratory Investigations

The diagnosis of toxoplasmic RC is primarily based on typical clinical findings, but laboratory testing may be required to confirm the diagnosis in atypical clinical presentations. A positive serological assay for IgG does not confirm the diagnosis of ocular toxoplasmosis, given the high rate of seropositivity in the normal population in most countries. The presence of IgM and/or IgA titer or a rising IgG titer indicates recent acquired infection. A negative serology can exclude the diagnosis of ocular toxoplasmosis [25].

The Goldmann-Witmer (GW) coefficient and the western blot technique are used to demonstrate local production of antibodies in aqueous humor or rarely in vitreous fluid. A GW coefficient of greater than three is considered highly suggestive of a diagnosis of active ocular toxoplasmic infection [26].

Detection of toxoplasma DNA in ocular fluids by PCR is helpful in the diagnosis of atypical clinical presentations, particularly in immunocompromised patients [27, 28].

12.1.1.6 Differential Diagnosis

Typical toxoplasmic RC can be easily differentiated for other infectious or noninfectious uveitic entities. Atypical clinical presentations should be differentiated from other infectious diseases, including necrotizing viral retinitis, tuberculosis, syphilis, bartonellosis, rickettsiosis, Lyme disease, fungal retinitis, bacterial retinitis, and toxocariasis [7, 8].

Toxoplasmic RC should also be differentiated from noninfectious entities including multifocal choroiditis, acute posterior multifocal placoid pigment epitheliopathy (APMPPE), serpiginous choroiditis, punctate inner choroidopathy, sarcoidosis, Behçet disease, ocular lymphoma, and other causes of optic nerve involvement [29].

Differential diagnosis of congenital ocular toxoplasmosis in newborns and young children mainly includes Rubella, CMV, Herpes, Syphilis, Toxocariasis, West Nile virus fever, acute lymphocytic choriomeningitis, macular coloboma, persistent hyperplastic vitreous, and neoplastic entities such as retinoblastoma and retinocytoma [29].

12.1.1.7 Treatment

Treatment of ocular toxoplasmosis remains controversial. However, the generally accepted criteria for treatment include the following: involvement of zone 1, especially in patients with active lesion affecting or threatening the fovea or optic nerve, lesion size >2 disk diameters, marked vitritis, retinal vascular occlusion, immunocompromised patients, elderly patients, and acquired toxoplasmosis [8, 9].

Some clinicians may elect to observe small lesions in the retinal periphery that are not associated with a significant decrease in vision or vitritis, while others treat virtually all patients in an effort to reduce the number of subsequent recurrences [9].

Numerous agents have been used to treat toxoplasmosis over the years [30, 31]. The standard treatment of ocular toxoplasmosis includes a combination of pyrimethamine, given in a loading dose of 100 mg on day 1 followed by 50 mg daily (25 mg in children), sulfadiazine 4 g/day, and corticosteroids (0.5–1 mg/Kg/day, depending on the severity of the inflammation). Folinic acid (25 mg per os two or three times a week) is added to prevent bone marrow suppression that may result from pyrimethamine therapy [30, 32, 33].

Corticosteroids should be used orally, always under anti-toxoplasmic therapy and begun within 48 h. The use of periocular or intravitreal corticosteroids should be avoided. Corticosteroids should also be avoided in immunocompromised patients. In general, treatment lasts from 4 to 6 weeks, at which time inflammation begins to subside and the retinal lesion shows signs of consolidation. This period may be extended if there is persistent disease activity.

Other alternatives include oral clindamycin, spiramycin, and azithromycin [9, 30]. The combination of pyrimethamine and azithromycin (500 mg on day 1, followed by 250 mg/day) is as effective, but less toxic, than the classic combination of pyrimethamine and sulfadiazine [8, 34].

Intravitreal clindamycin injection to treat toxoplasmosis RC is a promising approach [35].

Newborns with congenital toxoplasmosis are commonly treated with pyrimethamine and sulfonamides for 1 year, in consultation with a pediatric specialist. In cases of newly acquired toxoplasmosis during pregnancy, spiramycin 400 mg three times daily may be used [36].

Pyrimethamine should be avoided or used in lower dosage for the management of ocular toxoplasmosis in patients with HIV/AIDS who receive highly active antiretroviral therapy. Atovaquone is an alternative in these patients [37].

Vitreoretinal surgery will be required for vitreous opacities and for tractional or rhegmatogenous retinal detachment.

CNV can nowadays be successfully treated with intravitreal injection of anti-vascular endothelial growth factor (VEGF) [38, 39].

Prevention of toxoplasmosis mainly consists of measures to avoid exposure to infectious agent. Long-term intermittent use of one tablet of trimethoprim (160 mg)/sulfamethoxazole (800 mg) every 3 days was shown to decrease the risk of reactivation among patients with recurrent toxoplasmic RC [40].

12.1.2 Toxocariasis

Toxocariasis is a zoonotic disease caused by the infestation of humans by second-stage larvae of the dog nematode *Toxocara canis* or the cat nematode *Toxocara cati*. Toxocariasis manifests itself in one of two disease states: visceral larva migrans, the systemic form of the disease, or ocular larva migrans, the ocular form. It is rare for ocular toxocariasis (OT) to coexist with visceral larva migrans.

12.1.2.1 Epidemiology

OT is a worldwide distributed infection. It is an uncommon disease, with a prevalence ranging between 0 and 3.1 % of all uveitis cases [41, 42]. OT is predominantly a unilateral condition that occurs primarily in childhood but also can affect adults. The median patient age was found to be 11.5 years (range, 1–66 years) [43]. OT affects females and males with approximately equal frequency.

12.1.2.2 Life Cycle and Pathogenesis

The definitive hosts of *Toxocara* are dogs and cats. When infected, these animals pass *Toxocara* eggs in their feces into the environment. Once in the environment, it takes 2–4 weeks for *Toxocara* larva to develop in the eggs and for the eggs to become infectious. In dogs and cats, the life cycle is completed when the eggs are ingested and the larvae develop into adult worms in the intestine. Humans and other animals become infected through the unintentional ingestion of infectious eggs, which are found in soil contaminated by dog and cat feces. Infection rarely may occur when a person ingests undercooked meat from an animal infected with the *Toxocara* parasite. Children who have close contact with dogs, especially puppies, are at high risk for infection.

Ocular disease is caused by the migration of *Toxocara* larva through blood vessels in the circulatory system into the posterior segment of the eye [42]. Tissue damage is due to the host inflammatory reaction more than the infection itself.

12.1.2.3 Clinical Features

Patients present with unilateral decreased vision that may be accompanied by pain, photophobia, floaters, strabismus, or leukocoria. The anterior segment is typically quiet. However, nongranulomatous anterior inflammation and posterior synechiae may be present with severe disease. Posterior segment findings include three recognizable ocular syndromes: peripheral granuloma, posterior pole granuloma, and chronic endophthalmitis [41].

Peripheral granuloma is the most common clinical presentation of OT, occurring in nearly half of patients. It usually appears as a focal, elevated, white peripheral nodule, surrounded by pigmentary changes and associated with traction vitreoretinal bands that may extend from the peripheral mass to the optic nerve head (Fig. 12.5).

Posterior pole involvement is observed in one quarter of cases. The retinochoroidal granuloma may vary in size from less than one to two disk diameters and may spare or involve the fovea [41].

OT presents in nearly one quarter of patients in the form of chronic endophthalmitis with anterior uveitis and diffuse vitritis with a poor view of the fundus. Hypopion and retinal detachment may occur in severe cases [43–47]. Other less common clinical presentations of OT are optic neuritis, neuroretinitis, and mobile living larva in the eye [46].

Complications of OT include macular heterotropia, amblyopia, cataract, secondary glaucoma, ERM, retinal folds and tractional retinal detachment, macular scar from macular granuloma, cystoid macular edema (CME), detachment of the ciliary body and anterior choroid with hypotony, neovascular membranes, and phthisis bulbi. Visual loss is commonly caused by inflammation of the vitreous and traction retinal detachment [41, 43].

12.1.2.4 Imaging

On FA, the granuloma is characterized by central hyperfluorescence with early-phase dye leakage

(Fig. 12.5). Diffuse ischemic area in the periphery has also been reported [48].

The most characteristic ultrasonographic findings include highly reflective peripheral mass, pseudocystic transformation of the peripheral vitreous, vitreous membranes or retinal fold extending from the mass to the posterior pole, and tractional retinal detachment [49].

Ultrasound biomicroscopy (UBM) may be also useful in patients with opaque media or hypotony by showing pseudocystic transformation of the peripheral vitreous, a highly sensitive, but not specific, finding [50, 51].

On OCT, posterior pole granuloma may appear as a highly reflective mass protruding above the retinal pigment epithelium (RPE) [52, 53]. OCT may also show most important vitreoretinal tractions on macular region and optic disk and subretinal fluid.

Computed tomography (CT) and magnetic resonance imaging (MRI) are helpful for the differential diagnosis with retinoblastoma [46].

12.1.2.5 Laboratory and Ancillary Tests

ELISA testing has a high sensitivity and specificity in patients with a presumptive diagnosis of OT [43]. Current serologic testing for antibody to the *Toxocara* parasite does not reliably indicate active infection. In fact, studies have shown that the immunoglobulin-G *Toxocara* antibody can remain detectable for years after treatment, which limits the applicability of the test to monitor treatment success [54]. GW coefficient analysis in aqueous humor or vitreous may help establish the diagnosis of OT [55].

12.1.2.6 Differential Diagnosis

The most important differential diagnosis of OT consideration is retinoblastoma. Other entities to consider include infectious endophthalmitis, toxoplasmosis, pars planitis, sarcoidosis, syphilis, and congenital retinovascular abnormalities such as retinopathy of prematurity, persistent fetal vasculature, Coats disease, and familial exudative vitreoretinopathy.

12.1.2.7 Treatment

Although there is no uniformly satisfactory treatment for OT, medical therapy with periocular and systemic corticosteroids continue to be the therapeutic mainstay for eyes with active vitritis to reduce the inflammatory response to prevent structural complications [46, 47]. The utility of antihelminthic therapy such as albendazole, thiabendazole, or mebendazole is still controversial. Vitreoretinal surgery has been successfully used to manage complications such as rhegmatogenous and tractional retinal detachments, ERM, and persistent vitreous opacification [56]. Prognosis depends on the age of presentation,

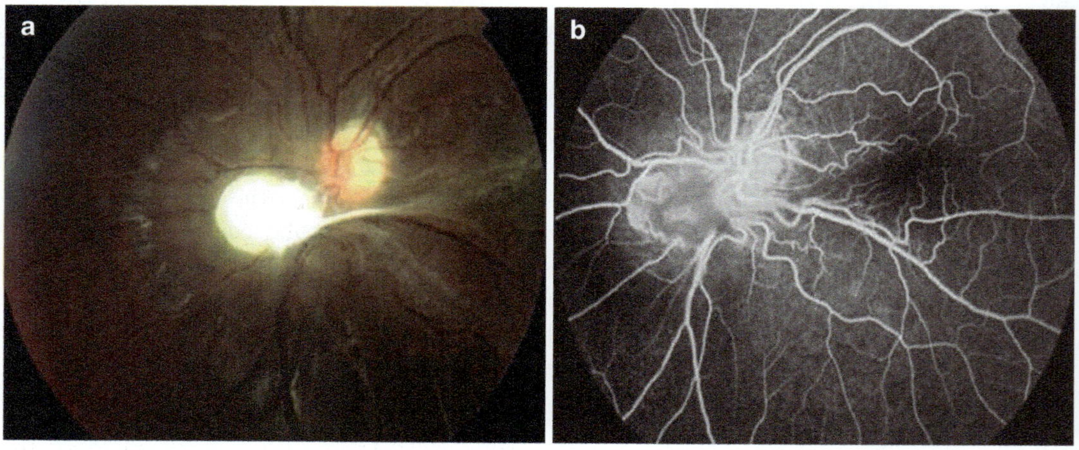

Fig. 12.5 (**a**) Fundus photograph shows a toxocara granuloma adjacent to the optic disk inferonasally with associated vitreoretinal traction (**b**) Late-phase fluorescein angiogram shows heterogeneous hyperfluorescence of the granuloma and associated retinal vascular tortuosity

location of toxocara lesion, and subsequent complications.

12.1.3 Diffuse Unilateral Subacute Neuroretinitis (DUSN)

Diffuse unilateral subacute neuroretinitis (DUSN), first described by Gass et al. in 1978 [57], is an infectious ocular disease caused by an unidentified motile nematode capable of infiltrating the subretinal space, causing inflammation and retinal degeneration that lead to profound vision loss [58].

12.1.3.1 Pathogenesis

Evidence to date suggests that DUSN is caused by solitary nematodes of two different sizes that migrate through the subretinal space. The smaller worm, measuring 400–1.000 μm in length, has been proposed to be either *Ancylostoma caninum* (the dog hookworm) or *Toxocara canis*, the latter being endemic to the southeastern United States, Caribbean islands, and Brazil. The larger worm is believed to be *Baylisascaris procyonis* (the raccoon roundworm), which measures 1.500–2.000 μm in length and has been found in the northern Midwestern United States and Canada [44, 46]. DUSN appears to involve an inflammatory or a local toxic tissue effect on the outer retina caused by the worm by-products left behind, as well as a more diffuse toxic reaction affecting both the inner and outer retina.

12.1.3.2 Epidemiology

Initially described in the Southeastern and Midwestern parts of the United States and the Caribbean islands, DUSN has also been reported in other parts of North America, in South America, in Northwestern Europe, China, and Africa [44, 46, 59, 60]. In Brazil, DUSN is considered an important cause of posterior uveitis in children and young healthy adults. The disease can affect children and young adults without gender preference or systemic problems. It is usually unilateral and occasionally is bilateral.

12.1.3.3 Clinical Features

The onset of DUSN is usually insidious. Some patients in the early stages of the disease complain of unilateral paracentral or central scotoma, ocular discomfort, or transient obscurations of vision [61]. Patients are usually in good general health. Clinical findings in patients with DUSN can be divided into two stages. The early stage is characterized by mild to moderate vitritis, mild optic disk edema, and recurrent crops of evanescent, multifocal, yellow-white lesions at the level of the outer retina and choroid with continued visual loss and central scotoma (Fig. 12.6). The white lesions are clustered within a small zone and fade over a few weeks leaving pigment mottling. Focal retinal hemorrhages and perivenous exudation may be rarely seen. Careful observation in the vicinity of the white lesions may show a small white nematode. Occasionally, a few patients may demonstrate mild anterior uveitis with cells, flare, and keratic precipitates. The late stage of the disease is characterized by optic disk atrophy, retinal vessel narrowing, and focal or diffuse RPE degeneration marked by profound visual loss. The worm can be identified at any stage of the disease [45].

12.1.3.4 Imaging

FA usually demonstrates mild leakage of dye from the capillaries on the optic disk and some of the retinal vessels. The gray-white lesions are

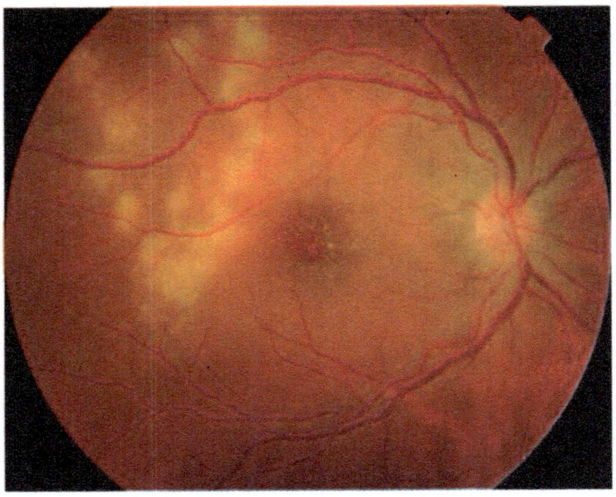

Fig. 12.6 Fundus photograph of a patient with DUSN shows a cluster of gray-white lesions (Courtesy, Carlos Pavesio)

nonfluorescent or hypofluorescent early and stain in the late phase of the angiogram.

ICGA may reveal hypofluorescent dark spots, and hyperfluorescence at the macular level [62]. ICGA could be a useful tool for the detection of subretinal nematodes [63].

Spectral domain OCT showed that RNFL and central retinal thickness were thinner in DUSN eyes compared to normal eyes. Late-stage disease had more pronounced thinning compared to early-stage patients. This thinning in retinal nerve fiber layer (RNFL) and central retinal thickness may reflect the low visual acuity in patients with DUSN [64].

Electroretinography in the affected eye is usually reduced quite early in the course of the disease and is more severely reduced with the b-wave being affected more than the a-wave in the later stage of the disease [44, 46]. Goldman perimetry is useful to evaluate remaining visual field before and after treatment of the disease.

12.1.3.5 Differential Diagnosis

Early signs of DUSN often are mistaken for multifocal choroiditis, sarcoidosis, acute posterior multifocal placoid pigment epitheliopathy, multiple evanescent white dot syndrome, serpiginous choroiditis, Behçet disease, ocular toxoplasmosis, nonspecific optic neuritis, and papillitis. Late features of the disease may be confused with posttraumatic chorioretinopathy, occlusive vascular disease, toxic retinopathy, unilateral optic atrophy, and retinitis pigmentosa [61].

12.1.3.6 Treatment

Therapy is limited in patients with DUSN. If the worm is visualized, laser treatment of the nematode with confluent laser burns 100–200 μ in size can be highly effective and may improve visual acuity and inflammatory ocular signs [46]. The worm can be induced to migrate away from the macula before treatment by directing a bright light on it. The worm may also be surgically removed for identification purposes. Chemotherapy with anthelmintic drugs, such as mebendazole, thiabendazole, or albendazole may be the only treatment available when a worm cannot be visualized, but success is often difficult to document. A treatment regimen of albendazole 400 mg daily for 4 weeks seems to be safe and beneficial for patients with DUSN [65].

Treatment with corticosteroids has shown transient suppression of the inflammation without altering the final outcome of the disease. Patients with retinal complications caused by the inflammation may benefit from surgical intervention in some cases.

12.2 Other Parasitic Diseases

12.2.1 Onchocerciasis

Onchocerciasis, also named river blindness or Robles disease, is a parasitic disease caused by the microfilariae *Onchocerca volvulus* [45]. *O. volvulus* is transmitted by the bite of the black Simulium fly, which breeds in rapidly flowing waters. The clinical manifestations of onchocerciasis range from no skin or eye lesions to very severe skin involvement and blindness.

12.2.1.1 Epidemiology

Onchocerciasis is endemic in many areas of sub-Saharan Africa and in isolated foci in Central and South America. It is rarely seen or diagnosed in the Western world. According to the World Health Organization, at least 18 million people are infected, of whom almost 300.000 are blind [66]. In hyperendemic areas, every one over the age of 15 is infected, and half will become blind before they die.

12.2.1.2 Pathogenesis

Humans are the only host for *O. volvulus*. The *O. volvulus* larvae are transmitted through the bite of female black flies of the *Simulium* genus. The larvae develop into mature adult worms that form subcutaneous nodules. The adult female releases millions of microfilariae that migrate throughout the body, particularly to the skin and the eye.

The ocular manifestations of onchocerciasis are caused by the presence of dead parasites within the eye. The microfilariae penetrate the eye by the bulbar conjunctiva at the limbus and then invade the cornea, aqueous humor, and iris.

They reach the posterior segment by the circulation or ciliary nerves, which supply the peripheral retina and choroid [46].

12.2.1.3 Clinical Features

Anterior segment involvement includes punctate keratitis, corneal opacity that turns to scar tissue, producing sclerosing keratitis in late stages [46]. An iridocyclitis also can be seen with atrophy of the iris, cataract, and glaucoma. Chorioretinal changes are also common. They typically begin in the periphery and vary widely in severity. Early disruption of the RPE is typical with pigment dispersion and focal areas of atrophy (Fig. 12.7). Later, severe chorioretinal atrophy occurs predominantly in the posterior pole with sheathing of the retinal vessels and visual field constriction. Optic disk atrophy is common in advanced disease. Macular edema can also be found.

12.2.1.4 Laboratory Investigations

Diagnosis of onchocerciasis is made by extraction of microfilariae or adult worms from skin or subcutaneous nodules by biopsy or by identification of live microfilariae in the aqueous humor [67].

12.2.1.5 Treatment

Ivermectin, given in a single oral dose of 150 μg/kg, is the first choice to treat onchocerciasis. Annual ivermectin therapy seems to improve intraocular inflammation [67]. Topical corticosteroids can be used to control any anterior uveitis. Vector control strategies tend to have limited success.

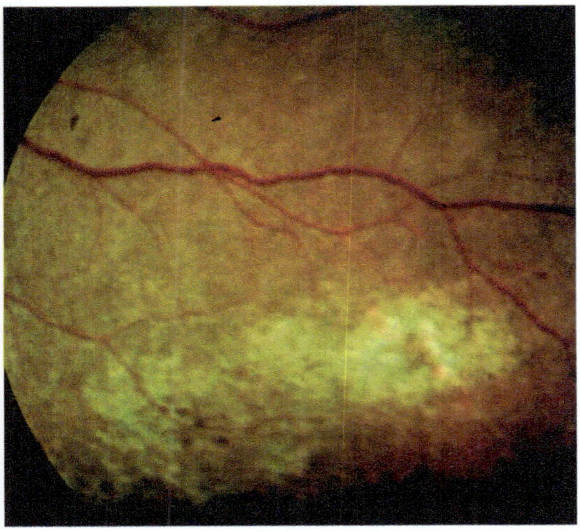

Fig. 12.7 Fundus photograph of a patient with onchocerciasis shows peripheral chorioretinal changes with pigment dispersion, and focal areas of atrophy (Courtesy, Aniki Rothova)

12.2.2 Cysticercosis

Cysticercosis is a systemic illness caused by the *Cysticercus cellulosae* larvae of the adult tapeworm *Taenia solium* and *Taenia saginata*. The most frequently reported locations are skin, skeletal muscle, heart, eye, and most importantly, the central nervous system.

12.2.2.1 Epidemiology

Cysticercosis is a common cause of ocular inflammation in some developing countries such as Central and South America, India, Southeast Asia, China, Eastern Europe, and certain parts of Africa [45, 68]. Ocular cysticercosis is a disorder of the young, occurring most frequently between the ages of 10 and 30 years, without gender predilection.

12.2.2.2 Pathogenesis

Human infection is caused by *Cysticercus cellulosae*, the larval stage of the cestode *Taenia solium*. Human cysticercosis is caused by ingestion of water or foods contaminated by the pork tapeworm. The eggs mature into larvae, penetrate the intestinal mucosa, and spread hematogenously to the eye via the posterior ciliary arteries into the subretinal space in the posterior pole [46].

12.2.2.3 Clinical Features

Although cysticercosis may involve any structure of the eye and its adnexae, the posterior segment is most often involved. Depending on the location of the intraocular cyst, patients may present asymptomatically with relatively good vision or may complain of floaters, moving sensations, ocular pain, photophobia, redness, and very poor visual acuity. Larvae within the subretinal space may cause an exudative retinal detachment or may perforate the retina, causing a retinal break that may be self-limiting or associated with

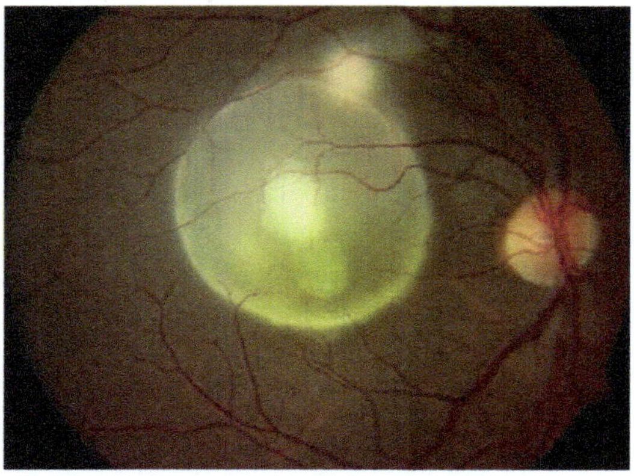

Fig. 12.8 Fundus photograph in a patient wit cystcercosis shows a live submacular translucent cyst with clear media (Courtesy, Amod Gupta)

retinal detachment and gain access to the vitreous cavity. The characteristic clinical appearance is that of a globular or spherical translucent white cyst (Fig. 12.8), with a head or scolex that undulates in response to the examining light within the vitreous or subretinal space [45]. The cyst itself varies in size from 1.5 to 6 disk diameters. RPE atrophy may be observed surrounding the presumptive entry site of the cysticercus into the subretinal space [46]. Larvae death produces a severe inflammatory reaction characterized by zonal granulomatous inflammation surrounding necrotic larvae on histologic examination.

12.2.2.4 Imaging

B-scan ultrasonography may also be helpful diagnostically in the presence intraocular cysticerci, revealing a characteristic picture of a sonolucent zone with a well-defined anterior and posterior margin. A central echo-dense, curvilinear, highly reflective structure within the cyst is suggestive of a scolex, further narrowing the diagnosis [46]. CT and MRI may reveal intracerebral calcification or hydrocephalus in the setting of neural cysticercosis. High-definition spectral-domain OCT of the cyst showed a hyperreflective coat [69].

12.2.2.5 Laboratory Investigations

Anticysticercus antibodies are detected by ELISA which was found to be highly sensitive [46]. Anterior chamber paracentesis may reveal a large number of eosinophils. Peripheral eosinophilia may also be present.

12.2.2.6 Differential Diagnosis

The differential diagnosis of ocular cysticercosis involving the posterior segment includes conditions associated with leukocoria (retinoblastoma, Coats disease, retinopathy of prematurity, persistent fetal vasculature, toxocariasis, and retinal detachment) and DUSN.

12.2.2.7 Treatment

Antihelminthic drugs such as praziquantel and albendazole have been used successfully in the medical management of active neural cysticercosis. However, these agents are generally not effective for intraocular disease. They are frequently used in combination with systemic corticosteroids, because larvae death is accompanied by worsening of the ocular disease and panuveitis [46]. Pars plana vitrectomy is usually required for posterior segment involvement. The cyst in vitreous can be removed through the sclerotomy site or can be aspired through the vitrector hand piece. In case of ruptured cyst, complete vitrectomy should be done to remove all the vitreous debris [70].

12.2.3 Gnathostomiasis

Human gnathostomiasis is mostly prevalent in Southeast Asia and Latin America, but there has been a progressive increase in its global frequency [71]. Although five different species of *Gnathostoma* are known to cause human disease, *Gnathostoma spinigerum* is the most common agent that involves the human eye. Humans become incidental hosts after intake of undercooked or raw meat of the host. After ingestion, the larvae cross the gastric or intestinal wall and migrate randomly throughout the body.

Ocular gnathostomiasis is a rare clinical condition, and intravitreal gnathostomiasis is an even rarer entity (Fig. 12.9). The route by which the worm can gain access to the eye and enter the subretinal space is not clear. It has been suggested that parasite may enter via the retinal arterioles or

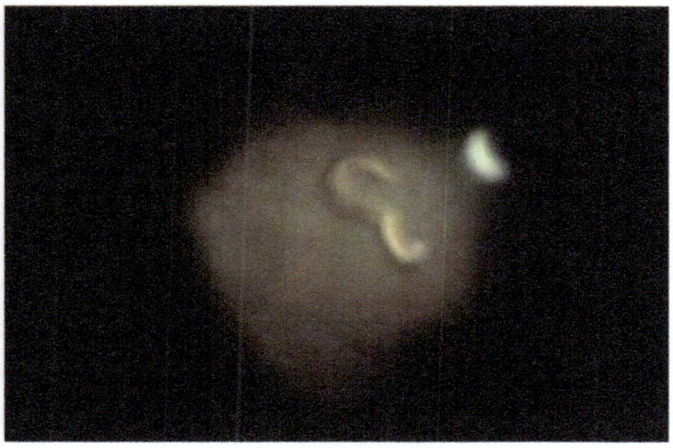

Fig. 12.9 Photograph showing intravitreal gnathostomiasis (Courtesy, Jyotirmay Biswas)

through the choroid and RPE after its passage through the ciliary circulation [72, 73]. The most common ocular clinical manifestation of gnathostomiasis is anterior uveitis. However, lid edema, conjunctival chemosis and orbital cellulitis, and retinochoroidal and vitreous hemorrhage associated with retinal tear or scarring close to the optic disk and blindness may also be presenting features [72, 74–77].

The treatment advocated for intracameral and intravitreal *Gnathostoma* is surgical removal of the entire worm which was found to be a safe and effective treatment modality. Laser photocoagulation has been advocated for subretinal worm distant from the center of the fovea [78].

12.2.4 Trichinellosis

Trichinellosis caused by *Trichinella spiralis* has a cosmopolitan distribution, but is generally less important as an infection of humans in the tropics than in more temperate regions of the world. Human transmission occurs by ingestion of infected meat containing larvae, either in typical cysts or unencapsulated in the case of several species [79]. The clinical course is characterized by a typical syndrome of fever, myalgia, periorbital and facial edema, and eosinophilia. Ocular involvement includes conjunctivitis, chemosis, macular and retinal hemorrhage, and atrophy of the RPE as larvae migrate through and into these ocular tissues [80, 81]. The diagnosis can be suggested from clinical history of ingesting raw or inadequately cooked meat and confirmed by specific serological tests. Treatment is based on albendazole and corticosteroids.

12.2.5 Schistosomiasis

Schistosomiasis caused by *Schistosoma mansoni* is a worldwide public health problem present in the Caribbean Isles, South America, Africa, and Arabia, with widespread geographical extension and an increase in prevalence. The parasite involves humans by attaching to the skin, penetrating it, and then migrating through the venous system to the portal veins where the parasites produce eggs.

Symptoms of acute or chronic systemic disease may include fever, cough, chills, blood in the urine, and painful urination, abdominal discomfort, bloody diarrhea or blood in stools, and renal, hepatic, and spleen failure. Ocular involvement in schistosomiasis includes keratouveitis, vascular changes such as retinal hemorrhages, cotton-wool spots, and hard exudates, optic disk atrophy, and choroiditis [82–85].

Diagnosis of schistosomiasis is based on isolation of *S. mansoni* eggs in stool examination. Blood tests and more recently PCR tests can aid in confirming the diagnosis, but positive results might only be an indication of past exposure. Currently, treatments for this disease include praziquantel (Biltricide®) and/or albendazole [86]. Ocular schistosomiasis should never be treated with praziquantel. In fact, parasite destruction within the eye may cause irreparable damage.

12.3 Fungal Infections

12.3.1 Ocular Histoplasmosis

12.3.1.1 Presumed Ocular Histoplasmosis Syndrome

Presumed ocular histoplasmosis syndrome (POHS) is a multifocal chorioretinitis presumed to be caused by infection with *Histoplasma capsulatum*, a dimorphic fungus with both yeast and filamentous forms early in life.

Epidemiology

POHS is most frequently found in endemic areas of the United States such as the Ohio and Mississippi River valleys, where 60 % of individuals react positively to histoplasmin skin testing. However, POHS has also been reported in nonendemic areas in this country (Maryland) and sporadically throughout Europe (the United Kingdom and the Netherlands) [87, 88]. Areas in South America, Africa, and Southeast Asia are also known to have a high prevalence of systemic histoplasmosis [89]. POHS occurs most frequently in the second to fifth decade of life. There is no gender preference, but the condition is found primarily in whites [88, 90, 91].

Pathogenesis

Primary infection occurs after inhalation of the fungal spores into the lungs. Acquired histoplasmosis is usually asymptomatic or may result in a benign illness, typically during childhood. Ocular disease is thought to arise as a consequence of hematogenous dissemination of the organism to the spleen, liver, and choroid following the initial pulmonary infection. The choroiditis may subside and leave an atrophic scar and depigmentation of the RPE, or it may result in disruption of the Bruch membrane, choriocapillaris, and RPE, with subsequent proliferation of subretinal vessels originating from the choroid. The initiating stimulus for the growth of new subretinal vessels is unknown. However, immune mechanisms in patients with an underlying genetic predisposition for the development of this disease have been implicated. A recent case-control study demonstrates significantly increased odds of CNV secondary to POHS in patients who smoke compared with patients who never smoked [92].

HLA-DRw2 is twice as common among patients with histo spots alone, whereas both HLA-B7 and HLA-DRw2 are two to four times more common among patients with disciform scars caused by POHS as compared to control subjects [93, 94].

Clinical Features

The diagnosis of POHS is based on the clinical triad of multiple white, atrophic choroidal scars (histo spots), peripapillary pigment changes, and a maculopathy caused by CNV in the absence of cellular reaction in the anterior chamber or vitreous cavity. Most often, both eyes are involved asymmetrically. Histo spots may appear in the macula or periphery, are discrete and punched out (arising from a variable degree of scarring in the choroid and adjacent outer retina), and are typically asymptomatic (Fig. 12.10). Histo spots are noted in 2.6 % of the population living in endemic areas and in 4.4 % of the endemic population with a positive histoplasmosis skin test [95]. Linear equatorial streaks can be seen in 5 % of patients. The histo spots are usually stable but may undergo changes in shape and size. They have been shown to become larger over time. The mechanism of change in size and shape of these lesions is unknown. Long-term follow-up has shown that 9–16 % of patients will develop new histo spots [96, 97]. It has also been shown that 50 % of eyes will have changes in atrophic scarring manifested by increased size or by formation of new scars in the peripapillary, macular, and peripheral regions.

A ring of peripapillary atrophy (Fig. 12.10) occurs in the majority of cases of POHS. This ring is characteristic, with a narrow inner pigment zone adjacent to the disk edge and a white depigmented zone away from the disk. CNV usually involves the macula (Fig. 12.10). Metamorphopsia and a profound reduction in central vision are the most common symptoms of macular involvement from CNV. On fundus examination, active neovascular membrane appears as a yellow-green subretinal lesion, frequently arising at the border of a histo spot, typically surrounded by a pigment ring and associated with overlying neurosensory detachment and subretinal hemorrhage. Cicatricial changes characterize advanced disease with subretinal fibrosis and disciform scarring of the macula. Over time, new choroidal scars develop in more than 20 % of patients. However, only 3.8 % of these progress to CNV. If histo spots appear in the macular area, the patient has a 25 % chance of developing CNV within 3 years. If no spots are observed, the chances fall to 2 %. The risk of developing CNV in the contralateral eye is high, ranging from 8 to 24 % over a 3-year period [98].

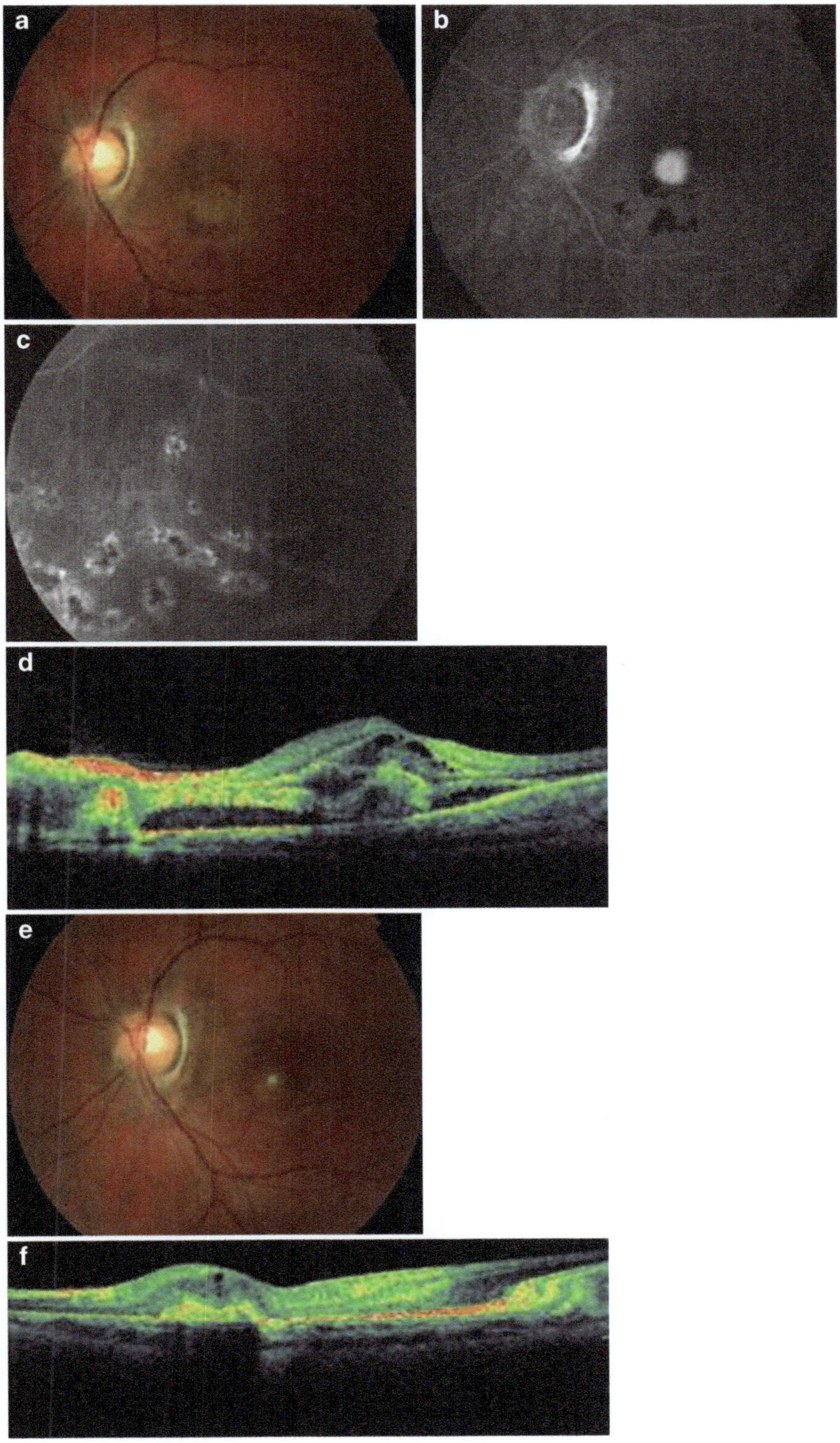

Fig. 12.10 (**a**) Color fundus photograph shows POHS related choroidal neovascular membrane with macular hemorrhages. (**b**) Late-phase fluorescein angiogram shows leakage of the choroidal neovascular membrane. (**c**) Mid-phase fluorescein angiogram shows peripheral histo spots. (**d**) OCT shows a subretinal hyperreflective lesion associated with SRD and cystoid spaces. (**e**) Color fundus photograph 12 months after a single intravitreal injection of Bevacizumab shows macular subretinal fibrotic lesion with resolution of SRD and persistence of some retinal cysts on OCT (**f**)

Ancillary Tests

Classic choroidal neovascularization is recognized on FA as discrete early hyperfluorescence with late leakage of dye into the overlying neurosensory retinal detachment. Occult CNV can occur in two forms: fibrovascular pigment epithelial detachments, which typically appear as stippled leakage associated with elevated RPE, and late leakage of undetermined source. A lacy pattern within classic CNV is observed more commonly in POHS than in other causes of CNV such as age-related macular degeneration (AMD) [95].

OCT is helpful in the diagnosis and follow-up of CNV.

The histoplasmin skin test is the most valuable laboratory test in the diagnosis of ocular histoplasmosis. Although 80 % of patients with POHS have a positive reactions to skin tests, this is not routinely used in clinical practice because in endemic regions up to two thirds of the population may be positive responders [98]. Serologic tests are generally not helpful in establishing causation because antibodies decline to low or undetectable levels 2–5 years after systemic infection [95].

Differential Diagnosis

The differential diagnosis of POHS includes entities other than AMD that is frequently associated with CNV including high myopia, angioid streaks, choroidal rupture, idiopathic CNV, multifocal choroiditis, punctate inner choroidopathy, and granulomatous fundus lesions that may mimic the scarring seen in POHS (as in toxoplasmosis, tuberculosis, coccidioidomycosis, syphilis, sarcoidosis, and toxocariasis). The atrophic spots and maculopathy of myopic degeneration and disciform scarring in AMD may also be confused with POHS.

Treatment

Treatment options for vision-threatening CNV include thermal laser photocoagulation, photodynamic therapy (PDT), submacular surgery for membrane removal, and intravitreal injection of triamcinolone or anti-VEGF agents [87].

Argon and krypton laser photocoagulation have proved their efficacy in the treatment of extrafoveal and juxtafoveal CNV in POHS. The proportion of eyes experiencing severe visual loss was significantly reduced with laser photocoagulation. Disease progression was seen in 12 % of treated individuals compared with 42 % of control patients. A high rate of persistent or recurrent CNV was observed following photocoagulation in 26 % of extrafoveal and in 33 % of juxtafoveal lesions [99].

PDT with verteporfin has been advocated for the treatment of subfoveal POHS-associated CNV based on small, prospective, uncontrolled case series [100–103].

Similarly, intravitreal triamcinolone was shown to be relatively safe and effective in the management of POHS-associated juxtafoveal and subfoveal CNV in small retrospective case studies [104].

More recently, intravitreal injection of anti-VEGF proved their efficacy in the management of CNV complicating POHS (Fig. 12.10) [105, 106]. A recent study showed that there is no significant difference in VA outcomes between intravitreal bevacizumab monotherapy versus intravitreal bevacizumab/PDT combination therapy after a follow-up of 2 years [107].

Submacular surgery for the removal of CNV lesions may be considered for patients with initial VA worse than 20/100 and in selected cases of extensive peripapillary CNV [108–114].

12.3.1.2 Histoplasmic Endophthalmitis

Histoplasmic endophthalmitis usually begins as a peripheral focal retinitis associated with vitritis and iridocyclitis [115]. Histoplasmic endophthalmitis is usually recognized in patients with disseminated histoplasmosis [116]. It is often seen in immunocompromised individuals and is becoming even more common as a result of the widespread use of chemotherapeutic agents. The diagnosis of histoplasmic endophthalmitis is made by cultures of the aqueous and vitreous. Treatment involves the use of systemic amphotericin B and ketoconazole. Intravitreal injections of amphotericin B are used in severe cases that are unresponsive to systemic treatment [115].

Compliance with Ethical Requirements

Conflict of Interest The authors declare that they have no conflict of interest.

Informed Consent No human studies were carried out by the authors for this article.

Animal Studies No animal studies were carried out by the authors for this article.

References

1. Nicolle C, Manceaux L. On a leishman body infection (or related organisms) of the gondi. CR Hebdomadaire Seances Acad Sci. 1908;146:207–9.
2. Petersen E, Kijlstra A, Stanford M. Epidemiology of ocular toxoplasmosis. Ocul Immunol Inflamm. 2012;20(2):68–75.
3. Holland GN. Ocular toxoplasmosis: a global reassessment. Part I: epidemiology and course of disease. Am J Ophthalmol. 2003;136(6):973–88.
4. Furtado JM, Winthrop KL, Butler NJ, Smith JR. Ocular toxoplasmosis I: parasitology, epidemiology and public health. Clin Experiment Ophthalmol. 2013;41(1):82–94.
5. Subauste CS, Ajzenberg D, Kijlstra A. Review of the series "Disease of the year 2011: toxoplasmosis" pathophysiology of toxoplasmosis. Ocul Immunol Inflamm. 2011;19(5):297–306.
6. Balasundaram MB, Andavar R, Palaniswamy M, Venkatapathy N. Outbreak of acquired ocular toxoplasmosis involving 248 patients. Arch Ophthalmol. 2010;128(1):28–32.
7. Delair E, Latkany P, Noble AG, Rabiah P, McLeod R, Brézin A. Clinical manifestations of ocular toxoplasmosis. Ocul Immunol Inflamm. 2011;19(2):91–102.
8. Butler NJ, Furtado JM, Winthrop KL, Smith JR. Ocular toxoplasmosis II: clinical features, pathology and management. Clin Experiment Ophthalmol. 2013;41(1):95–108.
9. Holland GN. Ocular toxoplasmosis: a global reassessment. Part II: disease manifestations and management. Am J Ophthalmol. 2004;137(1):1–17.
10. Bosch-Driessen LE, Berendschot TT, Ongkosuwito JV, Rothova A. Ocular toxoplasmosis: clinical features and prognosis of 154 patients. Ophthalmology. 2002;109(5):869–78.
11. Tan HK, Schmidt D, Stanford M, Teär-Fahnehjelm K, Ferret N, Salt A, Gilbert R, European Multicentre Study on Congenital Toxoplasmosis (EMSCOT). Risk of visual impairment in children with congenital toxoplasmic retinochoroiditis. Am J Ophthalmol. 2007;144(5):648–53.
12. Mets MB, Holfels E, Boyer KM, Swisher CN, Roizen N, Stein L, Stein M, Hopkins J, Withers S, Mack D, Luciano R, Patel D, Remington JS, Meier P, McLeod R. Eye manifestations of congenital toxoplasmosis. Am J Ophthalmol. 1996;122(3):309–24.
13. Kodjikian L, Wallon M, Fleury J, Denis P, Binquet C, Peyron F, Garweg JG. Ocular manifestations in congenital toxoplasmosis. Graefes Arch Clin Exp Ophthalmol. 2006;244(1):14–21.
14. Smith JR, Cunningham Jr ET. Atypical presentations of ocular toxoplasmosis. Curr Opin Ophthalmol. 2002;13(6):387–92.
15. Kahloun R, Mbarek S, Khairallah-Ksiaa I, Jelliti B, Ben Yahia S, Khairallah M. Branch retinal artery occlusion associated with posterior uveitis. J Ophthal Inflamm Infect. 2013;3(1):16.
16. Auer C, Bernasconi O, Herbort CP. Indocyanine green angiography features in toxoplasmic retinochoroiditis. Retina. 1999;19(1):22–9.
17. Khairallah M, Yahia SB, Zaouali S, Jenzeri S, Attia S, Messaoud R. Acute choroidal ischemia associated with toxoplasmic retinochoroiditis. Retina. 2007; 27(7):947–51.
18. Khairallah M, Kahloun R, Ben Yahia S, Jelliti B. Clinical, tomographic, and angiographic findings in patients with acute toxoplasmic retinochoroiditis and associated serous retinal detachment. Ocul Immunol Inflamm. 2011;19(5):307–10.
19. Diniz B, Regatieri C, Andrade R, Maia A. Evaluation of spectral domain and time domain optical coherence tomography findings in toxoplasmic retinochoroiditis. Clin Ophthalmol. 2011;5:645–50.
20. Oréfice JL, Costa RA, Scott IU, Calucci D, Oréfice F, Grupo Mineiro de Pesquisa em Doenças Oculares Inflamatórias (MINAS). Spectral optical coherence tomography findings in patients with ocular toxoplasmosis and active satellite lesions (MINAS Report 1). Acta Ophthalmol. 2013;91(1):e41–7.
21. Oréfice JL, Costa RA, Campos W, Calucci D, Scott IU, Oréfice F. Third-generation optical coherence tomography findings in punctate retinal toxoplasmosis. Am J Ophthalmol. 2006;142(3):503–50.
22. Oréfice JL, Costa RA, Orefice F, Campos W, da Costa-Lima Jr D, Scott IU. Vitreoretinalmorphology in active ocular toxoplasmosis: a prospective study by optical coherence tomography. Br J Ophthalmol. 2007;91:773–80.
23. Saxena S, Rastogi RA, Vishvkarma K, Hansraj S, Meyer CH. Spectral-domain optical coherence tomography in healed ocular toxoplasmosis. J Ocul Biol Dis Infor. 2010;3(3):109–11.
24. Stanford MR, Tomlin EA, Comyn O, Holland K, Pavesio C. The visual field in toxoplasmic retinochoroiditis. Br J Ophthalmol. 2005;89(7):812–4.
25. Papadia M, Aldigeri R, Herbort CP. The role of serology in active ocular toxoplasmosis. Int Ophthalmol. 2011;31(6):461–5.
26. Garweg JG, de Groot-Mijnes JD, Montoya JG. Diagnostic approach to ocular toxoplasmosis. Ocul Immunol Inflamm. 2011;19(4):255–61.

27. Fardeau C, Romand S, Rao NA, Cassoux N, Bettembourg O, Thulliez P, Lehoang P. Diagnosis of toxoplasmic retinochoroiditis with atypical clinical features. Am J Ophthalmol. 2002;134(2):196–203.
28. Montoya JG, Parmley S, Liesenfeld O, Jaffe GJ, Remington JS. Use of the polymerase chain reaction for diagnosis of ocular toxoplasmosis. Ophthalmology. 1999;106(8):1554–63.
29. Vasconcelos-Santos DV, Dodds EM, Oréfice F. Review for disease of the year: differential diagnosis of ocular toxoplasmosis. Ocul Immunol Inflamm. 2011;19(3):171–9.
30. de-la-Torre A, Stanford M, Curi A, Jaffe GJ, Gomez-Marin JE. Therapy for ocular toxoplasmosis. Ocul Immunol Inflamm. 2011;19(5):314–20.
31. Koo L, Young LH. Management of ocular toxoplasmosis. Int Ophthalmol Clin. 2006;46(2):183–93.
32. Stanford MR, See SE, Jones LV, Gilbert RE. Antibiotics for toxoplasmic retinochoroiditis: an evidence-based systematic review. Ophthalmology. 2003;110(5):926–31.
33. Soheilian M, Sadoughi MM, Ghajarnia M, Dehghan MH, Yazdani S, Behboudi H, Anisian A, Peyman GA. Prospective randomized trial of trimethoprim sulfamethoxazole versus pyrimethamine and sulfadiazine in the treatment of ocular toxoplasmosis. Ophthalmology. 2005;112(11):1876–82.
34. Bosch-Driessen LH, Verbraak FD, Suttorp-Schulten MS, van Ruyven RL, Klok AM, Hoyng CB, Rothova A. A prospective, randomized trial of pyrimethamine and azithromycin vs pyrimethamine and sulfadiazine for the treatment of ocular toxoplasmosis. Am J Ophthalmol. 2002;134(1):34–40.
35. Soheilian M, Ramezani A, Azimzadeh A, Sadoughi MM, Dehghan MH, Shahghadami R, Yaseri M, Peyman GA. Randomized trial of intravitreal clindamycin and dexamethasone versus pyrimethamine, sulfadiazine, and prednisolone in treatment of ocular toxoplasmosis. Ophthalmology. 2011;118(1):134–41.
36. Kump LI, Androudi SN, Foster CS. Ocular toxoplasmosis in pregnancy. Clin Experiment Ophthalmol. 2005;33(5):455–60.
37. Pearson PA, Piracha AR, Sen HA, Jaffe GJ. Atovaquone for the treatment of toxoplasma retinochoroiditis in immunocompetent patients. Ophthalmology. 1999;106:148–53.
38. Ben Yahia S, Herbort CP, Jenzeri S, Hmidi K, Attia S, Messaoud R, Khairallah M. Intravitreal bevacizumab (Avastin) as primary and rescue treatment for choroidal neovascularization secondary to ocular toxoplasmosis. Int Ophthalmol. 2008;28(4):311–6.
39. Rishi P, Venkataraman A, Rishi E. Combination photodynamic therapy and bevacizumab for choroidal neovascularization associated with toxoplasmosis. Indian J Ophthalmol. 2011;59(1):62–4.
40. Silveira C, Belfort Jr R, Muccioli C, Holland GN, Victora CG, Horta BL, Yu F, Nussenblatt RB. The effect of long-term intermittent trimethoprime sulfamethoxazole treatment on recurrences of toxoplasmic retinochoroiditis. Am J Ophthalmol. 2002;134(1):41–6.
41. Stewart JM, Cubillan LD, Cunningham Jr ET. Prevalence, clinical features, and causes of vision loss among patients with ocular toxocariasis. Retina. 2005;25(8):1005–13.
42. Taylor MR. The epidemiology of ocular toxocariasis. J Helminthol. 2001;75:109–18.
43. Woodhall D, Starr MC, Montgomery SP, Jones JL, Lum F, Read RW, Moorthy RS. Ocular toxocariasis: epidemiologic, anatomic, and therapeutic variations based on a survey of ophthalmic subspecialists. Ophthalmology. 2012;119(6):1211–7.
44. Sabrosa NA, de Souza EC. Nematode infections of the eye: toxocariasis and diffuse unilateral subacute neuroretinitis. Curr Opin Ophthalmol. 2001;12(6):450–4.
45. Ament CS, Young LH. Ocular manifestations of helminthic infections: onchocersiasis, cysticercosis, toxocariasis, and diffuse unilateral subacute neuroretinitis. Int Ophthalmol Clin. 2006;46(2):1–10.
46. Sabrosa NA, Zajdenweber M. Nematode infections of the eye: toxocariasis, onchocerciasis, diffuse unilateral subacute neuroretinitis, and cysticercosis. Ophthalmol Clin North Am. 2002;15(3):351–6.
47. Arevalo JF, Espinoza JV, Arevalo FA. Ocular toxocariasis. J Pediatr Ophthalmol Strabismus. 2012;28:1–11.
48. Verallo O, Fragiotta S, Verboschi F, Vingolo EM. Diagnostic aspects and retinal imaging in ocular toxocariasis: a case report from Italy. Case Rep Med. 2012;2012:984512.
49. Wan WL, Cano MR, Pince KJ, Green RL. Echographic characteristics of ocular toxocariasis. Ophthalmology. 1991;98(1):28–32.
50. Tran VT, Lumbroso L, LeHoang P, Herbort CP. Ultrasound biomicroscopy in peripheral retinovitreal toxocariasis. Am J Ophthalmol. 1999;127:607–9.
51. Cella W, Ferreira E, Torigoe AM, Macchiaverni-Filho N, Balarin V. Ultrasound biomicroscopy findings in peripheral vitreoretinal toxocariasis. Eur J Ophthalmol. 2004;14(2):132–6.
52. Suzuki T, Joko T, Akao N, Ohashi Y. Following the migration of a Toxocara larva in the retina by optical coherence tomography and fluorescein angiography. Jpn J Ophthalmol. 2005;49(2):159–61.
53. Higashide T, Akao N, Shirao E, Shirao Y. Optical coherence tomographic and angiographic findings of a case with subretinal toxocara granuloma. Am J Ophthalmol. 2003;136(1):188–90.
54. Małafiej E, Spiewak E. The significance of the level of antibodies in the evaluation of the effects of treatment of toxocariasis. Wiad Parazytol. 2001;47:805–10.
55. de Visser L, Rothova A, de Boer JH, et al. Diagnosis of ocular toxocariasis by establishing intraocular antibody production. Am J Ophthalmol. 2008;145:369–74.
56. Giuliari GP, Ramirez G, Cortez RT. Surgical treatment of ocular toxocariasis: anatomic and functional results in 45 patients. Eur J Ophthalmol. 2011;21(4):490–4.
57. Gass JD, Gilbert Jr WR, Guerry RK, Scelfo R. Diffuse unilateral subacute neuroretinitis. Ophthalmology. 1978;85(5):521–45.

58. Gass JD, Braunstein RA. Further observations concerning the diffuse unilateral subacute neuroretinitis syndrome. Arch Ophthalmol. 1983;101(11):1689–97.
59. Rasquin F, Waterschoot MP, Termote H, Carlier Y. Diffuse unilateral subacute neuroretinitis in Africa. Ocul Immunol Inflamm. 2006;14(1):59–62.
60. Harto MA, Rodriguez-Salvador V, Aviñó JA, Duch-Samper AM, Menezo JL. Diffuse unilateral subacute neuroretinitis in Europe. Eur J Ophthalmol. 1999;9(1):58–62.
61. de Amorim Garcia Filho CA, Gomes AH, de A Garcia Soares AC, de Amorim Garcia CA. Clinical features of 121 patients with diffuse unilateral subacute neuroretinitis. Am J Ophthalmol. 2012;153(4):743–9.
62. Vianna RN, Onofre G, Ecard V, Muralha L, Muralha A, de A Garcia CA. Indocyanine green angiography in diffuse unilateral subacute neuroretinitis. Eye (Lond). 2006;20(9):1113–6.
63. Jesús MR, Isabel RC. Indocyanine green angiography for the detection of subretinal nematodes in diffuse unilateral subacute neuroretinitis (DUSN). Int Ophthalmol. 2004;25(5–6):295–7.
64. Garcia Filho CA, Soares AC, Penha FM, Garcia CA. Spectral domain optical coherence tomography in diffuse unilateral subacute neuroretinitis. J Ophthalmol. 2011;2011:285296.
65. Souza EC, Casella AM, Nakashima Y, Monteiro ML. Clinical features and outcomes of patients with diffuse unilateral subacute neuroretinitis treated with oral albendazole. Am J Ophthalmol. 2005;140(3):437–45.
66. Rathinam SR, Cunningham ET. Infectious causes of uveitis in the developing world. Int Ophthalmol Clin. 2000;40:137–52.
67. Thylefors B. Onchocerciasis: an overview. Int Ophthalmol Clin. 1990;30:21–3.
68. Wittig EO. Ocular cysticercosis: an epidemiological study. Arq Neuropsiquiatr. 2001;59(3-B):696–701.
69. Mahendradas P, Avadhani K, Yadav NK, Vinekar A, Shetty R, Shetty BK. High-definition spectral-domain optical coherence tomography of intravitreal and subretinal cysticercus cysts in intraocular cysticercosis. Retina. 2011;31(10):2132–3.
70. Yadav SK, Winter I, Singh SK. Management of intravitreal cysticercosis. Nepal J Ophthalmol. 2009;1(2):143–5.
71. Herman JS, Chiodini PL. Gnathostomiasis, another emerging imported disease. Clin Microbiol Rev. 2009;22:484–92.
72. Bhattacharjee H, Bas D, Medhi J. Intravitreal gnathostomiasis and review of the literature. Retina. 2007;27:67–73.
73. Del Piero EJ, Cunningham ET, Sabrosa N, Khairallah M, Kahloun R. Diagnostic and therapeutic challenges. Retina. 2011;31(7):1428–34.
74. Biswas J, Gopal L, Sharma T, Badrinath SS. Intraocular Gnathostoma spinigerum. Clinicopathological study of two cases with review of literature. Retina. 1994;14:438–44.
75. Bathrick ME, Mango CA, Mueller JF. Intraocular gnathostomiasis. Ophthalmology. 1981;8:1293–5.
76. Funata M, Cutis P, de la Cruz Z, de Juan E, Green WR. Intraocular gnathostomiasis. Retina. 1993;13:240–4.
77. Sasona K, Ando F, Nagasaka T, Kidokoro T, Kawamoto F. A case of uveitis due to gnathostoma migration into the vitreous cavity. Nippon Ganka Gakkai Zasshi. 1994;98:1136–40.
78. Sabrosa NA, Cunningham Jr ET, Arevalo JF. Ocular nematode and trematode infections in the developing world. Int Ophthalmol Clin. 2010;50:71–85.
79. Otranto D, Eberhard ML. Zoonotic helminths affecting the human eye. Parasit Vectors. 2011;4:41.
80. Kociecki J, Kociecka W. Visual system involvement in selected zoonotic diseases. II. Trichinellosis. Klin Oczna. 2004;106(3):371–5.
81. Behrens-Baumann W, Freissler G. Retinochoroidopathy in a patient with seropositive trichinosis. Klin Monbl Augenheilkd. 1991;199(2):114–7.
82. Bialasiewicz AA, Hassenstein A, Schaudig U. Subretinal granuloma, retinal vasculitis and keratouveitis with secondary open-angle glaucoma in schistosomiasis. Ophthalmologe. 2001;98(10):972–5.
83. Oréfice F, Simal CJ, Pittella JE. Schistosomotic choroiditis. I. Funduscopic changes and differential diagnosis. Br J Ophthalmol. 1985;69(4):294–9.
84. Dickinson AJ, Rosenthal AR, Nicholson KG. Inflammation of the retinal pigment epithelium: a unique presentation of ocular schistosomiasis. Br J Ophthalmol. 1990;74(7):440–2.
85. Creed TD. Unilateral optic atrophy presumed secondary to schistosomiasis of the optic nerve. J Am Optom Assoc. 1993;64(6):440–5.
86. Olds GR, King C, Hewlett J, et al. Double-blind placebo-controlled study of concurrent administration of albendazole and praziquantel in schoolchildren with schistosomiasis and geohelminths. J Infect Dis. 1999;179(4):996–1003.
87. Oliver A, Ciulla TA, Comer GM. New and classic insights into presumed ocular histoplasmosis syndrome and its treatment. Curr Opin Ophthalmol. 2005;16(3):160–5.
88. Suttorp-Schulten MS, Bollemeijer JG, Bos PJ, Rothova A. Presumed ocular histoplasmosis in the Netherlands: an area without histoplasmosis. Br J Ophthalmol. 1997;81:7–11.
89. Sinha R, Raju S, Garg SP, Venkatesh P, Talwar D. Presumed ocular histoplasmosis syndrome in India. Ocul Immunol Inflamm. 2007;15:315–7.
90. Lewis ML, Schiffman JC. Long term follow up of the second eye in ocular histoplasmosis. Int Ophthalmol Clin. 1983;23:125–35.
91. Smith RE, Ganley JP. An epidemiologic study of presumed ocular histoplasmosis. Trans Am Acad Ophthalmol Otolaryngol. 1971;75:994–1005.
92. Chheda LV, Ferketich AK, Carroll CP, Moyer PD, Kurz DE, Kurz PA. Smoking as a risk factor for choroidal neovascularization secondary to presumed ocular histoplasmosis syndrome. Ophthalmology. 2012;119(2):333–8.

93. Braley RE, Meredith TA, Aaberg TM, Koethe SM, Witkowski JA. The prevalence of HLA-B7 in presumed ocular histoplasmosis. Am J Ophthalmol. 1978;85(6):859–61.
94. Meredith TA, Smith RE, Dueqesnoy RJ. Association of HLA-DR2 antigen with presumed ocular histoplasmosis. Am J Ophthalmol. 1980;89(1):70–6.
95. Ciulla TA, Piper HC, Xiao M, Wheat LJ. Presumed ocular histoplasmosis syndrome: update on epidemiology, pathogenesis, and photodynamic, antiangiogenic, and surgical therapies. Curr Opin Ophthalmol. 2001;12(6):442–9.
96. Lewis ML, Van Newkirk MR, Gass JD. Follow-up study of presumed ocular histoplasmosis syndrome. Ophthalmology. 1980;87(5):390–9.
97. Watzke RC, Claussen RW. The long-term course of multifocal choroiditis (presumed ocular histoplasmosis). Am J Ophthalmol. 1981;91(6):750–60.
98. Prasad AG, Van Gelder RN. Presumed ocular histoplasmosis syndrome. Curr Opin Ophthalmol. 2005; 16(6):364–8.
99. Five-year follow-up of fellow eyes of individuals with ocular histoplasmosis and unilateral extrafoveal or juxtafoveal choroidal neovascularization. Macular Photocoagulation Study Group. Arch Ophthalmol 1996;114(6):677–88.
100. Saperstein DA, Rosenfeld PJ, Bressler NM, Rosa RH, et al. Verteporfin therapy for CNV secondary to OHS. Ophthalmology. 2006;113(12):2371.e 1–3.
101. Rosenfeld PJ, Saperstein DA, Bressler NM, et al. Photodynamic therapy with verteporfin in ocular histoplasmosis: uncontrolled, open-label 2-year study. Ophthalmology. 2004;3(9):1725–33.
102. Postelmans L, Pasteels B, Coquelet P, Caspers L, Verougstraete C, Leys A, Wirix M, Mauget-Faÿsse M, Quanranta M, Snyers B, Smets E. Photodynamic therapy for subfoveal classic choroidal neovascularization related to punctate inner choroidopathy (PIC) or presumed ocular histoplasmosis-like syndrome (POHS-like). Ocul Immunol Inflamm. 2005;13(5):361–6.
103. Shah GK, Blinder KJ, Hariprasad SM, Thomas MA, Ryan Jr EH, Bakal J, Sharma S. Photodynamic therapy for juxtafoveal choroidal neovascularization due to ocular histoplasmosis syndrome. Retina. 2005; 25(1):26–32.
104. Rechtman E, Allen VD, Danis RP, Pratt LM, Harris A, Speicher MA. Intravitreal triamcinolone for choroidal neovascularization in ocular histoplasmosis syndrome. Am J Ophthalmol. 2003;136(4):739–41.
105. Mansour AM, Arevalo JF, Fardeau C, Hrisomalos EN, Chan WM, Lai TY, Ziemssen F, Ness T, Sibai AM, Mackensen F, Wolf A, Hrisomalos N, Heiligenhaus A, Spital G, Jo Y, Gomi F, Ikuno Y, Akesbi J, LeHoang P, Adan A, Mahendradas P, Khairallah M, Guthoff R, Ghandour B, Küçükerdönmez C, Kurup SK. Three-year visual and anatomic results of administrating intravitreal bevacizumab in inflammatoryocular neovascularization. Can J Ophthalmol. 2012;47(3):269–74.
106. Nielsen JS, Fick TA, Saggau DD, Barnes CH. Intravitreal anti-vascular endothelial growth factor therapy for choroidal neovascularization secondary to ocular histoplasmosis syndrome. Retina. 2012;32(3):468–72.
107. Cionni DA, Lewis SA, Petersen MR, Foster RE, Riemann CD, Sisk RA, Hutchins RK, Miller DM. Analysis of outcomes for intravitreal bevacizumab in the treatment of choroidal neovascularization secondary to ocular histoplasmosis. Ophthalmology. 2012;119(2):327–32.
108. de Juan E, Machemer R. Vitreous surgery for hemorrhagic and fibrous complications of age-related macular degeneration. Am J Ophthalmol. 1988;105: 25–9.
109. Thomas MA, Kaplan HJ. Surgical removal of subfoveal neovascularization in the presumed ocular histoplasmosis syndrome. Am J Ophthalmol. 1991;111:1–7.
110. Berger AS, Kaplan HJ. Clinical experience with the surgical removal of subfoveal neovascular membranes. Ophthalmology. 1992;99:969–76.
111. Submacular Surgery Trials Research Group. Surgical removal vs observation for subfoveal choroidal neovascularization, either associated with the ocular histoplasmosis syndrome or idiopathic: II. Quality-of-life findings from a randomized clinical trial: SST group H trial: SST report no. 10. Arch Ophthalmol. 2004;122:1616–28.
112. Bass EB, Gilson MM, Mangione CM, Hawkins BS, Miskala PH, Mann AL, Bressler NM. Surgical removal vs observation for idiopathic or ocular histoplasmosis syndrome-associated subfoveal choroidal neovascularization: Vision Preference Value Scale findings from the randomized SST Group H Trial: SST Report No. 17. Arch Ophthalmol. 2008;126(12):1626–32.
113. Hawkins BS, Bressler NM, Bressler SB, Davidorf FH, Hoskins JC, Marsh MJ, Miskala PH, Redford M, Sternberg Jr P, Thomas MA, Toth CA, Submacular Surgery Trials Research Group. Surgical removal vs observation for subfoveal choroidal neovascularization, either associated with the ocular histoplasmosis syndrome or idiopathic: II. Quality-of-life findings from a randomized clinical trial: SST group H trial: SST report no. 10. Arch Ophthalmol. 2004;122:1616–28.
114. Almony A, Thomas MA, Atebara NH, Holekamp NM, Del Priore LV. Long-term follow-up of surgical removal of extensive peripapillary choroidal neovascularization in presumed ocular histoplasmosis syndrome. Ophthalmology. 2008;115(3):540–45.e5.
115. Gonzales CA, Scott IU, Chaudhry NA, Luu KM, Miller D, Murray TG, Davis JL. Endogenous endophthalmitis caused by Histoplasma capsulatum var. capsulatum: a case report and literature review. Ophthalmology. 2000;107(2):725–9.
116. Goldstein BG, Buettner H. Histoplasmic endophthalmitis. A clinicopathologic correlation. Arch Ophthalmol. 1983;101(5):774–7.

13 Infections of the Posterior Segment: Acute Retinal Necrosis

Hani S. Al-Mezaine, Marwan Abouammoh, and Ahmed M. Abu El-Asrar

13.1 Introduction

Acute retinal necrosis (ARN) is a rare, but potentially a blinding disease, characterized by progressive peripheral necrotizing retinitis. The first report in the medical literature of this entity was published by Akira Urayama and his colleagues in Japan in 1971 [1]. The initial report that implicated human herpes virus as the etiological agent of ARN was published in 1982 [2]. Since then, varicella zoster virus (VZV), herpes simplex virus (HSV) type 1 and type 2, and, very rarely, cytomegalovirus (CMV) and Epstein-Barr (EB) virus have been definitively implicated as an etiological agents of ARN [3, 4].

In the United Kingdom, two nationwide surveillances estimated the incidence of ARN to be approximately one case per 1.6–2.0 million population per year [5, 6]. Goto H et al. [7] conducted an epidemiological survey of intraocular inflammation at the uveitis clinic of university hospitals in Japan during 2002 and showed that ARN is diagnosed in only 1.3 % of endogenous uveitis patients. Recently, Al-Mezaine et al. [8] showed that ARN has been diagnosed in 2.8 % from all uveitis patients admitted at a referral university hospital in Saudi Arabia.

13.2 Clinical Manifestations

Although ARN syndrome may occur in immunocompromised such as patients with acquired immunodeficiency syndrome (AIDS) [9, 10], the disease usually occurs suddenly and without any warning signs in healthy immunocompetent persons.

The onset of ARN is generally unilateral. Fellow eye involvement occurs in approximately one third of patients, typically within 6 weeks of the initial involvement [11]. Second eye involvement decades following an initial infection has been also reported [12, 13].

The most common complaints at presentation were red eye, blurred vision, decreased vision, and ocular pain. Biomicroscopic examination of the anterior segment may reveal episcleritis, scleritis, keratitis, and/or anterior chamber inflammation, which may be either non-granulomatous or granulomatous manifested by mutton fat-like keratic precipitates (Fig. 13.1). However, hypopyon, iris atrophy, and adhesion of anterior and posterior iris are extremely rare. Examination of the posterior segment may show vitreous inflammation, arteritis, patchy full thickness peripheral necrotizing retinitis (Fig. 13.2), and in some cases, involvement of the optic disk [14]. Typically, the retinitis presents as multifocal,

H.S. Al-Mezaine, MD (✉) • M. Abouammoh, MD
A.M. Abu El-Asrar, MD, PhD
Department of Ophthalmology,
College of Medicine, King Saud University,
KAUH, Old Airport Road, 245,
Riyadh 11411, Saudi Arabia
e-mail: halmezaine@ksu.edu.sa;
mabouammoh@ksu.edu.sa; abuasrar@ksu.edu.sa

K. Tabbara et al. (eds.), *Ocular Infections*, Essentials in Ophthalmology,
DOI 10.1007/978-3-662-43981-4_13, © Springer-Verlag Berlin Heidelberg 2014

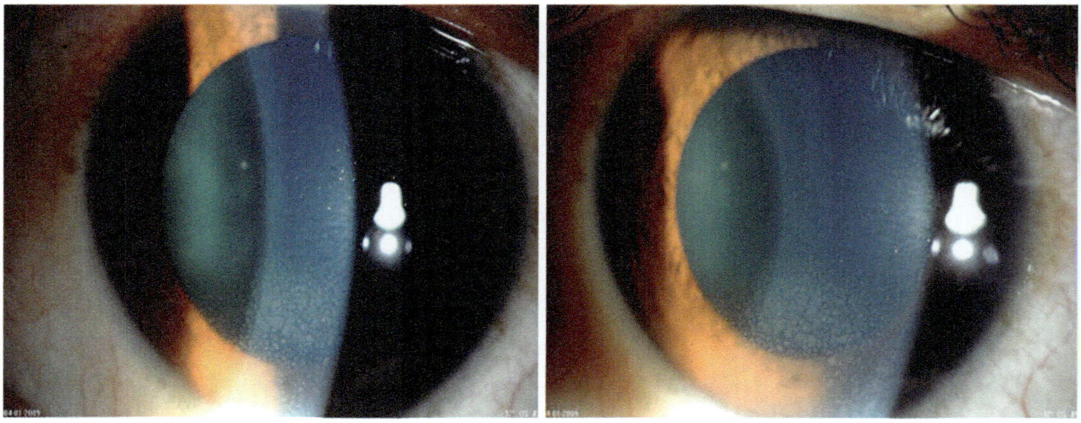

Fig. 13.1 Anterior segment photography of a patient with acute retinal necrosis showing a mutton fat-like keratic precipitates

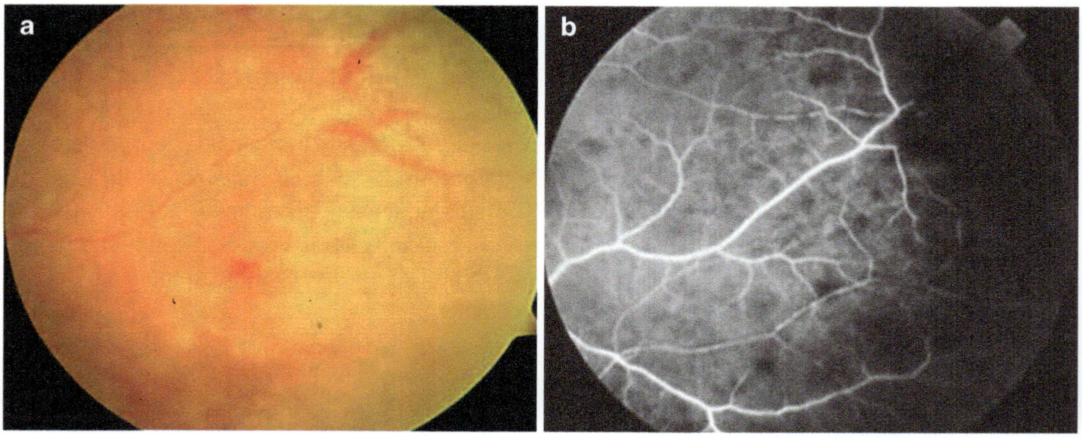

Fig. 13.2 (a) Peripheral retina of a patient with acute retinal necrosis showing periarterial vascular sheathing and necrotizing retinitis. (b) Fluorescein angiogram showing peripheral occlusive vasculopathy

small, patchy, white-yellow granular lesions in the peripheral retina gradually enlarge circumferentially and fuse to form dense geographic opaque lesions and eventually spreading toward the posterior pole. Vitreous organization and traction may progress during this phase, producing retinal breaks. Retinal detachment corresponding to the site of necrosis occurs at a very high rate, ranging from 50 to 75 % during the course of the disease [15].

Delayed complications of ARN may include chronic vitritis, macular edema, optic atrophy, epiretinal membrane formation, proliferative vitreoretinopathy, viral relapse with cessation of antiviral medication, and phthisis bulbi [16].

13.3 Diagnosis

In 1994, the American Uveitis Society established the standard clinical criteria for the diagnosis of ARN [17]. According to the criteria, the diagnosis of ARN syndrome should be generally based on clinical appearance and the course of infection. These criteria are (1) focal well-demarcated areas of retinal necrosis with discrete borders in the peripheral retina, (2) rapid circumferential progression of necrosis in the absence of antiviral therapy, (3) evidence of occlusive vasculopathy, and (4) prominent inflammation in the vitreous and anterior chamber. However, even with these specific diagnostic criteria, much ambiguity can still exist in assaying a definite etiology for many cases of posterior uveitis.

In the last decade, great advances have been made in the diagnosis of ARN syndrome, such as detection of viral DNA in intraocular fluids using polymerase chain reaction (PCR). PCR analysis of aqueous humor can be especially helpful and clinically important for cases of posterior uveitis of unknown etiology. In 2003, Tran et al. [18] performed PCR on aqueous humor for the detection of viral DNA in patients with necrotizing herpetic retinitis. Specific viral DNA was detected in the aqueous humor of 86.4 % of cases. Although more invasive than anterior chamber paracentesis, vitreous sampling obtained at the time of vitrectomy can also be used for the diagnosis of ARN [19].

PCR analysis of ocular fluids can also be supplemented with calculation of a Goldmann-Witmer coefficient (GWC) in the diagnosis of ARN. The GWC is a method of comparing intraocular antibody production to serum antibody production to diagnose ocular infections. The addition of a GWC to PCR can add additional diagnostic information in cryptic cases of posterior uveitis in which PCR is inconclusive [20, 21]. However, there are some drawbacks to this indirect method. Intraocular antibody production is not adequate during the early phase after onset, and therefore the GWC value cannot be calculated.

13.4 Management

13.4.1 Systemic Antiviral Therapy

After discovering the causative association between herpes viruses and ARN, the only available antiviral agent was intravenous acyclovir. The typical induction dose for intravenous acyclovir is 10–15 mg/kg given three times a day for 7–10 days. This should be followed by oral acyclovir 800 mg five times a day for 3–4 months [22–24]. Newer oral agents such as valacyclovir, famciclovir, and valganciclovir have greater bioavailability than oral acyclovir and can produce systemic concentrations nearly equal to those obtained with intravenous acyclovir [25].

13.4.2 Intravitreal Antiviral Therapy

Foscarnet is an inhibitor of viral DNA polymerase, is not dependent on viral kinases for activation, and therefore can be used against acyclovir-resistant herpes viruses. Multiple case reports describe the successful use of intravitreal foscarnet either as salvage therapy for cases of ARN not responding to standard therapy or as an adjuvant to IV acyclovir administered at the time of initial diagnosis [26, 27]. Most recently, a retrospective case series demonstrated a non-statistically significant 40 % reduction in the rate of retinal detachments in VZV-associated ARN patients treated with intravitreal foscarnet [28].

Ganciclovir can be given intravitreally or with the help of a surgically implanted device to release a sustained intravitreal concentration of 1 μg per hour over an 8-month period for patients with ARN related to CMV [29, 30].

Considering the high frequency of significant inflammation associated with ARN that contribute to the vision loss—such as moderate to severe vitritis, serous retinal detachment involving or threatening the macula, or retinitis or occlusive vasculitis involving or threatening the optic nerve or macula—it should be recommended to initiate a relatively a high dose of systemic corticosteroids (almost 1 mg/kg/day) together with antiviral drug at the onset of disease [23, 31]. The dosage of corticosteroid should be tapered in accordance with the clinical findings. Topical 1 % prednisolone acetate and a cycloplegic agent can be added to treat anterior chamber inflammation [32]. The use of oral antiplatelet agents, such as aspirin (100 mg/day), to help prevent retinal vascular occlusion has been suggested as well [23, 31], however the use of such agents remains controversial [32].

13.4.3 Prophylactic Laser Photocoagulation

The aim of prophylactic photocoagulation in ARN is to prevent retinal detachments and the associated poor visual outcomes. However, the use of photocoagulation in patients with ARN is controversial and the level of evidence supporting its use is generally weak [33]. Still, some authors believe that prophylactic laser treatment delivered posterior to active retinitis may help prevent progression to retinal detachment [34–36]. In the absence of a randomized study, the decision to apply laser must be individualized for each patient.

13.4.4 Surgery

Rhegmatogenous retinal detachment, often complicated by proliferative vitreoretinopathy, occurs in up to three-quarters of patients with ARN [34, 36–38]. When retinal detachments do occur in the setting of ARN, there are often both rhegmatogenous and tractional components, and management should address both of these contributing factors. Vitrectomy, lensectomy, endolaser, and long-acting gas or silicone oil tamponade have shown success in retinal reattachment repair and recovery of vision [39–42]. Recently, some investigators have advocated for early vitrectomy surgery in ARN patients before the appearance of a retinal detachment. Ishida et al. [42] reviewed the outcomes of patients with ARN who underwent a prophylactic vitrectomy; the surgery was not helpful in preventing detachments in eyes with posterior pole involvement. However, the rate of retinal detachment was lower in patients with mid-peripheral involvement that received the prophylactic surgery. Another study also found that early vitrectomy might prevent retinal detachments, but there was no clear benefit in the final visual outcome [41].

Compliance with Ethical Requirements

Conflict of Interest The authors declare that they have no conflict of interest.

Informed Consent No human studies were carried out by the authors for this article.

Animal Studies No animal studies were carried out by the authors for this article.

References

1. Urayama A, Yamada N, Sasaki T, et al. Unilateral acute uveitis with retinal periarteritis and detachment. Jpn J Clin Ophthalmol. 1971;25:607–19.
2. Culbertson WW, Blumenkranz MS, Haines H, et al. The acute retinal necrosis syndrome. Part 2: histopathology and etiology. Ophthalmology. 1982;89:1317–25.
3. Ganatra JB, Chandler D, Santos C, et al. Viral causes of the acute retinal necrosis syndrome. Am J Ophthalmol. 2000;129:166–72.
4. Walters G, James TE. Viral causes of the acute retinal necrosis syndrome. Curr Opin Ophthalmol. 2001;12:191–5.
5. Muthiah MN, Michaelides M, Child CS, et al. Acute retinal necrosis: a national population-based study to assess the incidence, methods of diagnosis, treatment strategies and outcomes in the UK. Br J Ophthalmol 2007;91:1452–5.
6. Cochrane TF, Silvestri G, McDowell C, et al. Acute retinal necrosis in the United Kingdom: results of a prospective surveillance study. Eye (Lond). 2012;26:370–7.
7. Goto H, Mochizuki M, Yamaki K, et al. Epidemiological survey of intraocular inflammation in Japan. Jpn J Ophthalmol. 2007;51:41–4.
8. Al-Mezaine HS, Kangave D, Abu El-Asrar AM. Patterns of uveitis in patients admitted to a University Hospital in Riyadh, Saudi Arabia. Ocul Immunol Inflamm. 2010;18:424–31.
9. Jabs DA, Schachat AP, Liss R, et al. Presumed varicella zoster retinitis in immunocompromised patients. Retina. 1987;7:9–13.
10. Friberg TR, Jost BF. Acute retinal necrosis in an immunosuppressed patient. Am J Ophthalmol. 1984;98:515–7.
11. Fisher JP, Lewis ML, Blumenkranz M, et al. The acute retinal necrosis syndrome. Part 1: clinical manifestations. Ophthalmology. 1982;89:1309–16.
12. Martinez J, Lambert HM, Capone A, et al. Delayed bilateral involvement in the acute retinal necrosis syndrome. Am J Ophthalmol. 1992;113:103–4.
13. Sergott RC, Belmont JB, Savino PJ, Fischer DH, Bosley TM, Schatz NJ. Optic nerve involvement in the acute retinal necrosis syndrome. Arch Ophthalmol. 1985;103:1160–2.
14. Okunuki Y, Usui Y, Kezuka T, et al. Four cases of bilateral acute retinal necrosis with a long interval after the initial onset. Br J Ophthalmol. 2011;95:1251–4.
15. Chang S, Young LH. Acute retinal necrosis: an overview. Int Ophthalmol Clin. 2007;47:145–54.
16. Fernando AEGD, Thi T, Nathalie C, et al. Long-term visual outcome of patients presenting with necrotizing viral retinopathies. ARVO Meeting Abstr. 2011;52:4268.
17. Holland GN. Standard diagnostic criteria for the acute retinal necrosis syndrome. Executive Committee of the American Uveitis Society. Am J Ophthalmol. 1994;117:663–7.

18. Tran TH, Rozenberg F, Cassoux N, et al. Polymerase chain reaction analysis of aqueous humour samples in necrotizing retinitis. Br J Ophthalmol. 2003;87:79–83.
19. Gargiulo F, De Francesco MA, Nascimbeni G, et al. Polymerase chain reaction as a rapid diagnostic tool for therapy of acute retinal necrosis. J Med Virol. 2003;69:397–400.
20. De Groot-Mijnes JD, Rothova A, Van Loon AM, et al. Polymerase chain reaction and Goldmann-Witmar coefficient analysis are complementary in the diagnosis of infectious uveitis. Am J Ophthalmol. 2006;141:313–8.
21. Abe T, Tsuchida K, Tamai M. A comparative study of the polymerase chain reaction and local antibody production in acute retinal necrosis and cytomegalovirus syndrome. Graefes Arch Clin Exp Ophthalmol. 1996;234:419–24.
22. Blumenkranz MS, Culbertson WW, Clarkson JG, et al. Treatment of the acute retinal necrosis syndrome with intravenous acyclovir. Ophthalmology. 1986;93:296–300.
23. Duker JS, Blumenkranz MS. Diagnosis and management of the acute retinal necrosis (ARN) syndrome. Surv Ophthalmol. 1991;35:327–43.
24. Morse LS, Mizoguchi M. Diagnosis and management of viral retinitis in the acute retinal necrosis syndrome. Semin Ophthalmol. 1995;10:28–41.
25. Weller S, Blum MR, Doucette M, et al. Pharmacokinetics of the acyclovir pro-drug valaciclovir after escalating single- and multiple-dose administration to normal volunteers. Clin Pharmacol Ther. 1993;54:595–605.
26. Patel P, Ahmed E, Subramanian ML. Intravitreal foscarnet therapy for acyclovir-resistant acute retinal necrosis after herpes simplex encephalitis. Ophthalmic Surg Lasers Imaging. 2010;9:1–3.
27. King J, Chung M, DiLoreto Jr DA. A 9 year-old girl with herpes simplex virus type 2 acute retinal necrosis treated with intravitreal foscarnet. Ocul Immunol Inflamm. 2007;15:395–8.
28. Wong R, Pavesio CE, Laidlaw DA, et al. Acute retinal necrosis: the effects of intravitreal foscarnet and virus type on outcome. Ophthalmology. 2010;117:556–60.
29. Kappel PJ, Charonis AC, Holland GN, et al. Outcomes associated with ganciclovir implants in patients with AIDS-related cytomegalovirus retinitis. Ophthalmology. 2006;113:683e1–8.
30. Martin DF, Dunn JP, Davis JL, et al. Use of the ganciclovir implant for the treatment of cytomegalovirus retinitis in the era of potent antiretroviral therapy: recommendations of the International AIDS Society-USA panel. Am J Ophthalmol. 1999;127:329–39.
31. Kawaguchi T, Spencer DB, Mochizuki M. Therapy for acute retinal necrosis. Semin Ophthalmol. 2008;23:285–90.
32. Wong RW, Jumper JM, McDonald HR, Johnson RN, Fu A, Lujan BJ, Cunningham Jr ET. Emerging concepts in the management of acute retinal necrosis. Br J Ophthalmol. 2013;97:545–52.
33. Park JJ, Pavesio C. Prophylactic laser photocoagulation for acute retinal necrosis. Does it raise more questions than answers? Br J Ophthalmol. 2008;92:1161–2.
34. Lau CH, Missotten T, Salzmann J, et al. Acute retinal necrosis features, management, and outcomes. Ophthalmology. 2007;114:756–62.
35. Han DP, Lewis H, Williams GA, et al. Laser photocoagulation in the acute retinal necrosis syndrome. Arch Ophthalmol. 1987;105:1051–4.
36. Sternberg Jr P, Han DP, Yeo JH, et al. Photocoagulation to prevent retinal detachment in acute retinal necrosis. Ophthalmology. 1988;95:1389–93.
37. Clarkson JG, Blumenkranz MS, Culbertson WW, et al. Retinal detachment following the acute retinal necrosis syndrome. Ophthalmology. 1984;91:1665–8.
38. Blumenkranz M, Clarkson J, Culbertson WW, et al. Visual results and complications after retinal reattachment in the acute retinal necrosis syndrome. The influence of operative technique. Retina. 1989;9:170–4.
39. McDonald HR, Lewis H, Kreiger AE, et al. Surgical management of retinal detachment associated with the acute retinal necrosis syndrome. Br J Ophthalmol. 1991;75:455–8.
40. Ahmadieh H, Soheilian M, Azarmina M, et al. Surgical management of retinal detachment secondary to acute retinal necrosis: clinical features, surgical techniques, and long-term results. Jpn J Ophthalmol. 2003;47:484–91.
41. Hillenkamp J, Nolle B, Bruns C, et al. Acute retinal necrosis: clinical features, early vitrectomy, and outcomes. Ophthalmology. 2009;116:1971–75e2.
42. Ishida T, Sugamoto Y, Sugita S, et al. Prophylactic vitrectomy for acute retinal necrosis. Jpn J Ophthalmol. 2009;53:486–9.

Infections of the Posterior Segment: Cytomegalovirus Retinitis

14

Marwan A. Abouammoh, Hani S. Al-Mezaine, and Ahmed M. Abu El-Asrar

14.1 Introduction

Cytomegalovirus is an omnipresent human virus of the *Herpesviridae* family. It is known to cause cytomegalovirus (CMV) retinitis which is an opportunistic ocular infection affecting immunosuppressed individuals, as seen in acquired immune deficiency syndrome (AIDS), or those with induced immunosuppression – by means of chemotherapy and immune modulators. This infection was common before the introduction of highly active antiretroviral therapy (HAART). But despite the decrease in incidence, it remains relatively important [1].

14.2 Epidemiology

CMV is a widely spread virus. A recent epidemiological study in the United States showed an overall age-adjusted CMV seroprevalence of 50.4 % [2]. CMV seroprevalence was higher in low socioeconomic groups, females, older age, and foreign birthplace [2]. Residents of developing countries have also higher CMV seroprevalence reaching up to 97 % [3, 4]. This virus is usually acquired via placental spread, breast-feeding, sexual contact, organ and bone marrow transplant, and blood transfusions. In healthy infected individuals, the virus remains quiescent until activation occurs by compromising or suppressing the immune system. Once immunity is suppressed, systemic infections of the lungs, central nervous system, gastrointestinal tract, and retina occur [1].

CMV retinitis occurs in 25–42 % of all patients who develop AIDS when $CD4^+$ T cell count is less than 50 cells/mm^3 [5–7]. These rates have decreased significantly in the HAART era [8, 9]. CMV retinitis was associated with higher mortality among AIDS patients prior to the introduction of HAART [10–12]. For those presumed to be on HAART, at least 20 % continue to be at risk of CMV retinitis due to poor response to HAART, do not tolerate the regimen, or are noncompliant [13, 14]. Patients on HAART who still develop CMV retinitis and have a detectable CMV viral load still have an increased risk of mortality [15].

In addition, CMV retinitis may still occur after reconstitution of $CD4^+$ T cell count to more than 500 cells/mm^3, which means there are other factors that might influence disease development, and continuous monitoring for such patients is needed [16].

14.3 Clinical Features

In early CMV retinitis with small peripheral retinal lesions, the disease may be asymptomatic or with minimal visual symptoms. The most common

M.A. Abouammoh, MD (✉) • H.S. Al-Mezaine, MD
A.M. Abu El-Asrar, MD, PhD
Department of Ophthalmology,
College of Medicine, King Saud University,
KAUH, Old Airport Road, 245,
Riyadh 11411, Saudi Arabia
e-mail: mabouammoh@ksu.edu.sa;
halmezaine@ksu.edu.sa; abuasrar@ksu.edu.sa

K. Tabbara et al. (eds.), *Ocular Infections*, Essentials in Ophthalmology,
DOI 10.1007/978-3-662-43981-4_14, © Springer-Verlag Berlin Heidelberg 2014

presenting symptoms were blurred vision, floaters, photopsia, and eye pain [17]. Floaters and photopsia were found to be significant predictors of CMV retinitis [18]. A recent study of 494 eyes in AIDS patients with CMV retinitis, 29 % had a visual acuity of 20/50 at the time of diagnosis and 15 % had 20/200 or worse [19]. A more recent study of 476 patients with AIDS and CMV retinitis and visual field data has shown that despite a six-fold reduction of incident visual field loss compared to the pre-HAART era, CMV retinitis still carries considerable risk of visual field loss [20]. Slit lamp examination of the anterior segment will usually reveal a white and quiet eye. Mild anterior chamber reaction and fine keratic precipitates may be seen. Vitreous reaction is typically negligible. Fundoscopic exam may show small white retinal infiltrates. These may resemble cotton wool spots and might be mistaken for HIV microangiopathy. Thus large – over 750 μm – cotton wool spots should be suspected as CMV retinitis.

Optic neuritis can occur in up to 4 % of patients with CMV retinitis. This occurs either through spread from adjacent retina or primary involvement of the optic nerve [21, 22]. It can lead to rapid irreversible visual loss, but early recognition and treatment has a better prognosis. CMV papillitis does not carry a worse prognosis for survival than CMV retinitis alone [21].

There are two characteristic clinical variants of CMV retinitis that have been described: (1) A fulminant edematous type, characterized by confluent areas of retinal whitening and marked edema that is usually accompanied with mild to moderate hemorrhagic necrotizing retinitis and vascular sheathing (Fig. 14.1) [23]. It has a slow persistent "brush fire"-like extension along the course of retinal vessels. (2) The second is the granular indolent type, more commonly starting in the retinal periphery as oval or round lesions surrounded by a granular border of punctate white lesions. This type is characterized by less retinal edema, fewer or no hemorrhages, and no vascular sheathing [24]. In selected patients, a perivascular CMV retinitis where vascular sheathing is the prominent finding can give an appearance similar to frosted branch angiitis (Fig. 14.2) [25].

This classification is somewhat abstruse as it is often seen when examining CMV retinitis patients in that they can harbor all these clinical forms concurrently.

Retinopathy lesion are generally plottes in one or more of three zones [26]. Zone 1 is the area within 1,500 mm of the optic nerve or 3,000 mm of the fovea. Zone 2 extends to the equator defined by ampullae vortex veins, and Zone 3 consists of the remaining anterior retina.

The median rate of progression for the retinal lesions towards the fovea without therapy is usu-

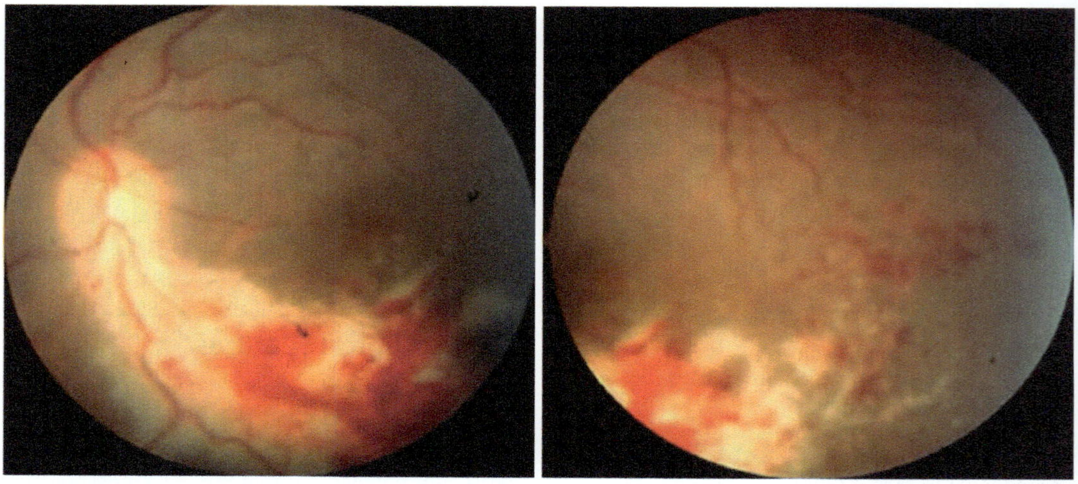

Fig. 14.1 Fulminant CMV retinitis

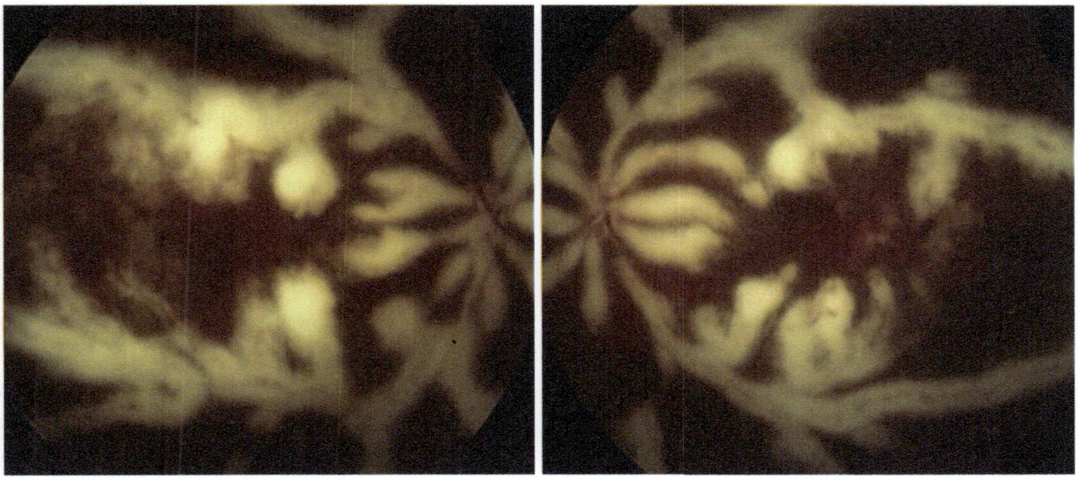

Fig. 14.2 Frosted branch angiitis due to perivascular CMV retinitis (Courtesy of Nicholas Jones)

ally slow at around 24 µm/day. Those on anti-CMV treatment have a therapeutic benefit with a median progression rate of 11.5 µm/day [27]. Due to the apparently slow evolution of retinal lesions, serial photographs are much more sensitive than fundoscopy or fundus drawings for the detection of relapsing CMV retinitis [1].

14.4 Diagnosis

CMV retinitis is diagnosed on the basis of clinical examination that reveals typical ophthalmoscopic findings in immunocompromised patients. Seropositivity is of no big value as it can be detected in the majority of normal individuals. Nevertheless, documented rising CMV DNA blood levels appear to be associated with active CMV retinitis in individuals with low $CD4^+$ T cell count [28]. In patients with active retinitis, there was a strong association between high tear levels of anti-CMV antibodies and active ocular infection [29]. PCR-based analysis of ocular fluids is of high sensitivity and specificity to aid in diagnosing critical cases to differentiate CMV from other causes of necrotizing retinitis like herpes viruses and toxoplasma retinochoroiditis in immunocompromised patients [30]. This is of utmost importance in patients who are not responsive to treatment, or in those with atypical lesions.

The differential diagnoses of CMV retinitis include those of cotton wool spots (CWS) in the early stage of the disease. In later disease, acute retinal necrosis (ARN) and progressive outer retinal necrosis (PORN) due to HSV or VZV, toxoplasma retinochoroiditis, syphilitic necrotizing retinitis, fungal infections, and intraocular lymphoma should be differentiated from CMV retinitis.

14.5 Treatment

Successful treatment of CMV retinitis requires both anti-CMV therapy and HAART. Therefore collaborating with the treating physician is a must in order to tailor the treatment plan as to get the most favorable response to anti-CMV therapy [31–33].

14.5.1 Ganciclovir

This is a virostatic antiviral agent that selectively inhibits CMV DNA polymerase. Due to its poor oral bioavailability, it is usually administered intravenously. Induction dose is 5–7.5 mg/kg twice daily for 2–4 weeks followed by 5 mg/kg/day for 5 days per week as a maintenance dose. Intravitreal route is an alternative means of delivery. Intravitreal injections are given at a dose of

200–2,000 mg/0.1 ml twice a week for 2–4 weeks as an induction dose. This is followed by a weekly injection as maintenance. The intravitreal implants – a polymer-based depot – provide a higher effective concentration at the site of action probably due to slow constant release of ganciclovir for up to 8 months and are exchangeable if empty or if infection recurs [34].

Intravitreal ganciclovir may be effective in cases of previously failed intravenous therapy to avoid serious systemic disadvantages and toxicity especially bone marrow suppression [35].

Valganciclovir is a prodrug of ganciclovir with better bioavailability after oral administration. Its effect and toxicity are similar to ganciclovir [36, 37]. The induction dose is 900 mg twice a day for 3 weeks followed by maintenance dose of 900 mg once a day [38].

14.5.2 Foscarnet

Foscarnet is a virostatic agent that inhibits CMV DNA polymerase. Due to its antiretroviral activity however, it results in decreased mortality when compared to ganciclovir [10]. Nevertheless, it is less tolerated by patients and highly nephrotoxic, but renal functions can revert to normal upon drug cessation [39].

Induction dose is 90 mg/kg intravenously twice a day for 2–3 weeks followed by 90–129 mg/kg once daily for maintenance. Intravitreal injections as an alternative can be given at a dose of 2.4 mg/0.1 ml twice a week for 2–3 weeks followed by maintenance injection once a week.

Foscarnet is usually used in ganciclovir-resistant cases [40]. In addition, combined therapy with both antiviral agents has been shown to decrease resistance [41].

14.5.3 Cidofovir

This drug suppresses viral replication by selectively inhibiting CMV DNA polymerase. Due to its toxic effects, it is administered along with probenecid and intravenous hydration. It may also cause severe anterior uveitis and inflammation leading to hypotony [42].

Induction dose is 5 mg/kg intravenous infusion given once weekly for 2 weeks, then every 2 weeks as a maintenance dose. Intravireal injections can be used to avoid systemic toxicity at a dose of 15–20 microgram (μg) every 6 weeks [43].

14.5.4 Fomivirsen

Fomivirsen binds the complementary sequence of mRNA and thus inhibits CMV replication [44]. It is only available as an intravitreal injection at a dose of 330 μg/week for 2 weeks as an induction regimen followed by the same dose every 4 weeks for maintenance. Side effects include anterior uveitis, vitritis, high intraocular pressure, retinal pigment epitheliopathy, and an increased risk of retinal detachment [45, 46].

Regardless of the antiviral agent, both intravitreal implants and injections are relatively safe in comparison to intravenous antiviral therapy. A recent study has shown that intravenous anti-CMV therapy seems to provide more benefits in terms of longer survival and decreased CMV dissemination. In addition, intraocular therapy had greater rates of retinitis progression and greater visual field loss. Hematologic and renal side effects were similar between systemic and intraocular anti-CMV therapy [47].

14.6 Complications

Rhegmatogenous retinal detachment is a serious complication of CMV retinitis occurring in 11–35 % of eyes [48, 49]. Such complication occurs due to necrotic breaks at the junction of healed retinitis and normal retina [50]. These breaks are usually multiple, irregular, and anterior in location which makes it difficult to visualize and increase the risk for retinal detachment [51].

The treatment of choice for rhegmatogenous retinal detachments associated with CMV retinitis is pars plana vitrectomy with silicone oil tamponade [52]. Relatively low redetachment rates have been shown after silicone oil removal [50, 53].

Prophylactic argon laser has been shown to reduce the risk of subsequent retinal detachments in patients treated medically for CMV retinitis [54].

Another recently described complication is immune reactivity uveitis (IRU). First described by Zegans and Karavellas [55, 56], this severe vitreous and anterior chamber inflammation is believed to occur in AIDS or immunocompromised patients with CMV retinitis who recover their immunity with HAART therapy. The postulated mechanism of IRU is believed to be due to immune reaction against CMV antigens [57–59]. Patients with IRU complain of blurred, decreased, or foggy vision and floaters. IRU can cause complications such as epiretinal membranes, cystoid macular edema, or vitreomacular traction [55, 60, 61]. The most common effective treatment for IRU is corticosteroids [62, 63]. Although continuing anti-CMV agents after immune reconstitution is not protective, it has been shown that aggressive anti-CMV administration before and early after starting HAART reduces incidence of IRU [55, 58, 60].

14.7 Prognosis

Although HAART has improved outcomes in CMV retinitis as compared to the pre-HAART era, a recent long-term study showed that AIDS patients with CMV retinitis are still at a high risk for mortality, retinitis progression, complications of the retinitis, and visual loss over a 5-year period [64]. Nevertheless, stopping anti-CMV agents after immune reconstitution did not increase possibility of poor outcome [15, 65].

14.8 Prevention

Before the advent of HAART, recommendations for ophthalmic screening in AIDS patients to rule out CMV retinitis were based on the $CD4^+$ T cell count: yearly screens in patients with a $CD4^+$ T cell count of >100 cells/ml, biannually for those with a $CD4^+$ T cell count ranging from 50 to 100 cells/ml, and every 3 months for those with <50 cells/ml [1, 18, 31]. Those at high risk can receive oral ganciclovir 1,000 mg three times daily and valaciclovir 2,000 mg four times a day as it will significantly reduce the risk of developing CMV disease, including CMV retinitis [66, 67]. This prophylaxis is not used in HIV-infected individuals who achieve immune reconstitution with HAART. Furthermore, patients with previous CMV retinitis should be examined regularly after immune reconstitution [68].

Compliance with Ethical Requirements

Conflict of Interest The authors declare that they have no conflict of interest.

Informed Consent No human studies were carried out by the authors for this article.

Animal Studies No animal studies were carried out by the authors for this article.

References

1. Wiegand TW, Young LHY. Cytomegalovirus retinitis. Int Ophthalmol Clin. 2006;46:91–110.
2. Bate SL, Dollard SC, Cannon MJ. Cytomegalovirus seroprevalence in the United States: the national health and nutrition examination surveys, 1988–2004. Clin Infect Dis. 2010;50:1439–47.
3. Ahmed SA, et al. The prevalence of human cytomegalovirus seropositivity among blood donors at the Unit of Blood Transfusion Medicine. Hospital Universiti Sains Malaysia. Southeast Asian J Trop Med Public Health. 2006;37:294–6.
4. Tabatabaee M, Tayyebi D. Seroepidemiologic study of human cytomegalovirus in pregnant women in Valiasr Hospital of Kazeroon, Fars, Iran. J Matern Fetal Neonatal Med. 2009;22:517–21.
5. Hoover DR, et al. Occurrence of cytomegalovirus retinitis after human immunodeficiency virus immunosuppression. Arch Ophthalmol. 1996;114:821–7.
6. Montaner JS, et al. The changing spectrum of AIDS index diseases in Canada. AIDS. 1994;8:693–6.
7. Pertel P, et al. Risk of developing cytomegalovirus retinitis in persons infected with the human immunodeficiency virus. J Acquir Immune Defic Syndr. 1992;5:1069–74.
8. Sugar EA, et al. Incidence of cytomegalovirus retinitis in the era of highly active antiretroviral therapy. Am J Ophthalmol. 2012;153:1016–24.e5.
9. Harooni M, Lashkari K, Freilich JM, Schepens CL. Cytomegalovirus retinitis. Int Ophthalmol Clin. 1996;36:131–40.

10. Mortality in patients with the acquired immunodeficiency syndrome treated with either foscarnet or ganciclovir for cytomegalovirus retinitis. Studies of Ocular Complications of AIDS Research Group, in collaboration with the AIDS Clinical Trials Group. N Engl J Med 1992;326:213–20.
11. Bowen EF, Griffiths PD, Davey CC, Emery VC, Johnson MA. Lessons from the natural history of cytomegalovirus. AIDS. 1996;10 Suppl 1:S37–41.
12. Gallant JE, Moore RD, Richman DD, Keruly J, Chaisson RE. Incidence and natural history of cytomegalovirus disease in patients with advanced human immunodeficiency virus disease treated with zidovudine. The Zidovudine Epidemiology Study Group. J Infect Dis. 1992;166:1223–7.
13. Lewis JS, Terriff CM, Coulston DR, Garrison MW. Protease inhibitors: a therapeutic breakthrough for the treatment of patients with human immunodeficiency virus. Clin Ther. 1997;19:187–214.
14. Le Moing V, et al. Predictors of long-term increase in CD4(+) cell counts in human immunodeficiency virus-infected patients receiving a protease inhibitor-containing antiretroviral regimen. J Infect Dis. 2002;185:471–80.
15. Jabs DA, et al. Risk factors for mortality in patients with AIDS in the era of highly active antiretroviral therapy. Ophthalmology. 2005;112:771–9.
16. Barrett L, Walmsley S. CMV retinopathy in the antiretroviral therapy era: prevention, diagnosis, and management. Curr Infect Dis Rep. 2012;14:435–44.
17. Wei LL, Park SS, Skiest DJ. Prevalence of visual symptoms among patients with newly diagnosed cytomegalovirus retinitis. Retina. 2002;22:278–82.
18. Hodge WG, et al. Clinical risk factors for cytomegalovirus retinitis in patients with AIDS. Ophthalmology. 2004;111:1326–33.
19. Thorne JE, et al. Incidence of and risk factors for visual acuity loss among patients with AIDS and cytomegalovirus retinitis in the era of highly active antiretroviral therapy. Ophthalmology. 2006;113:1432–40.
20. Thorne JE, Van Natta ML, Jabs DA, Duncan JL, Srivastava SK. Visual field loss in patients with cytomegalovirus retinitis. Ophthalmology. 2011;118:895–901.
21. Mansour AM. Cytomegalovirus optic neuritis. Curr Opin Ophthalmol. 1997;8:55–8.
22. Patel SS, et al. Cytomegalovirus papillitis in patients with acquired immune deficiency syndrome. Visual prognosis of patients treated with ganciclovir and/or foscarnet. Ophthalmology. 1996;103:1476–82.
23. Foscarnet-Ganciclovir Cytomegalovirus Retinitis Trial: 5. Clinical features of cytomegalovirus retinitis at diagnosis. Studies of ocular complications of AIDS Research Group in collaboration with the AIDS Clinical Trials Group. Am J Ophthalmol 1997;124:141–57.
24. Henderly DE, Freeman WR, Causey DM, Rao NA. Cytomegalovirus retinitis and response to therapy with ganciclovir. Ophthalmology. 1987;94:425–34.
25. Spaide RF, Vitale AT, Toth IR, Oliver JM. Frosted branch angiitis associated with cytomegalovirus retinitis. Am J Ophthalmol. 1992;113:522–8.
26. Holland GN, Buhles WC, Mastre B, Kaplan HJ. A controlled retrospective study of ganciclovir treatment for cytomegalovirus retinopathy. Use of a standardized system for the assessment of disease outcome. UCLA CMV Retinopathy. Study Group. Arch Ophthalmol. 1989;107:1759–66.
27. Holland GN, Shuler JD. Progression rates of cytomegalovirus retinopathy in ganciclovir-treated and untreated patients. Arch Ophthalmol. 1992;110:1435–42.
28. Tufail A, et al. Quantitative cytomegalovirus DNA level in the blood and its relationship to cytomegalovirus retinitis in patients with acquired immune deficiency syndrome. Ophthalmology. 1999;106:133–41.
29. Rozanova EB, Teplinskaia LE, Kaliberdina AF, Barisani-Asenbauer T. Cytomegalovirus antibodies in tear fluid of patients with retinitis. Arch Virol. 2006;151:2407–17.
30. McCann JD, et al. A sensitive and specific polymerase chain reaction-based assay for the diagnosis of cytomegalovirus retinitis. Am J Ophthalmol. 1995;120:219–26.
31. Dunn JP. Cessation of anti-CMV therapy in patients with CMV retinitis. Hopkins HIV Rep. 1998;10:11.
32. Kedhar SR, Jabs DA. Cytomegalovirus retinitis in the era of highly active antiretroviral therapy. Herpes. 2007;14:66–71.
33. Kempen JH. Medical management of human immunodeficiency virus infection. Indian J Ophthalmol. 2008;56:385–90.
34. Martin DF, et al. Ganciclovir implant exchange. Timing, surgical procedure, and complications. Arch Ophthalmol. 1997;115:1389–94.
35. Hatton MP, Duker JS, Reichel E, Morley MG, Puliafito CA. Treatment of relapsed cytomegalovirus retinitis with the sustained-release ganciclovir implant. Retina. 1998;18:50–5.
36. Lalezari J, et al. A safety study of oral valganciclovir maintenance treatment of cytomegalovirus retinitis. J Acquir Immune Defic Syndr. 2002;30:392–400.
37. Martin DF, et al. A controlled trial of valganciclovir as induction therapy for cytomegalovirus retinitis. N Engl J Med. 2002;346:1119–26.
38. Segarra-Newnham M, Salazar MI. Valganciclovir: a new oral alternative for cytomegalovirus retinitis in human immunodeficiency virus-seropositive individuals. Pharmacotherapy. 2002;22:1124–8.
39. Morbidity and toxic effects associated with ganciclovir or foscarnet therapy in a randomized cytomegalovirus retinitis trial. Studies of ocular complications of AIDS Research Group, in collaboration with the AIDS Clinical Trials Group. Arch Intern Med 1995;155:65–74.
40. Ohta H, et al. Foscarnet therapy for ganciclovir-resistant cytomegalovirus retinitis after stem cell transplantation: effective monitoring of CMV infection by quantitative analysis of CMV mRNA. Bone Marrow Transplant. 2001;27:1141–5.
41. Bacigalupo A, et al. Combined foscarnet-ganciclovir treatment for cytomegalovirus infections after

allogeneic hemopoietic stem cell transplantation. Transplantation. 1996;62:376–80.
42. Akler ME, Johnson DW, Burman WJ, Johnson SC. Anterior uveitis and hypotony after intravenous cidofovir for the treatment of cytomegalovirus retinitis. Ophthalmology. 1998;105:651–7.
43. Kirsch LS, et al. Intravitreal cidofovir (HPMPC) treatment of cytomegalovirus retinitis in patients with acquired immune deficiency syndrome. Ophthalmology. 1995;102:533–42. discussion 542–3.
44. Detrick B, et al. Inhibition of human cytomegalovirus replication in a human retinal epithelial cell model by antisense oligonucleotides. Invest Ophthalmol Vis Sci. 2001;42:163–9.
45. Stone TW, Jaffe GJ. Reversible bull's-eye maculopathy associated with intravitreal fomivirsen therapy for cytomegalovirus retinitis. Am J Ophthalmol. 2000;130:242–3.
46. Vitravene Study Group. Safety of intravitreous fomivirsen for treatment of cytomegalovirus retinitis in patients with AIDS. Am J Ophthalmol. 2002;133:484–98.
47. Jabs DA, Ahuja A, Van Natta M, Dunn JP, Yeh S. Comparison of treatment regimens for cytomegalovirus retinitis in patients with AIDS in the era of highly active antiretroviral therapy. Ophthalmology. 2013. doi:10.1016/j.ophtha.2012.11.023.
48. Freeman WR, et al. Risk factors for development of rhegmatogenous retinal detachment in patients with cytomegalovirus retinitis. Am J Ophthalmol. 1993; 116:713–20.
49. Sandy CJ, et al. Retinal detachment in AIDS-related cytomegalovirus retinitis. Eye (Lond). 1995;9(Pt 3):277–81.
50. Dave VP, Mathai A, Pappuru RR. Results of silicone oil removal in post-cytomegalovirus retinitis-related retinal detachment. J Ophthalmic Inflamm Infect. 2012;2:153–5.
51. Jabs DA, Enger C, Haller J, De Bustros S. Retinal detachments in patients with cytomegalovirus retinitis. Arch Ophthalmol. 1991;109:794–9.
52. Irvine AR, et al. Retinal detachment in AIDS: long-term results after repair with silicone oil. Br J Ophthalmol. 1997;81:180–3.
53. Morrison VL, Labree LD, Azen SP, Goldberg DE, Freeman WR. Results of silicone oil removal in patients with cytomegalovirus retinitis related retinal detachments. Am J Ophthalmol. 2005;140:786–93.
54. Althaus C, Loeffler KU, Schimkat M, Hudde T, Sundmacher R. Prophylactic argon laser coagulation for rhegmatogenous retinal detachment in AIDS patients with cytomegalovirus retinitis. Graefes Arch Clin Exp Ophthalmol. 1998;236:359–64.
55. Karavellas MP, Song M, Macdonald JC, Freeman WR. Long-term posterior and anterior segment complications of immune recovery uveitis associated with cytomegalovirus retinitis. Am J Ophthalmol. 2000; 130:57–64.
56. Zegans ME, et al. Transient vitreous inflammatory reactions associated with combination antiretroviral therapy in patients with AIDS and cytomegalovirus retinitis. Am J Ophthalmol. 1998;125:292–300.
57. Holland GN. Immune recovery uveitis. Ocul Immunol Inflamm. 1999;7:215–21.
58. Kuppermann BD, Holland GN. Immune recovery uveitis. Am J Ophthalmol. 2000;130:103–6.
59. Nussenblatt RB, Lane HC. Human immunodeficiency virus disease: changing patterns of intraocular inflammation. Am J Ophthalmol. 1998;125: 374–82.
60. Nguyen QD, Kempen JH, Bolton SG, Dunn JP, Jabs DA. Immune recovery uveitis in patients with AIDS and cytomegalovirus retinitis after highly active antiretroviral therapy. Am J Ophthalmol. 2000;129: 634–9.
61. Canzano JC, Reed JB, Morse LS. Vitreomacular traction syndrome following highly active antiretroviral therapy in AIDS patients with cytomegalovirus retinitis. Retina. 1998;18:443–7.
62. Hu J, Coassin M, Stewart JM. Fluocinolone acetonide implant (Retisert) for chronic cystoid macular edema in two patients with AIDS and a history of cytomegalovirus retinitis. Ocul Immunol Inflamm. 2011;19:206–9.
63. Morrison VL, et al. Intravitreal triamcinolone acetonide for the treatment of immune recovery uveitis macular edema. Ophthalmology. 2007;114:334–9.
64. Jabs DA, et al. Course of cytomegalovirus retinitis in the era of highly active antiretroviral therapy: five-year outcomes. Ophthalmology. 2010;117:2152–61. e1–2.
65. Holbrook JT, et al. Evaluation of the United States public health service guidelines for discontinuation of anticytomegalovirus therapy after immune recovery in patients with cytomegalovirus retinitis. Am J Ophthalmol. 2011;152:628–37.e1.
66. Spector SA, et al. Oral ganciclovir for the prevention of cytomegalovirus disease in persons with AIDS. Roche Cooperative Oral Ganciclovir Study Group. N Engl J Med. 1996;334:1491–7.
67. Feinberg JE, et al. A randomized, double-blind trial of valaciclovir prophylaxis for cytomegalovirus disease in patients with advanced human immunodeficiency virus infection. AIDS Clinical Trials Group Protocol 204/Glaxo Wellcome 123–014 International CMV Prophylaxis Study G. J Infect Dis. 1998;177:48–56.
68. Jabs DA, et al. Course of cytomegalovirus retinitis in the era of highly active antiretroviral therapy: 1. Retinitis progression. Ophthalmology. 2004;111:2224–31.

Emergent Ocular Infections

15

Moncef Khairallah, Salim Ben Yahia,
and Sana Khochtali

15.1 Introduction

Arthropod vector-borne diseases are among the most important emergent and resurgent infections that are mostly prevalent in tropical and subtropical areas, tending to expand worldwide, mainly due to climate changes and globalization. They are caused by viruses, bacteria, and parasites and are transmitted by the bite of hematophagous arthropods, mainly ticks and mosquitoes. Most vector-borne diseases are subclinical or manifest as a mild febrile illness, but a severe, potentially lethal systemic involvement also can occur. Specific viral and bacterial arthropod vector-borne diseases including West Nile virus (WNV) infection, Rift Valley fever (RVF), dengue fever (DF), Chikungunya, and rickettsioses have been recently associated with uveitis and other ocular manifestations [1–3].

M. Khairallah, MD (✉) • S. Ben Yahia, MD
S. Khochtali, MD
Department of Ophthalmology, Fattouma Bourguiba University Hospital, Monastir, Tunisia

Faculty of Medicine, University of Monastir, Monastir, Tunisia
e-mail: moncef.khairallah@rns.tn

15.2 West Nile Virus Infection

15.2.1 Introduction

WNV is a single-stranded RNA virus belonging to the genus *Flavivirus*, family *Flaviviridae*. It is a member of the Japanese encephalitis serocomplex [4]. Wild birds are the primary natural hosts, and virus is transmitted between birds by the bite of mosquitoes (primarily the Culex species) which may pass the virus to humans and other mammals. Less common modes of transmission include blood transfusion, organ transplantation, transplacental transmission, laboratory transmission, and breast feeding [5, 6].

The virus has been first identified in the West Nile District of Uganda in 1937. It is widely distributed in Africa, Europe, Australia, and Asia, and since its appearance in New York City in 1999, it has spread rapidly throughout the Western hemisphere, including the USA, Canada, Mexico, and the Caribbean and into parts of Central and South America. The disease, which causes both sporadic infection and outbreaks, may occur anytime between July and December, with a peak onset in late summer [4, 6].

The WNV infection is often asymptomatic, but systemic disease may vary from mild febrile illness to very severe neurologic disease. Ocular involvement has been recently characterized, and a typical multifocal chorioretinitis was highlighted as the most common manifestation [5, 7–26].

K. Tabbara et al. (eds.), *Ocular Infections*, Essentials in Ophthalmology,
DOI 10.1007/978-3-662-43981-4_15, © Springer-Verlag Berlin Heidelberg 2014

15.2.2 Clinical Symptoms and Signs

15.2.2.1 Systemic Disease

The incubation period for WNV infection ranges from 3 to 14 days. Human infections are often asymptomatic. Only approximately 20 % of infected persons develop symptoms, with a self-limiting flu-like syndrome in most cases [4, 5]. Severe neurologic disease may develop in less than 1 % of cases [6]. WNV infection neurologic manifestations mainly include meningitis, encephalitis, and poliomyelitis-like disease. Findings in encephalitis and/or meningitis typically include a headache of rapid onset, photophobia, back pain, confusion, and continued fever. Asymmetric paralysis of acute onset and absence of reflexes without pain are characteristic of WNV poliomyelitis-like syndrome [6]. Neuroinvasive disease is associated with high rates of morbidity and mortality, especially in patients with advanced age or diabetes [6].

15.2.2.2 Ocular Disease

A bilateral or rarely unilateral multifocal chorioretinitis is the most common ocular manifestation of WNV infection, occurring in almost 80 % of patients with acute WNV infection associated with neurologic illness [11]. Most patients are above 50 years in age, suffer from diabetes mellitus, and have no ocular symptoms or present with mildly reduced vision or floaters [5, 11, 15]. Active chorioretinal lesions appear as circular, deep, yellowish lesions on ophthalmoscopy, showing early hypofluorescence and late staining on fluorescein angiography (FA). Inactive chorioretinal lesions present in the form of round atrophic lesions with or without central pigmentation (Fig. 15.1a), and they usually exhibit a typical "targetlike appearance" on FA: central hypofluorescence and peripheral hyperfluorescence (Fig. 15.1b) [5, 11].

Chorioretinal lesions may vary in number and size, involving the midperiphery, with or without associated posterior pole involvement [5]. Linear clustering of chorioretinal lesions is a prominent feature of WNV-associated chorioretinitis. Streaks are oriented radially in the nasal and peripheral fundus and in a curvilinear pattern in the temporal posterior fundus. The linear pattern of chorioretinitis follows the course of retinal nerve fibers, suggesting a contiguous spread of central nervous system disease [27]. Indocyanine green (ICG) angiography reveals well-delineated hypofluorescent choroidal lesions, which are more numerous than those appreciated by FA or clinically [28].

A case of reactivation of WNV infection-related chorioretinitis has been recently reported,

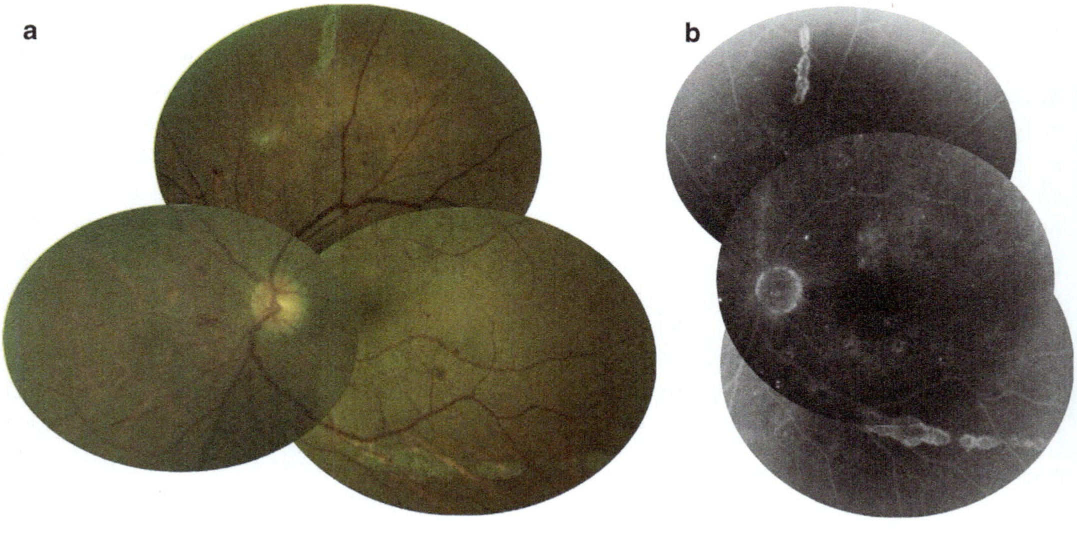

Fig. 15.1 (**a**) Color fundus photograph of the left eye of a diabetic patient with West Nile virus infection shows inactive multifocal chorioretinitis with a linear clustering of chorioretinal lesions. (**b**) Fluorescein angiogram of the same eye shows central hypofluorescence and peripheral hyperfluorescence of chorioretinal lesions, arranged in linear/curvilinear streaks. There are also features of nonproliferative diabetic retinopathy

with appearance of new active lesions exhibiting a typical pattern almost 1 year after the initial diagnosis was made [29].

Although multifocal chorioretinitis is the most common ocular manifestation of WNV infection, other findings can occur including anterior uveitis, retinal vasculitis, which may be occlusive in nature, retinitis, segmental zones of atrophy and mottling of the retinal pigment epithelium, optic nerve involvement, ocular nerve palsy, nystagmus, and congenital chorioretinal scarring [5, 7–26].

WNV-associated ocular disease usually has a self-limited course, and visual acuity returns to baseline in most patients. However, persistent visual impairment can occur due to a foveal chorioretinal scar, choroidal neovascularization, vitreous hemorrhage secondary to retinal neovascularization, severe ischemic maculopathy, macular edema, optic atrophy, or retrogeniculate damage [5, 14–16, 18–21, 25].

15.2.3 Laboratory Diagnosis

Antibody-capture enzyme-linked immunosorbent assay (MAC-ELISA) for the detection of WNV-specific IgM antibody in serum and/or cerebrospinal fluid is a very sensitive diagnostic method. Almost all patients have detectable IgM antibodies by 7–8 days after the onset of the disease, whereas WNV-specific serum IgG antibodies are detectable only by 3 weeks after the infection. The plaque-reduction neutralization test can help distinguish false-positive results of MAC-ELISA or other assays, and serologic cross-reactions among the flaviviruses. A fourfold or greater increase serum antibody titer in serum samples collected 2–3 weeks apart may be used to confirm the diagnosis of WNV infection, as IgM may persist in the serum for more than a year [30].

Furthermore, detection of viral nucleic acid by real-time reverse transcription polymerase chain reaction (RT-PCR) is highly specific for WNV infection, but it is less sensitive than serology. PCR test is mostly used in the screening of blood products. Viremia often lasts for several days and the virus itself is usually no longer detectable in the serum by the time WNV-specific serum IgM appears [4, 30].

15.2.4 Management

There is currently no effective treatment for WNV infection. In cases of severe systemic disease, intensive supportive therapy is indicated, often involving hospitalization, intravenous fluids, respiratory support, prevention of secondary infections, and good nursing care [6]. Antiviral agents such as ribavirin, interferon α 2b and interferon β, and intravenous immunoglobulins have shown to reduce viral replication in vitro or in animal models [6, 31–34]. However, their efficacy is still to be proven in humans.

Prevention remains the mainstay of WNV infection control. Measures to reduce the number of mosquitoes (draining standing water, larvicides) as well as personal protection (repellents, window screens, protective clothing) are recommended [35]. Widespread vaccination of horses in the USA has led to decreasing the incidence of equine infections [6]. Vaccine for human use is still in the research phase.

Specific ophthalmic treatment may be required including topical steroids for anterior uveitis, peripheral scatter retinal photocoagulation for neovascularization secondary to occlusive retinal vasculitis, pars plana vitrectomy for non-clearing vitreous hemorrhage or tractional retinal detachment, and intravitreal injection of anti-VEGF for choroidal neovascularization or macular edema [16, 36].

15.3 Dengue Fever

15.3.1 Introduction

Dengue fever (DF) is caused by any of the four immunologically related serotypes of the dengue virus, which belongs to the genus *Flavivirus* of the family *Flaviviridae*. It is transmitted through the bite of an infected female *Aedes aegypti/albopictus* mosquito. *Aedes albopictus* vector seems to produce a slow-moving outbreak by contrast to the sharp epidemics associated with *Aedes aegypti* [37].

DF is considered to be one of the most important arthropod-borne disease in the tropical and subtropical regions, being endemic in more than 100 countries, including America, Southeast

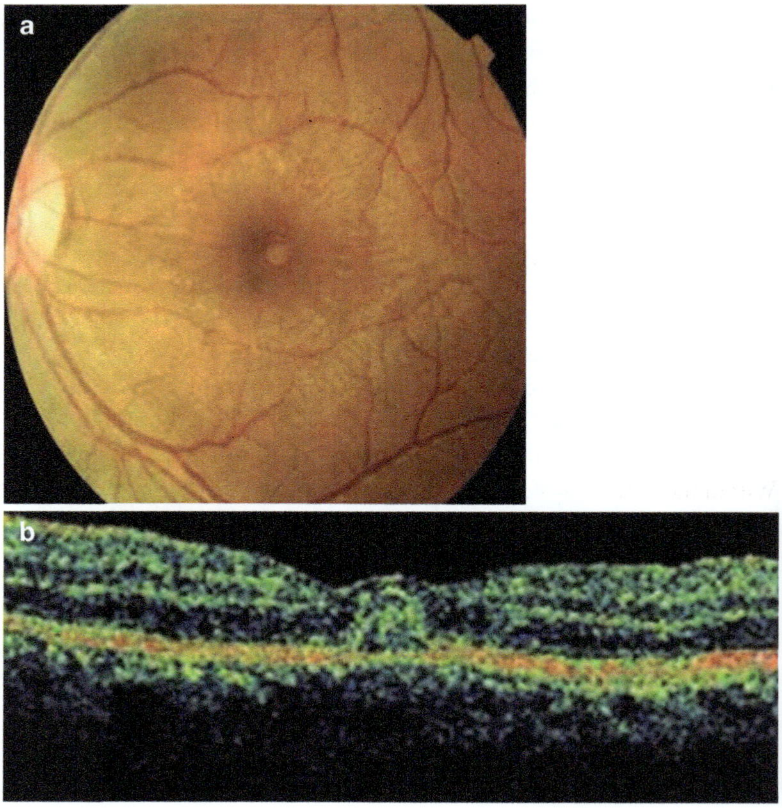

Fig. 15.2 (**a**) Color fundus photograph of the left eye of a patient with dengue fever shows a round yellowish lesion at the foveal center. (**b**) OCT of the same eye reveals a corresponding focal thickening of outer neurosensory retina – retinal pigment epithelium. These findings are consistent with foveolitis (Courtesy, Soon Phaik Chee)

Asia, Western pacific, Africa, and the Eastern Mediterranean [38]. The spectrum of systemic disease may range from mild flulike illness to life-threatening clinical presentations. Ocular involvement was found to occur in 10 % of patients hospitalized for serologically confirmed DF [39–43].

15.3.2 Clinical Symptoms and Signs

15.3.2.1 Systemic Disease

The incubation period for DF varies from 3 to 14 days. The initial infection may be asymptomatic, may result in a nonspecific febrile illness, or may produce features of classic DF including sudden onset of high fever, severe headache, myalgias, arthralgias, nausea, vomiting, and a maculopapular rash. The majority of DF cases are self-limiting. A small proportion of affected patients may develop life-threatening dengue hemorrhagic fever syndrome, which is characterized by increased capillary permeability and hemostatic disturbances, or dengue shock syndrome, which is characterized by severe systemic hypotension. DF is often associated with a bleeding tendency secondary to thrombocytopenia [37, 44].

15.3.2.2 Ocular Disease

The ocular involvement usually occurs within 1 month after the onset of symptoms of DF and is often bilateral. The patients may present with a sudden decrease in vision, a central scotoma, or floaters [45]. A subconjunctival hemorrhage, petechial in type and associated with a platelet count of less than 50.000/µl, was the most common ocular manifestation in an East Indian population with DF [46]. Numerous posterior segment changes have been associated with DF including retinal hemorrhages, retinal vasculitis, yellow subretinal dots, retinal pigment epithelium mottling, and foveolitis, seen clinically as a round yellowish lesion at the fovea with corresponding focal outer neurosensory retina – retinal pigment epithelium thickening on OCT (Fig. 15.2). Other findings include macular edema, serous retinal detachment, retinal vascular occlusion, choroidal changes, optic disk swelling, optic neuritis, and neuroretinitis [1–3, 41, 42, 44, 45, 47–56].

Dengue-associated ocular disease usually has a self-limited course, with a significant improvement of visual acuity in 2–4 weeks. However, persistent visual impairment may occur in a subset of patients with maculopathy or neuropathy [41, 42, 45, 51, 56, 57].

15.3.3 Laboratory Diagnosis

Within the first 2 days of fever, diagnosis is possible only by detecting virion, RNA, or dengue proteins, such as nonstructural protein 1 (NS1). In fact, NS1 antigen is usually detected in blood, from day 1 to day 9 of infection [37, 58].

Detection of newly formed antibodies (IgM) usually is not possible until after viremia ends or after fever subsides. MAC-ELISA has become a widely used assay, but it seems to have a high rate of false-positive results [59]. Other tests including immunochromatographic assay, complement fixation, neutralization test, hemagglutination inhibition, and IgG enzyme-linked immunosorbent assay (ELISA) are also helpful to confirm the diagnosis of DF [58].

Apart from the dengue-specific parameters, platelet count is a simple and available laboratory test that can support the diagnosis of dengue hemorrhagic fever or dengue shock syndrome.

15.3.4 Management

To date, there is no specific treatment available for dengue virus infection. Fever can be treated by antipyretics, but drugs such as acetylsalicylic acid and other nonsteroidal anti-inflammatory drugs should be avoided as they may worsen the bleeding tendency. Any medicine that decreases the platelet level should be avoided [37, 42]. In cases of dengue hemorrhagic fever, hospitalization, prompt treatment with intravenous fluids and close monitoring of vital signs, as well as hematologic parameters are indicated [37].

Preventive measures by avoiding contact with infected mosquitoes are required to decrease the infection incidence. Vaccines targeting all the four serotypes of dengue virus hopefully will be available in the near future [60].

There is no established treatment for ocular manifestations of DF. Topical, periocular, intravitreal, oral, and intravenous steroids, as well as intravenous immunoglobulins, have been advocated for the management of dengue ocular complications, based on the postulated immune-mediated pathogenesis of the disease. Indications for treatment may include dengue-associated uveitis and optic neuritis, visual acuity worse than 20/40, and deterioration of vision [45, 46].

15.4 Chikungunya

15.4.1 Introduction

Chikungunya virus is a single-stranded RNA virus of the genus *Alphavirus* of the family *Togaviridae* which is transmitted to humans by the bite of infected *Aedes* mosquitoes (*A. Aegypti* and *A. albopictus*). Since its first isolation in Tanzania in 1953, the virus has been associated with many epidemics in tropical regions of Africa, India, Southeast Asia, and South America. The infection which is endemoepidemic typically consists of an acute illness with fever, severe arthralgia, and skin rash [61]. Ocular involvement is relatively uncommon. The main ocular manifestations associated with Chikungunya virus infection are anterior uveitis and retinitis.

15.4.2 Clinical Symptoms and Signs

15.4.2.1 Systemic Disease

The incubation period ranges from 1 day to 12 days, with an average of 2–4 days. Onset of the disease is abrupt and is characterized by high fever, severe arthralgia and myalgia, along with headache and skin rash. Asymptomatic infections are rare (3–25 % of serologically proven infections) [62]. The debilitating polyarthralgia is very characteristic of Chikungunya. Joint pain often disappears in few weeks, but may persist for months or years in some patients [63, 64]. Skin lesions may be seen in almost one half of the patients. A pruriginous maculopapular rash, lasting for 2–3 days, is the most common feature [63–65]. Rarely, severe infection associated with multiorgan failure, central neurological involvement, neonatal infection, and death occurs [63, 64, 66].

15.4.2.2 Ocular Disease

Ocular manifestations associated with Chikungunya may be concomitant of the systemic disease or may follow its resolution [67]. Ocular involvement can be unilateral or bilateral. Ocular symptoms include redness, blurred vision, floaters, pain, irritation, photophobia, and diplopia. Acute anterior uveitis and retinitis are the most common ocular findings in Chikungunya. The anterior uveitis is nongranulomatous or granulomatous and can be associated with increased intraocular pressure. Posterior synechiae are not common [67–69]. The clinical course is typically benign.

Chikungunya retinitis presents in the form of areas of retinal whitening in the posterior pole with surrounding retinal and macular edema and associated mild vitritis (Fig. 15.3) [67]. FA usually shows early hypofluorescence and late hyperfluorescence of retinal lesions, along with focal areas of retinal vascular leakage and capillary non-perfusion [70].

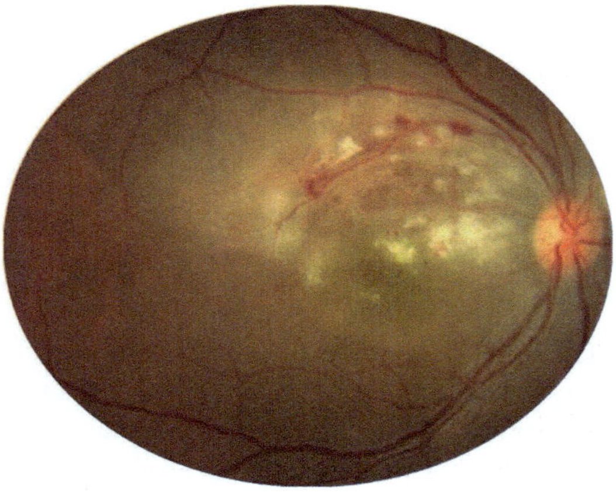

Fig. 15.3 Color fundus photograph of the right eye of a patient with Chikungunya shows confluent areas of retinitis associated with retinal hemorrhages, retinal edema, and foveal hard exudates (Courtesy, Padmamalini Mahendradas)

OCT reveals increased reflectivity in the nerve fiber layer zone with after shadowing corresponding to the areas of retinitis. It also helps in the detection and evaluation of associated retinal edema and exudative retinal detachment. Retinitis resolves gradually over a period of several weeks.

Other ophthalmic manifestations of Chikungunya have been reported including conjunctivitis, episcleritis, keratitis, panuveitis, multifocal choroiditis, optic neuritis, neuroretinitis, central retinal artery occlusion, panophthalmitis, lagophthalmos, and sixth nerve palsy [67, 68, 71].

Chikungunya-associated ocular disease is usually self-limiting, with most patients recovering good vision. However, permanent visual loss may occur mainly due to optic neuropathy.

Chikungunya virus has been recently detected in the human cornea. It has been suggested that cornea donation may be a route for the disease transmission, especially in endemic areas [72].

15.4.3 Laboratory Diagnosis

Chikungunya infection is suspected on the basis of clinical and epidemiological findings. However, confirmation of the diagnosis is important. In the acute phase of illness, it is based on the detection of viral nucleic acid in serum samples by RT-PCR, isolation of the virus, or detection of an antibody response. After resolution of the acute disease, the diagnosis is confirmed by the presence of an immune response. RT-PCR can detect viral nucleic acid from one day before the onset of symptoms, up to day 7 after the beginning of the disease. Antigen capture ELISA may detect viral antigens as early as day 2 after onset. Indirect immunofluorescence and ELISA are rapid and sensitive techniques for the screening of IgM or IgG immune reaction. IgM antibody and IgG antibody responses have been described to begin both by day 2 after the onset [66].

15.4.4 Management

Nonsteroidal anti-inflammatory drugs are currently recommended for Chikungunya-induced arthralgia. Ribavirin and interferon-α may inhibit viral replication [73, 74], but further studies are needed to assess their efficacy in humans. Another potential treatment for Chikungunya is chloroquine, but results of different studies have been inconclusive [75, 76].

Efforts are to be made to prevent transmission of the virus and to develop efficient and safe vaccines [62].

Topical steroids and cycloplegic agents are used for anterior uveitis. Associated ocular hypertension is managed with topical beta-blockers and oral or topical carbonic anhydrase inhibitors. Systemic steroids may be used to control the inflammation in posterior uveitis, panuveitis, and optic neuritis [67]. The use of acyclovir in association with corticosteroids has been described in some cases of Chikungunya retinitis [67], but its efficacy remains doubtful.

15.5 Rift Valley Fever

15.5.1 Introduction

Rift Valley fever (RVF) is an emerging arthropod-borne zoonotic disease caused by RVF virus, which belongs to the *Bunyaviridae* family. It is transmitted to humans through the bite of infected mosquitoes or through direct contact with blood, body fluids, or tissues of infected animals. RVF virus was first isolated in Kenya in 1930. It has been responsible of outbreaks in sub-Saharan African countries and in the Arabian Peninsula. Virus replication in the cattle gives high rates of mortality and abortion. RVF virus infection in humans usually causes a self-limiting, acute, and febrile illness, but severe potentially lethal forms may develop [77]. Macular or paramacular retinitis is the most common ocular complication, often resulting in permanent visual impairment.

15.5.2 Clinical Symptoms and Signs

15.5.2.1 Systemic Disease

After an incubation period of 3–6 days, RVF virus is often responsible for influenza like symptoms including fever, headache, arthralgias, myalgias, and gastrointestinal disturbances. The temperature curve usually shows a biphasic pattern, with an initial elevation lasting 2–3 days, followed by a remission and then a second febrile episode. Convalescence is typically rapid. Major life-threatening complications such as hepatic syndromes, hemorrhagic manifestations, or meningoencephalitis may rarely occur [78].

15.5.2.2 Ocular Disease

Ocular involvement has been reported to occur in 1–20 % of RVF infections [1–3, 79], usually 4–15 days after the onset of RVF. Prevalent symptoms at presentation include blurred vision, floaters, and scotomas. Unilateral or bilateral retinitis is the most common finding. It typically presents in the form of a large, single area of necrotizing retinitis, macular, or paramacular in location (Fig. 15.4a). Retinal lesions show early hypofluorescence and late staining on FA. Associated posterior segment changes include severe retinal vasculitis, retinal hemorrhages, vitritis, and optic disk edema [1–3, 79, 80]. Nongranulomatous anterior uveitis has also been described in association with posterior uveitis in patients with RVF. Anterior chamber inflammation disappears spontaneously within 2–3 weeks from the onset of systemic symptoms and is unlikely to result in complications such as glaucoma, posterior synechiae, or cataract. Retinitis usually recovers within 10–12 weeks. Permanent visual loss is common, mainly due to macular or paramacular scarring (Fig. 15.4b), retinal vascular occlusion, or optic atrophy [1–3, 79].

15.5.3 Laboratory Diagnosis

Once an outbreak is recognized and early cases are diagnosed, it becomes easier to suspect further cases of RVF. The most popular method of laboratory diagnosis is based on serologic testing to detect anti-RVF virus IgM antibodies or a rising titer of IgG antibodies in the serum by ELISA technique. Furthermore, laboratory detection of RVF virus antigen by antigen capture ELISA or

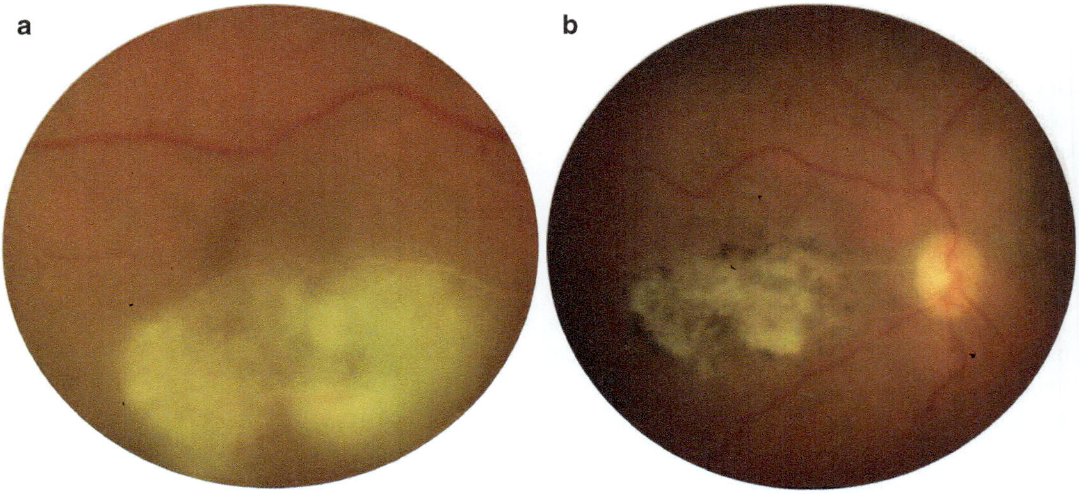

Fig. 15.4 (**a**) Color fundus photograph of the right eye of a patient with Rift Valley fever shows a large area of macular necrotizing retinitis associated with retinal vascular sheathing. (**b**) Color fundus photograph of the same eye after healing of the active retinitis shows a large atrophic retinochoroidal scar resulting in permanent severe visual loss (Courtesy, Emad Abboud)

viral RNA by RT-PCR in serum or other tissue samples confirms the diagnosis of RVF [81].

15.5.4 Management

The current treatment of RVF is only supportive with intravenous fluids and, when indicated, blood transfusion, hemodialysis, or mechanical ventilation. There is no antiviral therapy with proven efficacy in this setting [78]. Preventive measures are recommended including mosquito control and protection against mosquito bites. Vaccination of livestock may be a key element in breaking the chain of human epidemics and could lead to control of this significant public health threat [78, 82].

15.6 Rickettsioses

15.6.1 Introduction

Rickettsioses are worldwide distributed zoonoses due to obligate intracellular small gram-negative bacteria. Most of them are transmitted to humans by the bite of contaminated arthropods, such as ticks. Rickettsial agents are classified into three major categories: the spotted fever group, the typhus group, and the scrub typhus [83, 84]. A rickettsial disease should be suspected, during spring or summer in the presence of the triad of high fever, headache and general malaise, and skin rash in a patient living in or traveling back from a region endemic for rickettsioses. Ocular involvement is common, with retinitis and retinal vascular changes being the most common features [84].

15.6.2 Clinical Symptoms and Signs

15.6.2.1 Systemic Disease

The incubation period for rickettsial disease varies between 2 and 21 days. The initial presentation typically includes high fever with abrupt onset, headache, and myalgia. A maculopapular skin rash usually appears 3–5 days after the onset of fever. The skin rash, involving also the palms of the hands and the soles of the feet, is a hallmark of rickettsial infection. However, its absence should not rule out a possible rickettsial infection, especially during the first week of illness. A local skin lesion, termed tache noire (black spot), at the inoculating site may be seen

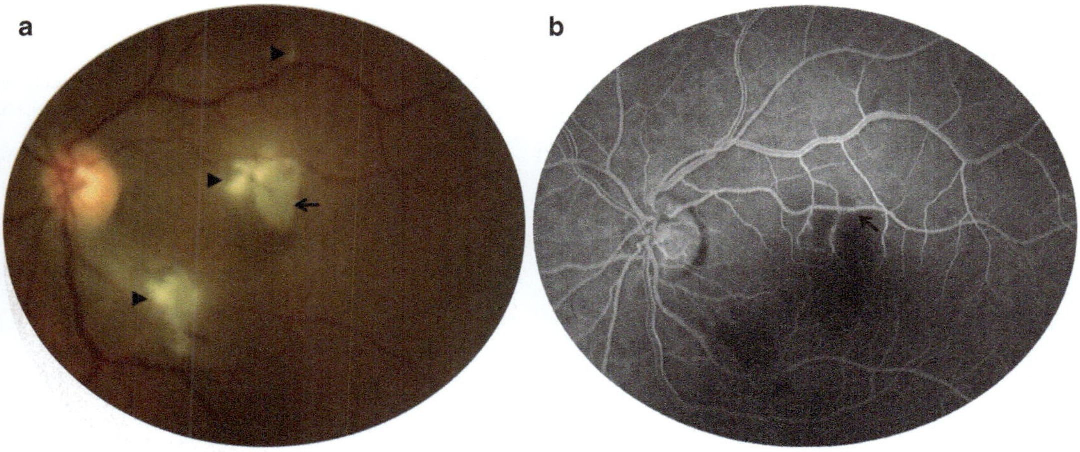

Fig. 15.5 (**a**) Color fundus photograph of the left eye of a patient with rickettsial disease shows white retinal lesions adjacent to retinal vessels (*arrowheads*). Note the presence of an associated triangular area of ischemic retinal whitening (*black arrow*). (**b**) Early fluorescein angiogram of the same eye shows hypofluorescence of areas of retinitis and confirms the diagnosis of occlusion of a small macular branch retinal artery (*black arrow*)

in several rickettsial infections, including Mediterranean spotted fever, caused by rickettsia conorii infection. Severe systemic complications may occur including interstitial pneumonitis, meningoencephalitic syndrome, acute renal failure, and disseminated intravascular coagulation [83, 84].

15.6.2.2 Ocular Disease

Ocular involvement is common in patients with rickettsiosis, but since it is frequently asymptomatic and self-limited, it may be easily overlooked [1–3, 84–86]. However, patients may present with ocular symptoms such as decreased vision, scotomas, floaters, or redness.

Bilateral or rarely unilateral non-necrotizing retinitis, with or without associated mild vitritis, is the most common ocular finding [1–3, 84–86]. It typically presents in the form of white retinal lesions infiltrating the inner retinal layers, located adjacent to retinal vessels, and varying in number, size, and location (Fig. 15.5a). Small retinal lesions in the posterior fundus may resemble cotton-wool spots, and large retinal lesions are usually associated with macular edema and exudative retinal detachment, which are accurately detectable by OCT. FA shows early hypofluorescence and late staining of large retinal lesions and slight hypofluorescence or isofluorescence of small retinal lesions [84, 85]. Retinal vascular lesions are a prominent feature of rickettsial disease. They may include focal or diffuse vascular sheathing, vascular leakage on FA, retinal hemorrhages, and retinal vascular occlusions, which mainly involve small branch retinal arteries (Fig. 15.5b) [1–3, 84–87]. A subclinical choroidal involvement only detectable by FA or ICGA is also common [84, 85].

Other reported ocular manifestations of rickettsiosis include conjunctivitis, keratitis, nongranulomatous anterior uveitis, panuveitis, optic disk edema, optic disk staining, optic neuritis, neuroretinitis, anterior ischemic optic neuropathy, and endophthalmitis [1–3, 84–88].

Ophthalmic involvement associated with rickettsial diseases often has a self-limited course. Areas of retinitis usually completely disappear without causing scarring in 3–10 weeks. Causes of persistent visual impairment include retinal pigment epithelial alterations due to resolved retinitis, macular edema, or exudative retinal detachment, branch retinal artery or vein occlusion, and optic neuropathy [1–3, 84–88].

15.6.3 Laboratory Diagnosis

Early diagnosis of rickettsial infection, primarily based on clinical features and epidemiologic data, is of utmost importance for early initiation of antibiotic therapy. Confirmation of diagnosis usually relies on positive indirect immunofluorescent antibody test results. Positive serologic criteria usually include either initial high antibody titer or a fourfold rise of the titer in the convalescent serum. Case confirmation with serology might take 2–3 weeks. Other laboratory tests, such as serologic testing using Western blot or detection of rickettsiae in blood or tissue using PCR, may be useful in selected cases [2, 83].

15.6.4 Management

Early treatment is required for a better outcome. Oral tetracyclines, particularly doxycycline (100 mg, twice a day for 7 to 10 days), are effective in the treatment of systemic rickettsial disease [1, 84, 85]. Fluoroquinolones are also effective. Macrolides, including clarithromycin, azithromycin, and particularly josamycin, can be used as alternative therapy in children and pregnant women.

Prevention includes personal protection against tick bites in endemic areas and improvement of sanitary conditions.

Specific ophthalmic therapy may be needed in patients with ocular involvement. It includes topical antibiotics for conjunctivitis and keratitis, topical corticosteroids and mydriatics for anterior uveitis, and systemic steroids in association with antibiotics in cases of severe ophthalmic involvement such as extensive retinitis threatening the macula or the optic disk, macular edema, exudative retinal detachment, severe vitritis, optic neuropathy, and retinal vascular occlusions [84].

Compliance with Ethical Requirements

Conflict of Interest The authors declare that they have no conflict of interest.

Informed Consent No human studies were carried out by the authors for this article.

Animal Studies No animal studies were carried out by the authors for this article.

References

1. Khairallah M, Jelliti B, Jenzeri S. Emergent infectious uveitis. Middle East Afr J Ophthalmol. 2009;16: 225–38.
2. Khairallah M, Chee SP, Rathinam SR, Attia S, Nadella V. Novel infectious agents causing uveitis. Int Ophthalmol. 2010;30:465–83.
3. Khairallah M, Ben Yahia S, Attia S. Arthropod vector-borne uveitis in the developing world. Int Ophthalmol Clin. 2010;50:125–44.
4. Petersen LR, Marfin AA. West Nile virus: a primer for the clinician. Ann Intern Med. 2002;137:173–9.
5. Garg S, Jampol LM. Systemic and intraocular manifestations of West Nile virus infection. Surv Ophthalmol. 2005;50:3–13.
6. Gyure KA. West Nile virus infections. J Neuropathol Exp Neurol. 2009;68:1053–60.
7. Bains HS, Jampol LM, Caughron MC, Parnell JR. Vitritis and chorioretinitis in a patient with West Nile virus infection. Arch Ophthalmol. 2003;121:205–7.
8. Vandenbelt S, Shaikh S, Capone Jr A, Williams GA. Multifocal choroiditis associated with West Nile virus encephalitis. Retina. 2003;23:97–9.
9. Adelman RA, Membreno JH, Afshari NA, Stoessel KM. West Nile virus chorioretinitis. Retina. 2003;23: 100–1.
10. Hershberger VS, Augsburger JJ, Hutchins RK, et al. Chorioretinal lesions in nonfatal cases of West Nile virus infection. Ophthalmology. 2003;110:1732–6.
11. Khairallah M, Ben Yahia S, Ladjimi A, et al. Chorioretinal involvement in patients with West Nile virus infection. Ophthalmology. 2004;111: 2065–70.
12. Shaikh S, Trese MT. West Nile virus chorioretinitis. Br J Ophthalmol. 2004;88:1599–600.
13. Eidsness RB, Stockl F, Colleaux KM. West Nile chorioretinitis. Can J Ophthalmol. 2005;40:721–4.
14. Myers JP, Leveque TK, Johnson MW. Extensive chorioretinitis and severe vision loss associated with West Nile virus meningoencephalitis. Arch Ophthalmol. 2005;123:1754–6.
15. Chan CK, Limstrom SA, Tarasewicz DG, Lin SG. Ocular features of west nile virus infection in North America: a study of 14 eyes. Ophthalmology. 2006;113:1539–46.
16. Seth RK, Stoessel KM, Adelman RA. Choroidal neovascularization associated with West Nile virus chorioretinitis. Semin Ophthalmol. 2007;22(2):81–4.
17. Kuchtey RW, Kosmorsky G, Martin D, Lee MS. Uveitis associated with West Nile virus infection. Arch Ophthalmol. 2003;121:1648–9.
18. Kaiser PK, Lee MS, Martin DA. Occlusive vasculitis in a patient with concomitant West Nile virus infection. Am J Ophthalmol. 2003;136:928–30.
19. Khairallah M, Ben Yahia S, Attia S, Jelliti B, Zaouali S, Ladjimi A. Severe ischemic maculopathy in a patient with West Nile virus infection. Ophthalmic Surg Lasers Imaging. 2006;37:240–2.

20. Teitelbaum BA, Newman TL, Tresley DJ. Occlusive retinal vasculitis in a patient with West Nile virus. Clin Exp Optom. 2007;90(6):463–7.
21. Gohari AZ, Willson RL, Gitter KA. West Nile virus occlusive retinal vasculitis. Retinal Cases Brief Rep. 2011;5:209–12.
22. Vaispapir V, Blum A, Soboh S, Ashkenazi H. West Nile virus meningoencephalitis with optic neuritis. Arch Intern Med. 2002;162:606–7.
23. Gilad R, Lampl Y, Sadeh M, Paul M, Dan M. Optic neuritis complicating West Nile virus meningitis in a young adult. Infection. 2003;31:55–6.
24. Anninger WV, Lomeo MD, Dingle J, Epstein AD, Lubow M. West Nile virus associated optic neuritis and chorioretinitis. Am J Ophthalmol. 2003;136:1183–5.
25. Anninger W, Lubow M. Visual loss with West Nile virus infection: a wider spectrum of a "new" disease. Clin Infect Dis. 2004;38:e55–6.
26. Alpert SG, Fergerson J, Noel LP. Intrauterine West Nile virus: ocular and systemic findings. Am J Ophthalmol. 2003;136:733–5.
27. Khairallah M, Ben Yahia S, Attia S, Zaouali S, Ladjimi A, Messaoud R. Linear pattern of West Nile virus-associated chorioretinitis is related to retinal nerve fibres organization. Eye (Lond). 2007;21:952–5.
28. Khairallah M, Ben Yahia S, Attia S, et al. Indocyanine green angiographic features in multifocal chorioretinitis associated with West Nile virus infection. Retina. 2006;26:358–9.
29. Beardsley R, McCannel C. Reactivation West Nile virus infection-related chorioretinitis. Semin Ophthalmol. 2012;27(3–4):43–5.
30. Shaikh NA, Ge J, Zhao YX, Walker P, Drebot M. Development of a novel, rapid, and sensitive immunochromatographic strip assay specific for West Nile Virus (WNV) IgM and testing of its diagnostic accuracy in patients suspected of WNV infection. Clin Chem. 2007;53(11):2031–4.
31. Jordan I, Briese N, Fischer N, Lau JY, Lipkin WI. Ribavirin inhibits West Nile virus replication and cytopathic effect in neutral cells. J Infect Dis. 2000;182:1214–7.
32. Samuel MA, Diamond MS. Alpha/beta interferon protects against lethal West Nile virus infection by restricting cellular tropism and enhancing neuronal survival. J Virol. 2005;79:13350–61.
33. Lazear HM, Pinto AK, Vogt MR, Gale Jr M, Diamond MS. Beta interferon controls West Nile virus infection and pathogenesis in mice. J Virol. 2011;85(14):7186–94.
34. Vogt MR, Moesker B, Goudsmit J, et al. Human monoclonal antibodies against West Nile virus induced by natural infection neutralize at a postattachment step. J Virol. 2009;83(13):6494–507.
35. Gibney KB, Colborn J, Baty S, et al. Modifiable risk factors for West Nile virus infection during an outbreak–Arizona, 2010. Am J Trop Med Hyg. 2012;86(5):895–901.
36. Afshar AR, Hariprasad SM, Jampol LM, Sheth VS. Use of intravitreous bevacizumab to treat macular edema in West Nile virus chorioretinitis. Arch Ophthalmol. 2012;130:396–8.
37. Halstead SB. Dengue. Curr Opin Infect Dis. 2002; 15:471–6.
38. World Health Organization. Dengue hemorrhagic fever: diagnosis, treatment and control. 2nd ed. Geneva: WHO; 1997.
39. Haritoglou C, Scholz F, Bialasiewicz A, Klauss V. Ocular manifestation in dengue fever. Ophthalmologe. 2000;97:433–6.
40. Haritoglou C, Dotse SD, Rudolp G, Stephan CM, Thurau SR, Klauss V. A tourist with dengue fever and visual loss. Lancet. 2002;360:1070.
41. Cruz-Villegas V, Berrocal AM, Davis JL. Bilateral choroidal effusions associated with dengue fever. Retina. 2003;23:576–8.
42. Lim WK, Mathur R, Koh A, Yeoh R, Chee SP. Ocular manifestations of dengue fever. Ophthalmology. 2004;111:2057–64.
43. Su DH, Bacsal K, Chee SP, et al. Prevalence of dengue maculopathy in patients hospitalized for dengue fever. Ophthalmology. 2007;114(9):1743–7.
44. Chan DP, Teoh SC, Tan CS, et al. Ophthalmic complications of dengue. Emerg Infect Dis. 2006;12:285–9.
45. Bacsal K, Chee SP, Cheng CL, Flores JV. Dengue-associated maculopathy. Arch Ophthalmol. 2007;125: 501–10.
46. Kapoor HK, Bhai S, John M, Xavier J. Ocular manifestations of dengue fever in an East Indian epidemic. Can J Ophthalmol. 2006;41:741–6.
47. Siqueira RC, Vitral NP, Campos WR, Orefice F, de Moraes Figueiredo LT. Ocular manifestations in dengue fever. Ocul Immunol Inflamm. 2004;12:323–7.
48. Chlebicki MP, Ang B, Barkham T, Lande A. Retinal hemorrhages in 4 patients with dengue fever. Emerg Infect Dis. 2005;11:770–1.
49. Loh BK, Bacsal K, Chee SP, Cheng BC, Wong D. Foveolitis associated with dengue fever: a case series. Ophthalmologica. 2008;222(5):317–20.
50. Kanungo S, Shukla D, Kim R. Branch retinal artery occlusion secondary to dengue fever. Indian J Ophthalmol. 2008;56(1):73–4.
51. Laurence B, Harold M, Thierry D. Ocular complications of dengue fever. Ophthalmology. 2008;115:1100–1.
52. De Amorim Garcia CA, Gomes AH, De Oliveira AG. Bilateral stellar neuroretinitis in a patient with dengue fever. Eye (Lond). 2006;20(12):1382–3.
53. Venkatramani J, Lim WK. Bilateral vitreous haemorrhage associated with dengue fever. Eye (Lond). 2006;20(12):1405–6.
54. Sanjay S, Wagle AM, Au Eong KG. Dengue optic neuropathy. Ophthalmology. 2009;116(1):170.
55. Tabbara K. Dengue retinochoroiditis. Ann Saudi Med. 2012;32(5):530–3.
56. Teoh SC, Chee CK, Laude A, Goh KY, Barkham T, Ang BS, Eye Institute Dengue-related Ophthalmic Complications Workgroup. Optical coherence tomography patterns as predictors of visual outcome in dengue-related maculopathy. Retina. 2010;30(3):390–8.

57. Chia A, Luu CD, Mathur R, Cheng B, Chee SP. Electrophysiological findings in patients with dengue-related maculopathy. Arch Ophthalmol. 2006;124(10):1421–6.
58. Blacksell SD, Newton PN, Bell D, et al. The comparative accuracy of 8 commercial rapid immunochromatographic assays for the diagnosis of acute dengue virus infection. Clin Infect Dis. 2006;42:1127–34.
59. Wichmann O, Lauschke A, Frank C, et al. Dengue antibody prevalence in German travelers. Emerg Infect Dis. 2005;11:762–5.
60. Sobia S, Ashfaq UA. A brief review on dengue molecular virology, diagnosis, treatment and prevalence in Pakistan. Genet Vaccines Ther. 2012;10(1):6.
61. Powers AM, Brault AC, Tesh RB, Weaver SC. Re-emergence of chikungunya and o'nyong-nyong viruses: evidence for distinct geographical lineages and distant evolutionary relationships. J Gen Virol. 2000;81:471–9.
62. Burt FJ, Rolph MS, Rulli NE, Mahalingam S, Heise MT. Chikungunya: a re-emerging virus. Lancet. 2012;379(9816):662–71.
63. Pialoux G, Gaüzère BA, Jauréguiberry S, Strobel M. Chikungunya, an epidemic arbovirosis. Lancet Infect Dis. 2007;7:319–27.
64. Chhabra M, Mittal V, Bhattacharya D, Rana U, Lal S. Chikungunya fever: a re-emerging viral infection. Indian J Med Microbiol. 2008;26:5–12.
65. Brighton SW, Prozesky OW, de la Harpe AL. Chikungunya virus infection. A retrospective study of 107 cases. S Afr Med J. 1983;63:313–5.
66. Sudeep AB, Parashar D. Chikungunya: an overview. J Biosci. 2008;33:443–9.
67. Mahendradas P, Ranganna S, Shetty R. Ocular manifestations associated with Chikungunya. Ophthalmology. 2008;115:287–91.
68. Lalitha P, Rathinam S, Banushree K, Maheshkumar S, Vijayakumar R, Sathe P. Ocular involvement associated with an epidemic outbreak of chikungunya virus infection. Am J Ophthalmol. 2007;144:552–6.
69. Mittal A, Mittal S, Bharathi JM, Ramakrishnan R, Sathe PS. Uveitis during outbreak of Chikungunya fever. Ophthalmology. 2007;114:1798.
70. Murthy KR, Venkataraman N, Satish V, Babu K. Bilateral retinitis following Chikungunya fever. Indian J Opthalmol. 2008;56:329–31.
71. Mittal A, Mittal S, Bharati MJ, Ramakrishnan R, Saravanan S, Sathe PS. Optic neuritis associated with Chikungunya virus infection in South India. Arch Ophthalmol. 2007;125:1381–6.
72. Couderc T, Gangneux N, Chrétien F, et al. Chikungunya virus infection of corneal grafts. J Infect Dis. 2012;206(6):851–9.
73. Ravichandran R, Manian M. Ribavirin therapy for Chikungunya arthritis. J Infect Dev Ctries. 2008;2:140–2.
74. Briolant S, Garin D, Scaramizzino N, Jouan A, Crance JM. In vitro inhibition of Chikungunya and Semliki forest viruses replication by antiviral compounds: synergistic effect of interferon-alpha and ribavirin combination. Antiviral Res. 2004;61:111–7.
75. Brighton SW. Chloroquine phosphate treatment of chronic Chikungunya arthritis. An open pilot study. S Afr Med J. 1984;66:217–8.
76. De Lamballerie X, Boisson V, Reynier JC, et al. On chikungunya acute infection and chloroquine treatment. Vector Borne Zoonotic Dis. 2008;8:837–9.
77. Ikegami T, Makino S. The pathogenesis of Rift Valley fever. Viruses. 2011;3(5):493–519.
78. Balkhy HH, Memish ZA. Rift Valley fever: an uninvited zoonosis in the Arabian peninsula. Int J Antimicrob Agents. 2003;21(2):153–7.
79. Al-Hazmi A, Al-Rajhi AA, Abboud EB, et al. Ocular complications of Rift Valley fever outbreak in Saudi Arabia. Ophthalmology. 2005;112:313–8.
80. Siam AL, Meegan JM, Gharbawi KF. Rift Valley fever ocular manifestations: observations during the 1977 epidemic in Egypt. Br J Ophthalmol. 1980;64(5):366–74.
81. Fukushi S, Nakauchi M, Mizutani T, Saijo M, Kurane I, Morikawa S. Antigen-capture ELISA for the detection of Rift Valley fever virus nucleoprotein using new monoclonal antibodies. J Virol Methods. 2012;180(1–2):68–74.
82. Bird BH, Maartens LH, Campbell S, et al. Rift Valley fever virus vaccine lacking the NSs and NSm genes is safe, nonteratogenic, and confers protection from viremia, pyrexia, and abortion following challenge in adult and pregnant sheep. J Virol. 2011;85(24):12901–9.
83. Rathi N, Rathi A. Rickettsial infections: Indian perspective. Indian Pediatr. 2010;47(2):157–64.
84. Khairallah M, Ladjimi A, Chakroun M, et al. Posterior segment manifestations of Rickettsia conorii infection. Ophthalmology. 2004;111:529–34.
85. Khairallah M, Ben Yahia S, Toumi A, et al. Ocular manifestations associated with murine typhus. Br J Ophthalmol. 2009;93:938–42.
86. Khairallah M, Ben Yahia S, Jelliti B, et al. Diagnostic value of ocular examination in Mediterranean spotted fever. Clin Microbiol Infect. 2009;15 Suppl 2:273–4.
87. Agahan AL, Torres J, Fuentes-Páez G, Martínez-Osorio H, Orduña A, Calonge M. Intraocular inflammation as the main manifestation of Rickettsia conorii infection. Clin Ophthalmol. 2011;5:1401–7.
88. Khairallah M, Zaouali S, Ben Yahia S, et al. Anterior ischemic optic neuropathy associated with rickettsia conorii infection. J Neuroophthalmol. 2005;25:212–4.

Endophthalmitis

16

Hani S. Al-Mezaine and Ahmed M. Abu El-Asrar

16.1 Introduction

Endophthalmitis is a devastating ocular inflammatory process that can lead to blindness. In endophthalmitis, there is inflammation of the vitreous cavity along with the retinal and uveal components of the eye. Endophthalmitis may be infectious or noninfectious, and the infectious cases may be a result of endogenous or exogenous sources. Endogenous endophthalmitis occurs secondary to a hematogenous dissemination and spread from a distant infective source in the body. Most cases of endophthalmitis are exogenous and occur after ocular surgery. Each type of infectious endophthalmitis differs in its microbial profile, symptoms, and clinical course as described herein.

16.2 Endogenous Endophthalmitis

Endogenous endophthalmitis as a result of hematogenous spread from other parts of the body makes up less than 2–8 % of cases [1]. Risk factors include a chronic disease state, invasive surgery, indwelling catheters, intravenous drug use, septicemia, and immunodeficiency. This type of endophthalmitis is rare in healthy individuals and is an indication for systemic investigations [2].

The presentation normally is acute and may be bilateral in 12 % of cases [3]. In one series, diabetes, intravenous drug abuse, and HIV/AIDS infection were the most influential risk factors, and liver abscesses, pneumonia, and endocarditis were the three most common sources of infection [3].

Both bacteria and fungi can cause endogenous endophthalmitis. The profile of bacteria that cause endogenous endophthalmitis differs according to geographical region. Gram-negative organisms, especially *Klebsiella*, predominate in East Asia [4]. *K. pneumoniae* genotype K1 is an emerging pathogen capable of causing catastrophic septic ocular or central nervous system complications from pyogenic liver abscess. Diabetes is a significant risk factor for the development of endogenous endophthalmitis and poor visual outcome in patients with *K. pneumoniae* liver abscess. Endogenous *K. pneumoniae* usually causes poor visual outcomes. Cases in Europe and North America are dominated by gram-positive organisms such as *Staphylococcus aureus*, *Staphylococcus epidermidis*, group B streptococci, *Streptococcus pneumoniae*, and *Listeria monocytogenes* [3, 5]. The most common cause of fungal endogenous endophthalmitis is *Candida* species, particularly *Candida albicans*,

H.S. Al-Mezaine, MD (✉)
A.M. Abu El-Asrar, MD, PhD
Department of Ophthalmology, King Abdulaziz University Hospital, College of Medicine, King Saud University, KAUH, Old Airport Road, 245 Riyadh 11411, Saudi Arabia
e-mail: halmezaine@ksu.edu.sa; abuasrar@ksu.edu.sa

K. Tabbara et al. (eds.), *Ocular Infections*, Essentials in Ophthalmology,
DOI 10.1007/978-3-662-43981-4_16, © Springer-Verlag Berlin Heidelberg 2014

followed by *Aspergillus*. The presentation usually is subacute and is associated with long-term intravenous catheters. Intravenous drug abusers with endocarditis are also at risk for endogenous fungal endophthalmitis.

16.3 Endophthalmitis After Cataract Surgery

Endophthalmitis, an infection of the vitreous compartment and the retinal and uveal coats of the eye, is a problematic complication associated with intraocular surgery. Because cataract surgery is the most frequently performed intraocular surgery, 90 % of postoperative endophthalmitis occurs following this procedure [6]. Post-cataract surgery endophthalmitis is divided into two types: acute-onset and chronic or delayed-onset endophthalmitis.

16.3.1 Acute-Onset Endophthalmitis

In this entity, the patient typically presents within the first week after cataract surgery. Patients presenting within 6 weeks of the surgery with reduced visual acuity and symptoms and signs of endophthalmitis should be managed as for acute endophthalmitis. The overall incidence of endophthalmitis after cataract operations has been estimated to be in the range of 0.04–0.2 % [7].

Improvements in modern cataract surgery have mainly involved a series of technical refinements. Most have concerned the evolution in the type of surgical incision being performed, beginning with the implementation of intracapsular cataract extraction, followed by extracapsular cataract extraction (ECCE), then small-incision scleral tunnel phacoemulsification, and, finally, clear corneal incision (CCI) phacoemulsification. The implementation of these technical refinements has resulted in simplified postoperative care and faster visual recovery and has been promoted from a safety standpoint. However, retrospective studies have recently suggested an association between an increased incidence of endophthalmitis following cataract surgery and the use of CCIs for cataract extraction [6–15].

Al-Mezaine et al. [15] showed that over a 10-year period, the incidence of acute-onset nosocomial endophthalmitis following cataract surgery was 0.068 % and that the risk of endophthalmitis was 1.73-fold higher for CCI phacoemulsification than ECCE. In their meta-analysis of studies addressing endophthalmitis following cataract surgery, Taban et al. [6] found that the incidence of endophthalmitis has varied over time—that is, from 0.087 % in the 1990s to 0.265 % in 2000/2003. For the time period between 1992 and 2003, they also determined that CCI phacoemulsification was a risk factor for endophthalmitis, with an increased rate of 0.189 % compared with 0.074 % for scleral tunnel incisions. Moreover, Cooper et al. determined that clear corneal incision was associated with a threefold greater risk of endophthalmitis than was scleral tunnel incision [11].

16.3.2 Clinical Features

Patients with acute endophthalmitis typically present with blurred vision (94.3 %), red eye (82.1 %), pain (74 %), and swollen lid (34.5 %) as it has been shown by the Endophthalmitis Vitrectomy Study (EVS) [9]. Other clinical signs might include conjunctival discharge; conjunctival and corneal edema; turbidity in the anterior chamber with cells, hypopyon, or fibrin clot; and/or vitritis that precludes a view of the posterior segment. Acute endophthalmitis is diagnosed by clinical means. Ocular echography is a valuable adjunctive tool in this type of clinical evaluation particularly in eyes with opaque media [16].

16.3.3 Etiology

The normal flora of the ocular surface comprises an array of bacteria that are believed to be a primary source of infection in endophthalmitis. Gram-positive bacteria are the most common cause of postoperative endophthalmitis [9, 17–19]. In the EVS [9], researchers found that 94.2 % of culture-positive endophthalmitis cases involved gram-positive bacteria: 70 % of isolates were gram-positive coagulase-negative staphylococci, 9.9 % were *Staphylococcus aureus*, 9.0 % were *Streptococcus* species, 2.2 % were *Enterococcus* species, and 3.0 % were other gram-positive species. Gram-negative species were involved in 5.9 % of cases.

16.3.4 Risk Factors

An increased intraocular exposure to the patient's own normal adnexal and ocular surface flora that occurs during cataract surgery might be the main risk factor for endophthalmitis. Intraoperative complications such as posterior capsular rupture and vitreous loss also increase the risk for endophthalmitis by tenfold [20]. In addition, several studies have suggested that the performance of CCIs is a risk factor for endophthalmitis [21–24]. Moreover, it has been shown that the use of silicone IOL optic material increased the risk of endophthalmitis by 3.3-fold compared to acrylic lenses [21]. Other factors that increase the risk for endophthalmitis include failure of sterile technique during intraocular surgery [25], preexisting periocular infections, advancing age (>85 years), and immunosuppressed status such as diabetes [26, 27].

16.3.5 Management

As put forth in the EVS [9], the initial treatment of endophthalmitis following cataract surgery involves a two-pronged approach: specimen collection and the administration of broad-spectrum antibiotics (such as a combination of vancomycin and ceftazidime). The diagnostic yield of vitreous specimen is roughly doubled that of an aqueous specimen (54.9 % vs 22.5 %, respectively) [28]. Polymerase chain reaction (PCR) amplification produces yields for aqueous and vitreous sampling that are the same [29], thus allowing the diagnosis to be made with the faster and more easily performed aqueous tap [30].

According to the EVS, the presenting visual acuity should form the basis of the decision between a vitreous tap and vitrectomy for patients, with the exception of those with diabetes [9]. For patients with a visual acuity better than light perception, either method can be used without affecting the final outcome. Whereas for patients with light perception vision, pars plana vitrectomy (PPV) should be performed because a threefold increase in the likelihood of achieving 20/40 final visual acuity occurs when this procedure is carried out [28]. The situation differs for patients with diabetes. Regardless of the presenting visual acuity, patients with diabetes have a greater likelihood of obtaining 20/40 acuity with PPV (57 %) compared with a simple tap (40 %) [31].

It has been demonstrated by the EVS group that poor visual outcome was associated with a presenting visual acuity of light perception, presence of afferent pupillary defect, corneal infiltrate or ring ulcer, hypopyon, abnormal IOP (<5 or >25 mmHg), rubeosis iridis, small pupil size after maximal dilatation, absent red reflex, and inability to see any retinal vessels by indirect ophthalmoscopy [9].

16.3.6 Prevention

Preoperative sterile preparation of the surgical site is one of the most common practice patterns employed to prevent postoperative endophthalmitis. This practice most often entails the instillation of povidone-iodine 5 % into the conjunctival sac, which, according to research studies, effectively decreases the bacterial load [32, 33]. A recent European survey by Ang and Barras [34] determined that 99.5 % of surgeons use povidone-iodine irrigation for prophylaxis. In their prospective study, Halachimi-Eyal et al. [35] compared the effects of the preoperative administration of topical moxifloxacin 0.5 % and povidone-iodine 5 % and that of povidone-iodine 5 % alone on conjunctival bacterial colonization. They found that the decrease in conjunctival bacterial colonization achieved with topical moxifloxacin 0.5 % and povidone-iodine 5 % did not exceed the effect of povidone-iodine 5 % alone.

Proper surgical draping is also critical. This practice involves using overhanging wraparound flaps from the drape (held securely in place by the speculum) to sequester the lashes and lid margins completely [36, 37].

Although topical perioperative antibiotic prophylaxis is generally performed, controversy surrounds this practice because its effectiveness is there [25]. Of these types of drugs, fourth-generation fluoroquinolones have become the most commonly prescribed owing to their broad-spectrum activity and enhanced ocular penetration [38, 39].

Of the various methods of antibiotic prophylaxis, the strongest support in the literature is for direct intracameral bolus injection at the conclusion of surgery. In their retrospective study, Montan et al. [40] found that the administration of a direct intracameral cefuroxime injection in more than 32,000 cases in Sweden resulted in an endophthalmitis rate of 0.06 %, which was significantly lower than those previously determined. (However, they also reported that 12 of the 13 culture-positive endophthalmitis organisms were cefuroxime resistant.) In addition, a lower rate of endophthalmitis was associated with the administration of intracameral cefuroxime compared with topical antibiotic use alone in a 3-year prospective, nonrandomized study of more than 225,000 cases in Sweden [41]. Furthermore, the value of intracameral antibiotic prophylaxis is underscored by the finding of a multicenter, prospective, randomized study by the European Society of Cataract and Refractive Surgeons (ESCRS) [21] showing that direct intracameral cefuroxime injections resulted in a 5.86-fold decreased (95 % confidence interval, 1.72–20.0) risk for culture-positive endophthalmitis [21, 42]. Although support exists in the literature regarding the safety of using intracameral preparations of vancomycin and cephalosporin [43–49], there are several risks associated with compounding medications for intraocular administration, including toxic anterior segment syndrome, retinal toxicity, ocular contamination, and dosing errors [50]. However, the need for the compounding of medications is eliminated when moxifloxacin is administered. In their study on the use of moxifloxacin for intracameral prophylaxis, O'Brien et al. [38] noted its potency and bacterial activity and described how the self-preserved commercial formulation negated the need for compounding. Although no prospective randomized studies have been conducted to support the use of subconjunctival antibiotic prophylaxis, research has indicated that it has a protective benefit [7].

16.4 Chronic (Delayed-Onset) Endophthalmitis

Chronic endophthalmitis is defined as an infection that occurs 6 weeks or more after cataract surgery and frequently persists, with recurrent low-grade inflammation, for months thereafter [51].

16.4.1 Incidence

Data regarding the incidence of chronic endophthalmitis following cataract surgery are scarce. Rogers et al. [52] estimated the ratio of acute to chronic postoperative endophthalmitis cases to be between 5:1 and 2:1, indicating that the incidence rate can be five cases per 10,000 individuals. Al-Mezaine et al. [53] determined the incidence of chronic endophthalmitis following cataract surgery in a tertiary care eye center to be 1.7 cases per 10,000 individuals. However, determining the real incidence of chronic endophthalmitis might be difficult because of the nature of the disease and its indolent course [53].

16.4.2 Etiology

In 1986, Meisler et al. [54] reported a syndrome of chronic indolent granulomatous uveitis that manifests weeks to months after cataract surgery. This uveitis improves initially with topical corticosteroid therapy but flares up whenever the administration of steroids is tapered or stopped. According to electron microscopy findings and its identification in anaerobic cultures, *Propionibacterium acnes* was determined to be a cause of this syndrome.

In addition to *P. acnes* [53, 55–58], which has been implicated in the majority of cases of chronic endophthalmitis (41–63 %), various

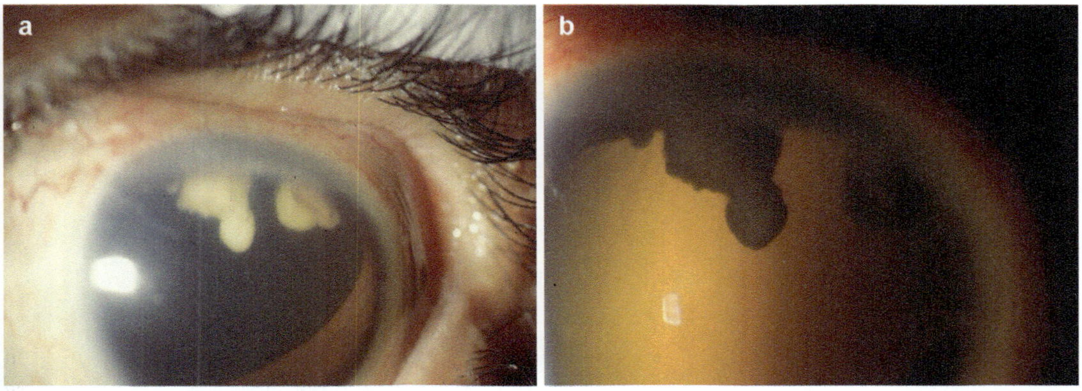

Fig. 16.1 Slit-lamp photograph showing (**a**) white plaque extending from the capsule equator "fluff balls" caused by *Aspergillus terreus*; (**b**) retroillumination (Adapted from Al-Mezaine et al. [53])

organisms have been associated with chronic endophthalmitis, including *Staphylococci* [59–61] (more frequently *S. epidermidis* but occasionally *S. aureus*), fungal organisms [62, 63], *Achromobacter* species [61], *Corynebacterium* species [61], *Mycobacterium chelonae* [64], *Cephalosporium* species [65], gram-negative bacteria (*Alcaligenes xylosoxidans*) [66, 67], and *Actinomyces* species [68], and polymicrobial or mixed infections [67, 69] have also been reported.

16.4.3 Clinical Presentation

Patients with chronic endophthalmitis usually present with low-grade and recurrent uveitis months or even years after cataract surgery. The inflammation starts at the anterior chamber and then progresses to the vitreous. Patients most frequently complain of decreased visual acuity and, to a lesser degree, mild pain, discomfort, and/or redness.

Clinical signs of chronic endophthalmitis might include the presence of cells and flare in the anterior chamber and granulomatous uveitis with precipitates on the cornea and intraocular lens. An infection is generally suspected when a white capsular plaque, representing retained lens particles and sequestered organisms, is present [70]. The endophthalmitis can develop or worsen following Nd-YAG laser posterior capsulotomy, presumably due to liberation of previously loculated organisms [71]. Although the plaque is indicative of *P. acnes* infiltrate, it is also observed with other bacterial and fungal infections [53, 72–74]. Vitritis is usually mild in cases of chronic endophthalmitis. The presence of "fluff balls" or "pearls on a string" in cases of chronic endophthalmitis is seen with fungal infections (Fig. 16.1). Moreover, sectoral iris infiltration by fungal element can occur before the infection developed into fulminant fungal endophthalmitis (Fig. 16.2) [53, 56, 70].

16.4.4 Diagnosis

Diagnosing chronic endophthalmitis poses a challenge. Any intraocular inflammation occurring at any time within several months of a breach of ocular integrity should prompt suspicion of the diagnosis. Anaerobic cultures of intraocular specimens should therefore be monitored for a period of 14 days. However, even after 14 days, these cultures are often negative because most of the organisms are usually sequestered within the capsular bag. Another challenge is the increased likelihood of false-negative culture results owing to the small number of microorganisms in the sample, the physiological requirements of fastidious organisms, and low pathogenicity [75]. Research has shown that PCR is more sensitive than culturing in the detection of chronic endophthalmitis caused by *P. acnes* [76].

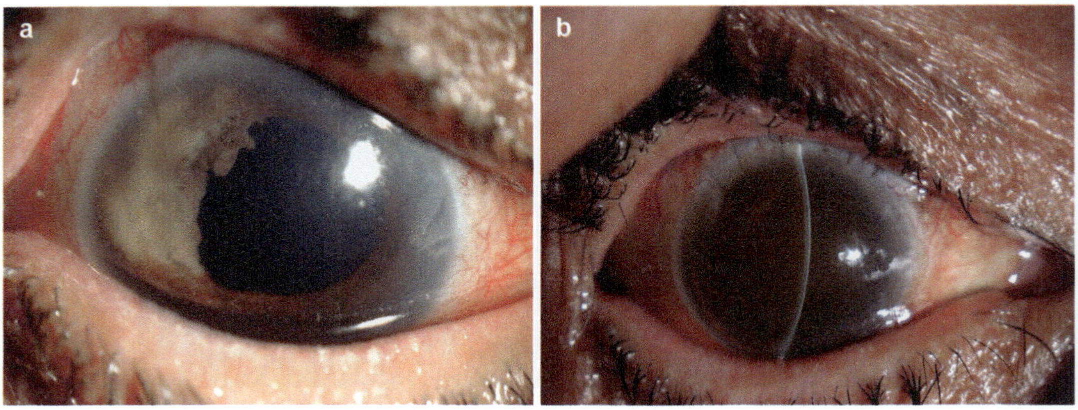

Fig. 16.2 Slit-lamp photograph showing (**a**) sectoral iris infiltration with *Aspergillus niger*; (**b**) fulminant fungal endophthalmitis 2 months later (Adapted from Al-Mezaine et al. [53])

16.4.5 Management

The indolent nature of the organisms and their sequestration within the capsule protects them from host defenses and their different virulence factors make it hard to define a treatment protocol for chronic postoperative endophthalmitis or extrapolate the guidelines set for acute endophthalmitis [70]. Clark et al. [57] and Aldare et al. [58] have proposed several management recommendations: the injection of intravitreal antibiotics alone, followed by PPV with partial capsulectomy, and, lastly, vitrectomy with total capsulotomy and intraocular lens (IOL) removal or exchange.

A cross-sectional review of the biggest case series [53, 57, 59, 77] on chronic endophthalmitis revealed varying results. Differences in causative organism, the type of initial therapeutic method performed, and the extent of the intervention [78] contribute to these varying results. From these series, a total of 98 patients with chronic endophthalmitis were studied. The overall visual outcome was 20/40 or better in about 46 % of the cases, whereas 54 % had varying degrees of visual impairment. An infection caused by *P. acnes* or gram-positive organisms was associated with a better visual outcome (better than 20/40 in more than 50 % of cases) than an infection caused by other types of bacteria. A fungal infection was associated with a more unfavorable prognosis. Those cases in which the initial treatment involved intravitreal injection alone had the highest rate of recurrence (90 %). The performance of PPV and the administration of intravitreal injections were associated with a decreased rate of recurrence in all series. The inclusion of partial capsulotomy to PPV and the administration of antibiotic injections further decreased the rate of recurrence to 42 % [78]. However, in all series, the overall calculated rate decreased to as low as 50 % when treatment involved PPV, intravitreal antibiotic injections, total capsulotomy, and removal or exchange of the IOL, whereas the rate of recurrence was 68 % when PPV was combined with only intravitreal antibiotic injection [78].

16.5 Posttraumatic Endophthalmitis

Infectious endophthalmitis is a devastating complication of open-globe injuries. It comprises approximately 25–30 % of all cases of infectious endophthalmitis. The incidence of culture-positive endophthalmitis after open-globe injuries varies between 0.5 and 17 % [79–93]. Previous reports have demonstrated that delayed primary repair, dirty wound, breach of lens capsule, retained intraocular foreign body (IOFB), grade 4 injury (presenting visual acuity of worse than 5/200 to light perception), placement of primary intraocular lens, needle injuries, and rural setting are associated with an increased risk of posttraumatic endophthalmitis [79, 81–84, 87, 88, 90–93]. Posttraumatic endophthalmitis is associated with its own microbiologic spectrum which is distinct from other subgroups of exogenous endophthalmitis. Gram-positive organisms such as *Bacillus*, *Staphylococci*, and *Streptococci* are frequently isolated pathogens [79–82, 94–101]. Posttraumatic endophthalmitis still carries a poor prognosis. When pooling data from previously reported studies of posttraumatic endophthalmitis, visual acuities of 20/40 or better were preserved only in 37 % of patients. Reasons for guarded prognosis include polymicrobial infection, the virulence of the infecting microorganisms, and possible delayed diagnosis and initiation of treatment. In addition, concomitant injuries may directly result in ocular damage that limits ultimate visual recovery [79–98, 101].

Useful clinical symptoms and signs in the diagnosis of endophthalmitis after open-globe injury include worsening vision and pain, hypopyon, vitritis, retinitis, periphlebitis, as well as corneal ring infiltrate. Diagnostic imaging in the setting of trauma helps in the detection of suspected IOFB or to rule out retinal and choroidal detachments. Axial computed tomography (CT) scans are most useful for localization of metallic IOFBs. Echography facilitates assessment of the degree of vitreous opacification, presence of IOFB, status of the posterior hyaloids face, as well as detection of either choroidal or retinal detachments.

Because of the substantial incidence of endophthalmitis after open-globe injuries, careful consideration should be given to the use of prophylactic antimicrobial therapy. The purpose of prophylaxis is to provide effective antibiotic level as rapidly as possible against a broad range of organisms. The use of systemic antibiotics in the prophylactic treatment of posttraumatic endophthalmitis has become the standard of care in patients with open-globe injuries, on the basis of clinical experience, but there is little experimental evidence that supports the efficacy of such therapy [79, 82, 95]. Ariyasu et al. [102] demonstrated microbial contamination of the anterior chamber at the time of repair in one-third of their eyes with open-globe injuries. None of these eyes developed clinical endophthalmitis. The incidence of positive anterior chamber culture was significantly lower in patients receiving intravenous antibiotics before wound repair compared with patients not receiving such therapy. These data support the prophylactic use of broad-spectrum intravenous antibiotics against the development of posttraumatic endophthalmitis by reducing the incidence of intraocular microbial contamination. Good coverage for most organisms is obtained with intravenous vancomycin coupled with a third-generation cephalosporin, such as ceftazidime, which can penetrate the vitreous cavity in effective levels in inflamed aphakic experimental eyes [103, 104]. Ceftazidime provides effective coverage for gram-negative intraocular infections [103, 105], and vancomycin provides coverage for gram-positive organisms [104, 105]. The beneficial role of prophylactic intravenous vancomycin coupled with ceftazidime was suggested [90, 92].

Animal models have demonstrated the efficacy of intravitreal antibiotics for prophylaxis of posttraumatic endophthalmitis [106, 107]. A small randomized trial showed that prophylactic intravitreal injection of vancomycin (1 mg) and ceftazidime (2.25 mg) decreases the risk of posttraumatic endophthalmitis [108]. Recently, a multicenter study provided strong evidence supporting the role of adjunct intraocular antibiotic injection at the time of primary repair in reducing the rate of posttraumatic endophthalmitis in open-globe injuries with retained IOFB [109]. Some authors recommended prophylactic intravitreal antibiotic administration in high-risk cases [81, 98, 110]. Therefore, it is crucial to identify these high-risk cases. Essex et al. [88] found that cases with ≥2 of the three risk factors (delay in primary repair of ≥24 h, dirty wound, and lens breach) had a relative risk of 5.1 for developing endophthalmitis. They therefore recommended intravitreal antibiotic injection for these cases at the time of primary repair. In a previous study, we identified clinical risk factors for the development of endophthalmitis after repair of open-globe injuries. Our logistic regression analysis indicated that dirty wound was an independent risk factor for the development of endophthalmitis with a relative risk of 11.6. In addition, the presence of retained IOFB in association with rural address or dirty wound was associated with a high risk for the development of posttraumatic endophthalmitis after primary repair. The relative risks were estimated to be 11.0 and 9.2, respectively, for developing endophthalmitis over those with none of these combinations. We therefore would consider prophylactic intravitreal administration of antibiotics in these high-risk groups at the time of primary repair [92]. The combination of vancomycin (1 mg/0.1 ml) and ceftazidime (2.25 mg/0.1 ml) can be considered in these cases.

Initial treatment of posttraumatic endophthalmitis includes intravitreal antibiotic injection. Directly injecting antibiotics into the globe affords highest drug concentration in the vitreous humor. One must cover gram-positive and gram-negative organisms when treating posttraumatic endophthalmitis. For initial therapy, we recommend intravitreal vancomycin (1 mg/0.1 ml) and ceftazidime (2.25 mg/0.1 ml). In addition to appropriate antibiotic treatment, early therapeutic vitrectomy is often indicated. The use of silicone oil tamponade in vitrectomy for posttraumatic endophthalmitis has been shown to be useful [111, 112].

16.6 Bleb-Associated Endophthalmitis

Bleb-associated infections are infrequent but potentially devastating complication after glaucoma-filtering surgery. The spectrum of disease severity ranges from infection limited to the filtering bleb to intraocular extension leading to endophthalmitis. Blebitis is defined as presumed infection in or around the filtering bleb without vitreous involvement. It may be associated with mild to moderate anterior chamber inflammation.

Bleb-associated endophthalmitis is a devastating complication of glaucoma-filtering surgery. It denotes bleb infection with involvement of the vitreous. The presence of inflammatory cells in the vitreous is a key for differentiating endophthalmitis from blebitis. It usually develops months or years after glaucoma-filtering surgery. Risk factors for its development include the use of an antifibrotic agent, an inferior bleb location, thin bleb, bleb leak, chronic use of antibiotics, blepharitis, prior conjunctivitis and upper respiratory infection, and a history of bleb infection.

The widespread introduction of antiproliferative agents such as 5-fluorouracil and mitomycin-C as an adjunct use in trabeculectomy has remarkably improved the success rate of filtration surgery. However, their use results in formation of thin, avascular blebs, increased risk of late bleb leaks, and a higher incidence of endophthalmitis. Lehmann et al. [113] reported the odds of endophthalmitis to be three times higher in patients who receive antiproliferatives versus those who do not. The reported incidence of bleb-associated endophthalmitis, after glaucoma-filtering procedures with adjunctive mitomycin-C, ranges from 2.1 to 3.2 %. This incidence is higher than the reported rate in eyes undergoing filtering surgery without the use of antifibrotic agents [114–116].

A different microbiological spectrum distinguishes this group from endophthalmitis observed in other clinical settings [114, 117–125]. Unlike acute postoperative endophthalmitis, which results from direct intraoperative inoculation of microorganisms, bleb-associated endophthalmitis follows transconjunctival migration of bacteria into the eye [117]. The poor visual outcome in bleb-associated endophthalmitis could be because of its association with the virulent *Streptococcus* species and gram-negative bacteria such as *Haemophilus influenzae*. Exotoxins produced by *Streptococcus* species might aid the organism in penetrating through intact conjunctiva overlying the bleb. Bleb-associated endophthalmitis is associated with its own microbiologic spectrum which is distinct from that of acute-onset endophthalmitis after cataract surgery. In acute-onset endophthalmitis after cataract surgery, the less virulent coagulase-negative staphylococci, predominantly *Staphylococcus epidermidis*, was the most common organism, accounting for 70 % of the isolates [105]. On the other hand, the more virulent streptococcal species and gram-negative bacteria such as *Haemophilus influenzae* are more common causes of delayed-onset bleb-associated endophthalmitis [114, 117–125]. Streptococcal species produce exotoxins and are capable of penetrating the intact conjunctiva overlying the bleb with rapid spread into the anterior chamber and vitreous. The most common isolates are *Streptococcus* species and gram-negative bacteria, predominantly *Haemophilus influenzae*, followed by *Staphylococcus epidermidis* [114, 117–125]. The rate of isolation of *Streptococcus* species in bleb-associated endophthalmitis is higher than the 9.0 % rate found in endophthalmitis after cataract surgery [105]. Endophthalmitis caused by *Streptococcus* species was reported to be associated with an aggressive clinical course and a correspondingly poor visual prognosis [126, 127]. Series of bleb-associated endophthalmitis reported that *Streptococcus* species was the organism most frequently associated with poor visual prognosis [114, 117–122, 124]. These findings are consistent with the results of the Endophthalmitis Vitrectomy Study showing that patients with growth of coagulase-negative *Staphylococci* achieved the best visual outcome and that *Streptococci* were associated with the poorest visual outcome [128]. Therefore, the favorable overall visual outcome in patients with endophthalmitis after cataract-related surgery relative to patients with bleb-associated endophthalmitis might be related to the high frequency of infection with coagulase-negative *Staphylococci* in endophthalmitis after cataract-related surgery [105].

Bleb-associated endophthalmitis still carries a poor prognosis. In combining previously reported studies, visual acuities of 20/400 or better were preserved in only 43 % of patients, and 24 % of patients had final visual acuity of no light perception. Reasons for guarded prognosis include the virulence of infecting organisms [114, 117–122, 124] and ocular comorbidities, such as the advanced stage of glaucoma in many of these patients. However, the poor outcome may also suggest the lack of an effective treatment regimen. In our series we identified a significant association between good visual outcome and better presenting visual acuity, shorter interval from onset of symptoms to treatment, and clear cornea at presentation in the univariate analysis. Shorter interval from onset of symptoms to treatment retained statistical significance in the multivariate analysis. In addition, univariate and multivariate analyses identified diabetes mellitus to be a negative predictor of good visual outcome [124].

Early diagnosis and prompt intensive treatment of blebitis are critical in view of rapid deterioration and potential risk of progression to endophthalmitis, which has relatively devastating outcome. In early stage, conjunctival injection localized to the region of filtering bleb may be noted. Later bleb appears milky, with loss of translucency. Turbid fluid inside bleb may be visible, possibly with frank purulent material in or leaking from the bleb. Inflammatory cells may spill over into the anterior chamber. Hypopyon in the presence of signs of external bleb infection indicates endophthalmitis until proven otherwise. The presence of inflammatory cells within the vitreous is key for differentiating endophthalmitis from blebitis. Slit-lamp biomicroscopy examination of the bleb and Seidel test to detect any bleb leak should be performed. Ultrasound examination of vitreous should be performed if fundus examination is obscured due to inflammation. A swab of conjunctiva over the bleb and an anterior chamber tap should be performed for Gram stain and culture sensitivity before starting antibiotic therapy. Vitreous tap also should be performed if a hypopyon is present or there is any indication of involvement of the vitreous.

Intensive topical broad-spectrum antibiotic regimen alone is appropriate for patients with blebitis, without evidence of vitreous involvement. After the antibiotics have been used for about 24 h and signs of improvement of blebitis become evident, topical steroid should be initiated to prevent scarring and preserve the filtration site. The EVS guidelines for the treatment of post-cataract surgery endophthalmitis [129] cannot be applied to bleb-associated endophthalmitis because it is different in its presentation, infective organisms, and prognosis. Bleb-associated endophthalmitis needs more aggressive treatment. Recent retrospective studies demonstrated that patients treated with initial vitrectomy had better visual outcome and a lower incidence of no light perception vision than those treated with tap and injection [122, 124]. On the other hand, other studies [121, 125] reported worse visual outcome with vitrectomy. In these studies, the patients who underwent initial vitrectomy had a more severe infection and poorer visual acuity at time of endophthalmitis diagnosis. Because of this selection bias, final visual outcomes would be expected to be worse in the vitrectomy group.

Compliance with Ethical Requirements

Conflict of Interest The authors declare that they have no conflict of interest.

Informed Consent No human studies were carried out by the authors for this article.

Animal Studies No animal studies were carried out by the authors for this article.

References

1. Okada AA, Johnson RP, Liles WC, D'Amico DJ, Baker AS. Endogenous bacterial endophthalmitis. Report of a ten-year retrospective study. Ophthalmology. 1994;101(5):832–8.
2. Chee SP, Jap A. Endogenous endophthalmitis. Curr Opin Ophthalmol. 2001;12(6):464–70.
3. Jackson TL, Eykyn SJ, Graham EM, Stanford MR. Endogenous bacterial endophthalmitis: a 17-year prospective series and review of 267 reported cases. Surv Ophthalmol. 2003;48(4):403–23.
4. Wong JS, Chan TK, Lee HM, Chee SP. Endogenous bacterial endophthalmitis: an east Asian experience and a reappraisal of a severe ocular affliction. Ophthalmology. 2000;107(8):1483–91.
5. Kresloff MS, Castellarin AA, Zarbin MA. Endophthalmitis. Surv Ophthalmol. 1998;43(3):193–224.
6. Taban M, Behrens A, Newcomb RL, Nobe MY, Saedi G, Sweet PM, McDonnell PJ. Acute endophthalmitis following cataract surgery; a systematic review of the literature. Arch Ophthalmol. 2005;123:613–20.
7. Miller JJ, Scott IU, Flynn Jr HW, Smiddy WE, Newton J, Miller D. Acute-onset endophthalmitis after cataract surgery (2000–2004): incidence, clinical settings, and visual acuity outcomes after treatment. Am J Ophthalmol. 2005;139:983–7.
8. Colleaux KM, Hamilton WK. Effect of prophylactic antibiotics and incision type on the incidence of endophthalmitis after cataract surgery. Can J Ophthalmol. 2000;35:373–8.
9. Endophthalmitis Vitrectomy Study Group. Results of the Endophthalmitis Vitrectomy Study; a randomized trial of immediate vitrectomy and of intravenous antibiotics for the treatment of postoperative bacterial endophthalmitis. Arch Ophthalmol. 1995;113:1479–96.
10. Maxwell Jr DP, Diamond JG, May DR. Surgical wound defects associated with endophthalmitis. Ophthalmic Surg. 1994;25:157–61.
11. Cooper BA, Holekamp NM, Bohigian G, Thompson PA. Case-control study of endophthalmitis after cataract surgery comparing sclera tunnel and clear corneal wounds. Am J Ophthalmol. 2003;136:300–5.
12. Nagaki Y, Hayasaka S, Kadoi C, Matsumoto M, Yanagisawa S, Watanabe K, Hayasaka Y, Ikeda N, Sato S, Kataoka Y, Togashi M, Abe T. Bacterial endophthalmitis after small-incision cataract surgery; effect of incision placement and intraocular lens type. J Cataract Refract Surg. 2003;29:20–6.
13. Lertsumitkul S, Myers PC, O'Rourke MT, Chandra J. Endophthalmitis in the western Sydney region: a case-control study. Clin Experiment Ophthalmol. 2001;29:400–5.
14. West ES, Behrens A, McDonnell PJ, Tielsch JM, Schein OD. The incidence of endophthalmitis after cataract surgery among the U.S. Medicare population increased between 1994 and 2001. Ophthalmology. 2005;112:1388–94.
15. Al-Mezaine HS, Kangave D, Al-Assiri A, Al-Rajhi AA. Acute-onset nosocomial endophthalmitis after cataract surgery: incidence, clinical features, causative organisms, and visual outcomes. J Cataract Refract Surg. 2009;35:634–49.
16. Miño de Kaspar H, Shriver EM, Nguyen EV, Egbert PR, Singh K, Blumenkranz MS, Ta CN. Risk factors for antibiotic resistant conjunctival bacterial flora in patients undergoing intraocular surgery. Graefes Arch Clin Exp Ophthalmol. 2003;241:730–3.
17. Aaberg TM, Flynn HW, Schiffman J, Newton J. Nosocomial acute-onset postoperative endophthalmitis survey; a 10-year review of incidence and outcomes. Ophthalmology. 1998;105:1004–10.
18. Morlet N, Li J, Semmens J, Ng J. The Endophthalmitis Population Study of Western Australia (EPSWA): first report; on behalf of team EPSWA. Br J Ophthalmol. 2003;87:574–6.
19. Mamalis N, Kearsley L, Brinton E. Postoperative endophthalmitis. Curr Opin Ophthalmol. 2002;13:14–8.
20. Hatch WV, Cernat G, Wong D, Devenyi R, Bell CM. Risk factors for acute endophthalmitis after cataract surgery: a population-based study. Ophthalmology. 2009;116:425–30.
21. ESCRS Endophthalmitis Study Group. Prophylaxis of postoperative endophthalmitis following cataract surgery: results of the ESCRS multicenter study and identification of risk factors. J Cataract Refract Surg. 2007;33:978–88.
22. Menikoff JA, Speaker MG, Marmor M, Raskin EM. A case-control study of risk factors for postoperative endophthalmitis. Ophthalmology. 1991;98:1761–8.

23. Lalwani GA, Flynn Jr HW, Scott IU, Quinn CM, Berrocal AM, Davis JL, Murray TG, Smiddy WE, Miller D. Acute-onset endophthalmitis after clear corneal cataract surgery (1996–2005); clinical features, causative organisms, and visual acuity outcomes. Ophthalmology. 2008;115:473–6.
24. Thoms SS, Musch DC, Soong HK. Postoperative endophthalmitis associated with sutured versus unsutured clear corneal cataract incisions. Br J Ophthalmol. 2007;91:728–30.
25. Ciulla TA, Starr MB, Masket S. Bacterial endophthalmitis prophylaxis for cataract surgery. An evidence-based update. Ophthalmology. 2002;109:13–24.
26. Kernt M, Kampik A. Endophthalmitis: pathogenesis, clinical presentation, management, and perspectives. Clin Ophthalmol. 2010;4:121–35.
27. Anijeet D. Endophthalmitis after cataract surgery [letter]. Ophthalmology. 2010;117:853.
28. Barza M, Pavan PR, Doft BH, Wisniewski SR, Wilson LA, Han DP, Kelsey SF. Evaluation of microbiological diagnostic techniques in postoperative endophthalmitis in the Endophthalmitis Vitrectomy Study; for the Endophthalmitis Vitrectomy Study Group. Arch Ophthalmol. 1997;115:1142–50.
29. Therese KL, Anand AR, Madhavan HN. Polymerase chain reaction in the diagnosis of bacterial endophthalmitis. Br J Ophthalmol. 1998;82:1078–82.
30. Sowmya P, Madhavan HN. Diagnostic utility of polymerase chain reaction on intraocular specimens to establish the etiology of infectious endophthalmitis. Eur J Ophthalmol. 2009;19:812–7.
31. Doft BH, Wisniewski SR, Kelsey SF, Fitzgerald SG. Diabetes and postoperative endophthalmitis in the Endophthalmitis Vitrectomy Study; the Endophthalmitis Vitrectomy Study Group. Arch Ophthalmol. 2001;119:650–6.
32. Ou JI, Ta CN. Endophthalmitis prophylaxis. Ophthalmol Clin North Am. 2006;19(4):449–56.
33. Carrim ZI, Mackie G, Gallacher G, Wykes WN. The efficacy of 5% povidone-iodine for 3 minutes prior to cataract surgery. Eur J Ophthalmol. 2009;19:560–4.
34. Ang GS, Barras CW. Prophylaxis against infection in cataract surgery: a survey of routine practice. Eur J Ophthalmol. 2006;16:394–400.
35. Halachimi-Eyal O, Lang Y, Keness Y, Miron D. Preoperative topical moxifloxacin 0.5% and povidone-iodine 5.0% versus povidone-iodine 5.0% alone to reduce bacterial colonization in the conjunctival sac. J Cataract Refract Surg. 2009;35:2109–14, errata 2010;36:535.
36. Chan DG, Francis IC. Effective draping for cataract surgery by using a relieving incision in the operative drape [letter]. Clin Experiment Ophthalmol. 2004; 32:656.
37. Buzard K, Liapis S. Prevention of endophthalmitis. J Cataract Refract Surg. 2004;30:1953–9.
38. O'Brien TP, Arshinoff SA, Mah FS. Perspectives on antibiotics for postoperative endophthalmitis prophylaxis: potential role of moxifloxacin. J Cataract Refract Surg. 2007;33:1790–800.
39. Moshirfar M, Feiz V, Vitale AT, Wegelin JA, Basavanthappa S, Wolsey DH. Endophthalmitis after uncomplicated cataract surgery with the use of fourth-generation fluoroquinolones: a retrospective observational case series. Ophthalmology. 2007;114: 686–91.
40. Montan PG, Wejde G, Koranyi G, Rylander M. Prophylactic intracameral cefuroxime; efficacy in preventing endophthalmitis after cataract surgery. J Cataract Refract Surg. 2002;28:977–81.
41. Wejde G, Montan P, Lundström M, Stenevi U, Thorburn W. Endophthalmitis following cataract surgery in Sweden: national prospective survey 1999–2001. Acta Ophthalmol Scand. 2005;83: 7–10.
42. Barry P, Seal DV, Gettinby G, Lees F, Peterson M, Revie CW. ESCRS study of prophylaxis of postoperative endophthalmitis after cataract surgery; preliminary report of principal results from a European multicenter study; the ESCRS Endophthalmitis Study Group. J Cataract Refract Surg. 2006;32: 407–10.
43. Montan PG, Wejde G, Setterquist H, Rylander M, Zetterström C. Prophylactic intracameral cefuroxime; evaluation of safety and kinetics in cataract surgery. J Cataract Refract Surg. 2002;28:982–7.
44. Gimbel HV, Sun R, DeBrof BM. Prophylactic intracameral antibiotics during cataract surgery: the incidence of endophthalmitis and corneal endothelial cell loss. Eur J Implant Refract Surg. 1994;6:280–5.
45. Espiritu CRG, Caparas VL, Bolinao JG. Safety of prophylactic intracameral moxifloxacin 0.5% ophthalmic solution in cataract surgery patients. J Cataract Refract Surg. 2007;33:63–8.
46. Lane SS, Osher RH, Masket S, Belani S. Evaluation of the safety of prophylactic intracameral moxifloxacin in cataract surgery. J Cataract Refract Surg. 2008;34:1451–9.
47. Arbisser LB. Safety of intracameral moxifloxacin for prophylaxis of endophthalmitis after cataract surgery. J Cataract Refract Surg. 2008;34:1114–20.
48. Yoeruek E, Spitzer MS, Saygili O, Tatar O, Biedermann T, Yoeruek E, et al. Comparison of in vitro safety profiles of vancomycin and cefuroxime on human corneal endothelial cells for intracameral use. J Cataract Refract Surg. 2008;34:2139–45.
49. Hui M, Lam PTH, Cheung S-W, Pang C-P, Chan C-Y, Lam DSC. In vitro compatibility study of cephalosporin with intraocular irrigating solutions and intracameral medications. Clin Experiment Ophthalmol. 2011;39:164–70.
50. Lockington D, Flowers H, Young D, Yorston D. Assessing the accuracy of intracameral antibiotic preparation for use in cataract surgery. J Cataract Refract Surg. 2010;36:286–9.
51. Mandelbaum S, Meisler DM. Postoperative chronic microbial endophthalmitis. Int Ophthalmol Clin. 1993;33:71–9.
52. Rogers NK, Fox PD, Noble BA, Kerr K, Inglis T. Aggressive management of an epidemic of

chronic pseudophakic endophthalmitis: results and literature survey. Br J Ophthalmol. 1994;78:115–9.
53. Al-Mezaine HS, Al-Assiri A, Al-Rajhi AA. Incidence, clinical features, causative organisms, and visual outcomes of delayed-onset pseudophakic endophthalmitis. Eur J Ophthalmol. 2009;19: 804–11.
54. Meisler DM, Palestine AG, Vastine DW, Demartini DR, Murphy BF, Reinhart WJ, Zakov ZN, McMahon JT, Cliffel TP. Chronic Propionibacterium endophthalmitis after extracapsular cataract extraction and intraocular lens implantation. Am J Ophthalmol. 1986;102:733–9.
55. Meisler DM, Mandelbaum S. Propionibacterium-associated endophthalmitis after extracapsular cataract extraction. Review of reported cases. Ophthalmology. 1989;96:54–61.
56. Zambrano W, Flynn Jr HW, Pflugfelder SC, Roussel TJ, Culbertson WW, Holland S, Miller D. Management options for Propionibacterium acnes endophthalmitis. Ophthalmology. 1989;96:1100–5.
57. Clark WL, Kaiser PK, Flynn Jr HW, Belfort A, Miller D, Meisler DM. Treatment strategies and visual acuity outcomes in chronic postoperative Propionibacterium acnes endophthalmitis. Ophthalmology. 1999;106:1665–70.
58. Aldave AJ, Stein JD, Deramo VA, Shah GK, Fischer DH, Maguire JI. Treatment strategies for postoperative Propionibacterium acnes endophthalmitis. Ophthalmology. 1999;106:2395–401.
59. Fox GM, Joondeph BC, Flynn Jr HW, Pflugfelder SC, Roussel TJ. Delayed-onset pseudophakic endophthalmitis. Am J Ophthalmol. 1991;111: 163–73.
60. Seedor JA, Koplin RS, Shah M, Almeda Jr EE, Perry HD. Chronic postoperative endophthalmitis from Staphylococcus aureus. J Cataract Refract Surg. 1990;16:512–3.
61. Ficker L, Meredith TA, Wilson LA, Kaplan HJ, Kozarsky AM. Chronic bacterial endophthalmitis. Am J Ophthalmol. 1987;103:745–8.
62. Stern WH, Tamura E, Jacobs RA, Pons VG, Stone RD, O'Day DM, Irvine AR. Epidemic postsurgical Candida parapsilosis endophthalmitis. Clinical findings and management of 15 consecutive cases. Ophthalmology. 1985;92:1701–9.
63. Pflugfelder SC, Flynn Jr HW, Zwickey TA, Forster RK, Tsiligianni A, Culbertson WW, Mandelbaum S. Exogenous fungal endophthalmitis. Ophthalmology. 1988;95:19–30.
64. El-Asrar AM, Tabbara KF. Chronic endophthalmitis after extracapsular cataract extraction caused by Mycobacterium chelonae subspecies abscessus. Eye. 1995;9:798–801.
65. Puliafito CA, Baker AS, Haaf J, Foster CS. Infectious endophthalmitis. Review of 36 cases. Ophthalmology. 1982;89:921–9.
66. Aaberg Jr TM, Rubsamen PE, Joondeph BC, Flynn Jr HW. Chronic post-operative gram-negative endophthalmitis. Retina. 1997;17:260–1.
67. Rahman MK, Holz ER. Alcaligenes xylosoxidans and post-operative endophthalmitis in a pseudophakic eye. Am J Ophthalmol. 2000;129:813–5.
68. Raman VS, Evans N, Shreshta B, Cunningham R. Chronic postoperative endophthalmitis caused by Actinomyces neuii. J Cataract Refract Surg. 2004; 30:2641–3.
69. Manners RM, Canning CR. Posterior lens capsule abscess due to Propioni-bacterium acnes and Staphylococcus epidermidis following extracapsular cataract extraction. Br J Ophthalmol. 1991;75:710–2.
70. Samson CM, Foster CS. Chronic postoperative endophthalmitis. Int Ophthalmol Clin. 2000;40: 57–67.
71. Meisler DM, Zakov ZN, Bruner WE, Hall GS, McMahon JT, Zachary AA, Barna BP. Endophthalmitis associated with sequestered intraocular Propionibacterium acnes. Am J Ophthalmol. 1987; 104:428–9.
72. Roussel TJ, Olson ER, Rice T, Meisler D, Hall G, Miller D. Chronic postoperative endophthalmitis associated with Actinomyces species. Arch Ophthalmol. 1991;109:60–2.
73. Pathengay A, Shah GY, Das T, Sharma S. Curvularia lunata endophthalmitis presenting with a posterior capsular plaque. Indian J Ophthalmol. 2006;54:65–6.
74. Chien AM, Raber IM, Fischer DH, Eagle RC, Naidoff MA. Propionibacterium acnes endophthalmitis after intracapsular cataract extraction. Ophthalmology. 1992;99:487–90.
75. Deramo VA, Ting TD. Treatment of Propionibacterium acnes endophthalmitis. Curr Opin Ophthalmol. 2001;12:225–9.
76. Lohmann C, Linde HJ, Reischl U. Improved detection of microorganisms by polymerase chain reaction in delayed endophthalmitis after cataract surgery. Ophthalmology. 2000;107:1047–51.
77. Shirodkar AR, Pathengay A, Flynn Jr HW, Albini TA, Berrocal AM, Davis JL, Lalwani GA, Murray TG, Smiddy WE, Miller D. Delayed versus acute-onset endophthalmitis after cataract surgery. Am J Ophthalmol. 2012;153:391–98.e2.
78. Maalouf F, Abdulaal M, Hamam RN. Chronic postoperative endophthalmitis: a review of clinical characteristics, microbiology, treatment, strategies, and outcomes. Int J Inflamm. 2012;2012: 313248.
79. Brinton GS, Topping TM, Hyndiuk RA, Aaberg TM, Reeser FH, Abrams GW. Posttraumatic endophthalmitis. Arch Ophthalmol. 1984;102:547–50.
80. Williams DF, Mieler WF, Abrams GW, Lewis H. Results and prognostic factors in penetrating ocular injuries with retained intraocular foreign bodies. Ophthalmology. 1988;95:911–6.
81. Boldt HC, Pulido JS, Blodi CF, Folk JC, Weingeist TA. Rural endophthalmitis. Ophthalmology. 1989; 96:1722–6.
82. Thompson JT, Parver LM, Enger CL, Mieler WF, Liggett PE. For the National Eye Trauma System. Infectious endophthalmitis after penetrating injuries

with retained intraocular foreign bodies. Ophthalmology. 1993;100:1468–74.
83. Verbraeken H, Rysselaere M. Post-traumatic endophthalmitis. Eur J Ophthalmol. 1994;4:1–5.
84. Thompson WS, Rubsamen PE, Flynn Jr HW, Schiffman J, Cousins SW. Endophthalmitis after penetrating trauma. Risk factors and visual acuity outcomes. Ophthalmology. 1995;102:1696–701.
85. Duch-Samper AM, Menezo JL, Hurtado-Sarriō M. Endophthalmitis following penetrating eye injuries. Acta Ophthalmol Scand. 1997;75:104–6.
86. Abu El-Asrar AM, Al-Amro SA, Khan NM, Kangave D. Visual outcome and prognostic factors after vitrectomy for posterior segment foreign bodies. Eur J Ophthalmol. 2000;10:304–11.
87. Sabaci G, Bayer A, Mutlu FM, Karagül S, Yildirim E. Endophthalmitis after deadly-weapon-related open-globe injuries: risk factors, value of prophylactic antibiotics, and visual outcomes. Am J Ophthalmol. 2002;133:62–9.
88. Essex RW, Yi Q, Charles PG, Allen PJ. Post-traumatic endophthalmitis. Ophthalmology. 2004;111:2015–22.
89. Chaudhry IA, Shamsi FA, Al-Harthi E, Al-Theeb A, Elzaridi E, Riley FC. Incidence and visual outcome of endophthalmitis associated with intraocular foreign bodies. Graefes Arch Clin Exp Ophthalmol. 2008;246:181–6.
90. Andreoli CM, Andreoli MT, Kloek CE, Ahuero AE, Vavvas D, Durand ML. Low rate of endophthalmitis in a large series of open globe injuries. Am J Ophthalmol. 2009;147:601–8.
91. Faghihi H, Hajizadeh F, Esfahani MR, Rasoulinejad SA, Lashay A, Mirshahi A, Karkhaneh R, Tabatabaey A, Khabazkhoob M, Faghihi S. Posttraumatic endophthalmitis. Report No. 2. Retina. 2012;32: 146–51.
92. Al-Mezaine HS, Osman EA, Kangave D, Abu El-Asrar AM. Risk factors for culture-positive endophthalmitis after repair of open globe injuries. Eur J Ophthalmol. 2010;20:201–8.
93. Zhang Y, Zhang MN, Jiang CH, Yao Y, Zhang K. Endophthalmitis following open globe injury. Br J Ophthalmol. 2010;94:111–4.
94. Affeldt JC, Flynn Jr HW, Forster RK, Mandelbaum S, Clarkson JG, Jarus GD. Microbial endophthalmitis resulting from ocular trauma. Ophthalmology. 1987;94:407–13.
95. Nobe JR, Gomez DS, Liggett P, Smith RE, Robin JB. Post-traumatic and postoperative endophthalmitis: a comparison of visual outcomes. Br J Ophthalmol. 1987;71:614–7.
96. Alfaro DV, Roth D, Liggett PE. Posttraumatic endophthalmitis: causative organisms, treatment, and prevention. Retina. 1994;14:206–11.
97. Abu El-Asrar AM, Al-Amro SA, Al-Mosallam AA, Al-Obeidan S. Post-traumatic endophthalmitis. Causative organisms and visual outcome. Eur J Ophthalmol. 1999;9:21–31.
98. Lieb DF, Scott IU, Flynn Jr HW, Miller D, Feuer WJ. Open globe injuries with positive intraocular cultures. Factors influencing final visual acuity outcomes. Ophthalmology. 2003;110:1560–6.
99. Kunimoto DY, Das T, Sharma S, Jalali S, Majji AB, Gopinathan U, Athmanathan S, Rao TN. Microbiologic spectrum and susceptibility of isolates: Part II. Posttraumatic endophthalmitis. Endophthalmitis Research Group. Am J Ophthalmol. 1999;128:242–4.
100. Chhabra S, Kunimoto DY, Kazi L, Regillo CD, Ho AC, Belmont J, Maguire J, Vander J, Brown GC. Endophthalmitis after open globe injury: microbiologic spectrum and susceptibilities of isolates. Am J Ophthalmol. 2006;142:852–4.
101. Al-Omran AM, Abboud EB, Abu El-Asrar AM. Microbiologic spectrum and visual outcome of posttraumatic endophthalmitis. Retina. 2007;27:236–42.
102. Ariyasu RG, Kumar S, LaBree LD, Wagner DG, Smith RE. Microorganisms cultured from the anterior chamber of ruptured globes at the time of repair. Am J Ophthalmol. 1995;119:181–8.
103. Meredith TA. Antimicrobial pharmacokinetics in endophthalmitis treatment: studies of ceftazidime. Trans Am Ophthalmol Soc. 1993;91:653–99.
104. Meredith TA, Aguilar HE, Shaarawy A, Kincaid M, Dick J, Niesman MR. Vancomycin levels in the vitreous cavity after intravenous administration. Am J Ophthalmol. 1995;119:774–8.
105. Han DP, Wisniewski SR, Wilson LA, Barza M, Vine AK, Doft BH, Kelsey SF. Spectrum and susceptibilities of microbiologic isolates in the Endophthalmitis Vitrectomy Study. Am J Ophthalmol. 1996;122:1–17.
106. Alfaro DV, Davis J, Kim S, Bia F, Bogard JF, Briggs JW, Liggett PE. Experimental *Bacillus cereus* posttraumatic endophthalmitis and treatment with ciprofloxacin. Br J Ophthalmol. 1996;80:755–8.
107. Alfaro 3rd DV, Hudson SJ, Kasowski EJ, Barton CP, Brucker AJ, Lopez JD, Beverly DT, King LP. Experimental pseudomonal posttraumatic endophthalmitis in a swine model. Treatment with ceftazidime, amikacin, and imipenem. Retina. 1997; 17:139–45.
108. Narang S, Gupta V, Gupta A, Dogra MR, Pandav SS, Das S. Role of prophylactic intravitreal antibiotics in open globe injuries. Indian J Ophthalmol. 2003;51: 39–44.
109. Soheilian M, Rafati N, Mohebbi MR, Yazdani S, Habibabadi HF, Feghhi M, Shahriary HA, Eslamipour J, Piri N, Peyman GA, Traumatic Endophthalmitis Trial Research Group. Prophylaxis of acute posttraumatic bacterial endophthalmitis: a multicenter, randomized clinical trial of intraocular antibiotic injection, report 2. Arch Ophthalmol. 2007;125:460–5.
110. Mieler WF, Ellis MK, Williams DF, Han DP. Retained intraocular foreign bodies and endophthalmitis. Ophthalmology. 1990;97:1532–8.
111. Azad R, Ravi K, Talwar D, Rajpal, Kumar N. Pars plana vitrectomy with or without silicone oil endotamponade in post-traumatic endophthalmitis. Graefes Arch Clin Exp Ophthalmol. 2003;241:478–83.

112. Yan H, Lu Y, Yu J, Han J, Zhang J, Chen S, Xu Y. Silicone oil in the surgical treatment of traumatic endophthalmitis. Eur J Ophthalmol. 2008;18:680–4.
113. Lehmann OJ, Bunce C, Matheson MM, Maurino V, Khaw PT, Wormald R, Barton K. Risk factors for development of post-trabeculectomy endophthalmitis. Br J Ophthalmol. 2000;84:1349–53.
114. Greenfield DS, Suñer IJ, Miller MP, Kangas TA, Palmberg PF, Flynn Jr HW. Endophthalmitis after filtering surgery with mitomycin. Arch Ophthalmol. 1996;114:943–9.
115. Higginbotham EJ, Stevens RK, Musch DC, Karp KO, Lichter PR, Bergstrom TJ, Skuta GL. Bleb-related endophthalmitis after trabeculectomy with mitomycin C. Ophthalmology. 1996;103:650–6.
116. Kuang TM, Lin YC, Liu CJ, Hsu WM, Chou CK. Early and late endophthalmitis following trabeculectomy in a Chinese population. Eur J Ophthalmol. 2008;18:66–70.
117. Mandelbaum S, Forster RK, Gelender H, Culbertson W. Late onset endophthalmitis associated with filtering blebs. Ophthalmology. 1985;92:964–72.
118. Ciulla TA, Beck AD, Topping TM, Baker AS. Blebitis, early endophthalmitis, and late endophthalmitis after glaucoma-filtering surgery. Ophthalmology. 1997;104:986–95.
119. Kangas TA, Greenfield DS, Flynn Jr HW, Parrish 2nd RK, Palmberg P. Delayed-onset endophthalmitis associated with conjunctival filtering blebs. Ophthalmology. 1997;104:746–52.
120. Waheed S, Ritterband DC, Greenfield DS, Liebmann JM, Seedor JA, Ritch R. New patterns of infecting organisms in late bleb-related endophthalmitis: a ten year review. Eye (Lond). 1998;12:910–5.
121. Song A, Scott IU, Flynn Jr HW, Budenz DL. Delayed-onset bleb-associated endophthalmitis. Clinical features and visual acuity outcomes. Ophthalmology. 2002;109:985–91.
122. Busbee BG, Recchia FM, Kaiser R, Nagra P, Rosenblatt B, Pearlman RB. Bleb-associated endophthalmitis: clinical characteristics and visual outcomes. Ophthalmology. 2004;111:1495–503.
123. Prasad N, Latina MA. Blebitis and endophthalmitis after glaucoma filtering surgery. Int Ophthalmol Clin. 2007;47:85–97.
124. Al-Turki TA, Al-Shahwan S, Al-Mezaine HS, Kangave D, Abu El-Asrar AM. Microbiology and visual outcome of bleb-associated endophthalmitis. Ocul Immunol Inflamm. 2010;18:121–6.
125. Leng T, Miller D, Flynn Jr HW, Jacobs DJ, Gedde SJ. Delayed-onset bleb-associated endophthalmitis (1996–2008): causative organisms and visual acuity outcomes. Retina. 2011;31:344–52.
126. Mao LK, Flynn Jr HW, Miller D, Pflugfelder SC. Endophthalmitis caused by Streptococcal species. Arch Ophthalmol. 1992;110:798–801.
127. Miller JJ, Scott IU, Flynn Jr HW, Smiddy WE, Corey RP, Miller D. Endophthalmitis caused by Streptococcus pneumoniae. Am J Ophthalmol. 2004;138:231–6.
128. The Endophthalmitis Vitrectomy Study Group. Microbiologic factors and visual outcome in the Endophthalmitis Vitrectomy Study. Am J Ophthalmol. 1996;122:830–46.
129. Results of the Endophthalmitis Vitrectomy Study. A randomized trial of immediate vitrectomy and of intravenous antibiotics for the treatment of postoperative bacterial endophthalmitis. Endophthalmitis Vitrectomy Study Group. Arch Ophthalmol 1995;113:1479–96.